COUNTLESS BLESSINGS

COUNTLESS BLESSINGS

A History of Childbirth and Reproduction in the Sahel

Barbara M. Cooper

INDIANA UNIVERSITY PRESS

This book is a publication of

Indiana University Press
Office of Scholarly Publishing
Herman B Wells Library 350
1320 East 10th Street
Bloomington, Indiana 47405 USA

iupress.indiana.edu

Manufactured in the United States of America

Library of Congress Cataloging-in-Publication Data

Names: Cooper, Barbara MacGowan, author.
Title: Countless blessings : a history of childbirth and reproduction in the
Sahel / Barbara M. Cooper.
Description: Bloomington, Indiana : Indiana University Press, 2019. |
Includes bibliographical references and index.
Identifiers: LCCN 2018031196 (print) | LCCN 2018035445 (ebook) | ISBN
9780253042033 (e-book) | ISBN 9780253042002 (hardback : alk. paper) | ISBN
9780253042019 (pbk. : alk. paper)
Subjects: LCSH: Childbirth—Niger. | Childbirth—Sahel. | Childbirth—Social
aspects—Niger. | Childbirth—Social aspects—Sahel. | Fertility,
Human—Niger. | Fertility, Human—Sahel. | Birth customs—Niger. | Birth
customs—Sahel. | Reproductive health—Niger. | Reproductive
health—Sahel. | Women, Hausa—Social conditions. | Hausa (African
people)—Social life and customs.
Classification: LCC GT2465.S15 (ebook) | LCC GT2465.S15 C66 2019 (print) |
DDC 392.1/20966—dc23
LC record available at https://lccn.loc.gov/2018031196

1 2 3 4 5   24 23 22 21 20 19

CONTENTS

Acknowledgments   *vii*

List of Ethnonyms, Foreign Terms, and Acronyms   *xi*

Introduction   *1*

1   Environment, Seduction, and Fertility   *36*

2   Tensions in the Wake of Conquest: Gender and Reproduction after Abolition   *62*

3   Personhood, Socialization, and Shame   *84*

4   Colonial Accounting   *115*

5   Perils of Pregnancy and Childbirth   *147*

6   Producing Healthy Babies and Healthy Laborers   *174*

7   Feminists, Islamists, and Demographers   *201*

8   Let's Talk about Bastards   *233*

9   Contemporary Sexuality and Childbirth   *261*

Conclusion: Traveling Companions and Entrustments in Contemporary Niger   *297*

Works Cited   *307*

Index   *339*

ACKNOWLEDGMENTS

I PROBABLY WOULDN'T HAVE TAKEN UP QUESTIONS OF the body, person-hood, and emotional ethics had I not had Julie Livingston as a colleague at Rutgers from 2003 to 2015. Her research, stimulating ideas, and lively intellect gave me the temerity to try my hand in domains far outside my comfort zone. I presented one of the earliest (and most tangled) pieces of this research at the Rutgers Center for Historical Analysis seminar on ver-nacular epistemologies that she cohosted with Indrani Chatterjee in 2010. Meredeth Turshen's passionate commitment to women's health in Africa and Ousseina Alidou's sensitive and nuanced attention to women's lives in Niger also informed my growing interest in the topics in this book. Later, Jo-hanna Schoen joined the Rutgers history department, bringing her insight into reproductive health ethics, her boundless enthusiasm, and her uncon-ditional support when my energies were beginning to flag. Plus she brought chocolate. The incomparable Dorothy Hodgson, fellow traveler the entire way, gently nudged me along over many lunches, dinners, and, yes, glasses of wine. Numerous graduate students assisted me in this work during its long gestation: Johanna Jochumsdottir, Christina Chiknas, Dale Booth, Taylor Moore, and Hillary Buxton. This is the quintessential Rutgers book.

This is also a Mellon New Directions book. It is hard to convey my heartfelt gratitude to Mellon for having faith in my project and for seeing me through some very difficult years. The Mellon Foundation has proved unstintingly supportive of scholars pursuing imaginative and risky ven-tures into topics outside their initial training. For a heavenly year, I was hosted by the Office of Population Research at Princeton, where I had the great good fortune to learn from Tom Espenshade, Jim Trussel, Betsy Arm-strong, Noel Cameron, and Keith Hansen. An intense summer course for nurse-midwifery training at the University of Pennsylvania School of Nurs-ing with Barbara Reale and Kate McHugh reinforced my conviction that nurse-midwives are the most fabulous people on the planet. In France, a variety of lively research institutions provided me with access to their li-braries and opportunities to exchange ideas with researchers, practition-ers, and scholars: the Institut Nationale d'Études Demographiques, Centre

Population et Développement at the Université de Paris–Descartes, and the Centre d'Études d'Afrique Noire at the Université de Bordeaux.

The Mellon grant also enabled me to begin reaching out to specialists in Niger who could orient me to research on population, health, and reproduction in Niamey. Of particular importance to gaining a sense for the existing research by Nigerien public health specialists was Madame Abdoulaye Amina, who provided me with access to the library of the École Nationale de Santé Publique de Niamey, where a multitude of theses I have cited in this book are housed. Zeinabou Hadari of the Centre Reines Daura was instrumental in making it possible for me to reach out to the networks of women activists and NGOs that are under the surface of my research. Her friendship, hospitality, and commitment to my project as a scholar and activist for women's education have been invaluable. Aissata Sidikou of the Coodination des Organisations Non Gouvernementales et Associations Féminines Nigérienne and the Association des Femmes Juristes du Niger welcomed me into the fold of a dynamic network of women in Niamey.

The importance of my work with Hawa Képine of the Association des Femmes Juristes du Niger during sabbatical fieldwork is evident throughout the book; I have come to think of her as my wise sister in pursuit of an understanding of the realities of women's lives in Niger. The congenial atmosphere of the Laboratoire d'Études et de Recherche sur les Dynamiques Sociales et le Développement Local stimulated me from the earliest stages of this research. It was there that I met the late Hadiza Moussa. I have had the great good fortune of benefiting from her magisterial study of infertility and contraceptive use in Niamey, *Entre Absence et Refus d'Enfant*. Hadiza died in a road accident in late 2013 to the great sorrow of her many friends, colleagues, and admirers. Her extraordinary research immeasurably enriches this book. Mahaman Tidjani Alou, Jean-Pierre Olivier de Sardan, and Aissa Diarra, among many others, provided valuable ideas and suggestions at different stages of the project.

As I have so often in the past, I found an intellectual home at the Institut de Recherches en Sciences Humaines in Niamey, directed by Abdou Bontiani. I imposed regularly on Seyni Moumouni in his office at the institute, where he generously offered a ready ear and the reassuring support of a fellow historian. At various moments my Boston University homie Sue Rosenfeld shared her home and her acerbic humor in the service of my research. Few friends are willing to host weekly djembe lessons and *ceebu jen*. Caroline Anderson Agalheir gave my daughter and me a home with all the amenities, including yoga, viewings of *Downton Abbey*, and opportunities to play "Just Dance."

Often finding the time to write up one's research is as hard as managing the actual research and fieldwork. Two residential fellowships enabled me to gain access to libraries and archives in France and, perhaps more crucially, to find time to think and write. I am grateful to Alan Roberts for making possible a magical semester as a visiting scholar with my daughter Rachel in Aix-en-Provence at the Institute for American Universities (IAU College) in 2014. While my daughter learned to paint at the Marchutz school of IAU, I perused documents at the Archives Nationales d'Outre-mer and drafted two chapters. This book also benefitted from a fellowship at the Paris Institute for Advanced Studies (France) in the spring of 2015, with the financial support of the French state program Investissements d'avenir, managed by the Agence Nationale de la Recherche (ANR-11-LABX-0027-01 Labex RFIEA+). A semester under the direction of Gretty Myrdal in the gorgeous Hotel de Lauzun provided me with unsurpassed bibliographic support, marvelous meals, stimulating discussion with colleagues (including Nancy Hunt), and a tantalizing view of the Seine.

During that year I was also able to get to know some of the scholars at Centre Population et Développement better, in particular Doris Bonnet, whose work I so admire. I began a fruitful collaboration with Catherine Baroin on an edited collection about shame in the Sahel; that project sharpened my thinking considerably and introduced me to the work of many other French and West African scholars. During my various trips through Paris, my friends Anne Hugon, Pascale Barthelemy, Odile Goerg, Tamara Gilles-Vernick, Myra Jehlen, and Camille Lefebvre could be counted on to give me a warm welcome and a respite from writing and archives. I am particularly indebted to Christelle Taraud for stimulating conversations about Islamic Africa and for accompanying me to many movies in the neighborhood of St. Michel.

This is in many ways a synthetic work pulling together insights scattered in research on a multitude of different ethnic groups in a range of settings: Susan Rasmussen on Tuareg women in Niger, Mohamed Ag Erless on Kel-Adagh Tuareg in Mali, Paul Riesman on Fulani in Burkina Faso, Jean-Pierre Olivier de Sardan on Songhai in Niger, Paul Stoller on Zarma in Niger, Adeline Masquelier on Mauri women and youth in Nigeria, Elisha Renne on Hausa and Yoruba in Nigeria, and Doris Bonnet on Mossi in Burkina Faso. Murray Last generously shared both published and unpublished work that helped me think about Hausa therapeutics, and Erin Pettigrew gave me her marvelous dissertation on Muslim healing in Mauritania. My role as historian has been to have the audacity to attempt to draw together themes in this rich body of work across national boundaries. Others can hardly be faulted for the failings that may have resulted from that audacity.

I ended up publishing major chunks of my work in article and chapter form—more amenable to "executive summary" for policy audiences—rather than attempt to integrate it all into a book oriented toward historians. Little of that work is reiterated here, but the process of getting feedback from editors and outside readers was immensely helpful. Readers of the full manuscript for Indiana University Press gave me crucial direction as well. Thank you, invisible friends. Both Julie Livingston and Johanna Schoen read the full manuscript and provided invaluable feedback and support.

Most of all my daughters Cara and Rachel Miller kept me going through many ups and downs on three continents. My strong and thoughtful girls are my own countless blessings. This book is for them.

ETHNONYMS, FOREIGN TERMS, AND ACRONYMS

Ethnonyms

Bella (also Buzu): Tamasheq speakers whose families had historically been captives of freeborn Tuareg

Fulani (also FulBe or Peul): freeborn speakers of the Fulfulde language

Hausa: speakers of the Hausa language

Kanuri (also Beriberi): speakers of the Kanuri language

RimaiBe: Fulfulde speakers whose families had been taken captive by Fulani communities

Zarma (also Djerma, Zerma, Sonrai, Songhai): speakers of the Zarma dialect of the Songhai languages

Tuareg (also Kel Tamasheq): freeborn speakers of the Tamasheq language

Tubu: speakers of the Tubu language (closely related to Kanembu)

Foreign Terms and Expressions

Afrique Occidentale Française (AOF): French West Africa, the federation of territories France took over in Western Africa (comprising Senegal, Mauritania, Mali, Niger, Burkina Faso (formerly Upper Volta), Benin, Guinea, and Côte d'Ivoire) ruled from Dakar

Al-azl (Ar): withdrawal prior to ejaculation

Assesseur (Fr): an adviser to the judge within the French-instituted courts who provides input on customary practice

Corvée (Fr): obligatory labor supplied for colonial projects or to colonial figures of authority

Entourage (Fr): one's family and close friends, particularly those who are consulted in the context of medical issues

Justice indigène (Fr): the evolving judicial system for the indigenous populations under French rule

Kafiri (Ar): someone who is pagan, non-Muslim, enslaveable

Kunya (Hausa): the affective complex of shame, restraint, modesty, and honor

Lycée (Fr): final secondary school within the French system

Matrone (Fr): an older woman who assists other women in childbirth who has been recruited to assist within the French-initiated medical system

Métis/métisse (Fr): an individual of mixed European and African ancestry

Prestation (Fr): obligatory labor tax

Qadi (Ar) or *kadi* (Hausa): a Muslim judge appointed by the local ruler

Sage-femme (Fr): biomedically trained midwife

Tirailleurs (Fr): African soldiers serving within the French colonial army

Tribunaux du premier degré (Fr): lowest and most local-level courts within the French-instituted judicial system

Zina (Ar): fornication, sex outside of marriage

Acronyms

ACT Association des Chefs Traditionnels

AFJN Association des Femmes Juristes du Niger

AFN Association des Femmes du Niger

AGEFOM Agence Économique de la France d'Outre-mer

AIN Association Islamique du Niger

AMI Assistance Médicale aux Indigènes

AOF Afrique Occidentale Française

ASFN Association des Sage-Femmes du Niger

CEDAW Convention for the Elimination of All Forms of Discrimination against Women

CONGAFEN Coordination des Organisations Non Gouvernementales et Associations Féminines Nigérienne

CONIPRAT Comité Nigérien sur les Pratiques Traditionnelles

CRC Convention on the Rights of the Child

FWA French West Africa or Afrique Occidentale Française

ICESCR International Covenant on Economic, Social and Cultural Rights

INSEE Institut National de la Statistique

SIM Sudan Interior Mission

UFMN Union des Femmes Musulmanes du Niger

UFN Union des Femmes du Niger

UNESCO United Nations Educational, Scientific, and Cultural Organization

UNFPA United Nations Population Fund

COUNTLESS BLESSINGS

INTRODUCTION

NIGER PRESENTS A STRIKING PARADOX. IT HAS ARGUABLY the highest total fertility rate in the world (at 7.6 children per woman in 2015), making it one of the very few countries in which fertility rates have gone up rather than down since 1980 (H. Issaka Maga and J.-P. Guengant 2017, 162). As a result, it also has a startlingly high population growth rate (3.9%); the size of the population rose from roughly 2.5 million in 1950 to almost 20 million (19.9 million, half of whom are under fifteen) in 2015.[1] The growth rate reflects a rising life expectancy and a declining infant mortality rate, both of which are to be celebrated and, if possible, accelerated (Keenan et al. 2018). But with such a high growth rate, the health, education, and bureaucratic infrastructure simply can't keep pace. As sociologist Issaka Maga Hamidu observes, Niger's population ought to be at the top of the political agenda, but it is not ("Niger: sleepwalking" 2016. Deutsche Welle, January 3).[2] Instead, the latest scandal in the capital is that prominent political couples desperate for children have allegedly "purchased" twin babies through an international "baby factory" network linking Nigeria, Benin, and Niger (Juompan-Yakam 2014; Abdou Assane 2017).

This book will explore the historical circumstances that have contributed to this pattern of high fertility, high infertility, and institutional inertia. I will trace the history of Niger over the long twentieth century through the lens of reproduction in the broadest sense: social (how societies at all scales ensure their own continuation), material (how the labor necessary to survival is secured and deployed), and biological (how a population, family, or individual replaces itself physically).[3] I will take up all these senses of reproduction because the three are entangled in Niger. Social status has historically been a function of one's capacity to attract material resources through the labor of others and to pass that status along to one's children. Every generation has been entrusted with the obligation to reproduce the heritage of the past, to provide for the day-to-day survival of family and workforce in the present, and to have children to ensure the perpetuation of the family line. To fail to make good on this debt is in effect to die a social death, betraying through negligence both ancestor and descendant while endangering the security of the community as a whole (Shipton 2007). It is not enough to simply reproduce, however—one must reproduce in the context of a "long and broad history of gendered and generational struggles over health, wealth, and power," which is to say that when and how one becomes pregnant matters a great deal (Thomas 2007, 51). Reproduction "gone awry" is the subject of ethical debate and gendered and generational violence. The female capacity to give birth renders women vulnerable both when they do manage to become pregnant and when they fail to do so.

I first became interested in the history of reproduction, thus broadly understood, at the time of the polio vaccination crisis of 2003, when rumors circulated that the vaccine would spread HIV and cause sterility in Muslim girls. Why, I wondered, were there perennial rumors about an alleged Western assault on African fertility? Why did fertility—or, to be more precise, the fear of infertility—seem to recur in moral panics in this region (Renne 1996, 2010)? It seemed to me that a historical approach to reproduction in Niger would enable me to discover the prior experience of medical and political intervention that might account for this "vaccine anxiety" (Leach and Fairhead 2007). I also hoped to rectify what I saw as a shortcoming of my previous work on marriage in the Hausa-speaking region of Maradi. When I conducted fieldwork for *Marriage in Maradi* (1997) I was relatively young and had no children. When the women I interviewed discovered that I had not yet given birth, they remarked dismissively of my marriage, "then it's not a marriage yet." I knew that this book would have to be about more than demography—it would have to take up what childbirth has meant to the men and women of Niger over time, and it would have to take up registers ranging from the intimacy of the individual body to the infrastructure of the state to the logic of the international NGO.

The arguments in this book build on but do not repeat observations I have articulated elsewhere focusing primarily on the Hausa-speaking region of Maradi. Demographic dynamics in southern Niger are profoundly influenced by proximity to Nigeria, where ethnoregional competition takes on significant religious overtones as Muslims in the north compete with Christians in the south for political ascendancy. Despite the tiny size of the Christian minority in Niger, the "fear of small numbers" that Arjun Appadurai describes so eloquently as a global phenomenon takes form in Niger as an anxiety among different subpopulations to produce more children *relative to one another* and to make the size of competing "communities" visible, often through celebratory rituals such as the baby naming ceremonies that are such a prominent part of life in the Sahel (Appadurai 2006; B. Cooper 2010c, 2011). Fertility, in other words, is always experienced and understood relative to others, which means that reproductive politics can be highly competitive at every scale (Johnson-Hanks 2006a). These dynamics do not necessarily respect national boundaries, even when the political contexts on either side of the border differ significantly. Yet demographic data is collected as if populations within these boundaries do not move, do not share languages and cultures, and do not carry ideas and practices as they travel.

Given the importance of competitive reproductive dynamics, it follows that understanding the history of childbirth and fertility in Niger also entails close attention to infertility. I have argued elsewhere that policy makers have given scant attention to the implications of the fear of infertility or subfertility. In Niger, as in much of Africa, sterility and secondary infertility are very significant dimensions of social and emotional life; altering reproductive behavior in ways that could slow the population growth rate will require much more serious attention to the profound problem of infertility. This simple observation flies in the face of the pervasive discourse of a crisis of overpopulation in the media and in a great deal of policy making (B. Cooper 2013). Finally, the tendency in contemporary media coverage of health in Niger to implicitly blame mothers for both overpopulation and infant malnutrition miscasts women as the problem rather than as savvy interpreters of the world around them operating under conditions and constraints not of their own choosing (B. Cooper 2007, 2009).

Accounting for Fertility

So whence comes this emphasis on overpopulation? A classic Malthusian model would posit that fertility must decline when population size outstrips the resources necessary to life; whether that decline occurs through famine or sexual restraint is a matter of history and policy. The key relationship in the Malthusian approach is productive capacity relative to consuming population under the assumption of fixed national boundaries and population immobility. If the capacity of the environment to produce more food does not grow at the same rate as the population, a dire outcome is easily predicted unless populations alter their consumption (Malthus 1798). Malthus criticized the English poor laws for limiting the mobility of laborers and for incentivizing marriage, thereby disinclining the poor to delay or entirely forgo childbearing.

Debates about population dominated the eighteenth- and nineteenth-century intellectual scene; however, a formal theory of demographic transition coalesced slowly. It was not until 1945 that demographer Frank Notestein articulated a general three-stage description of demographic transition, drawing from the contemporary understanding of the history of Western Europe.[4] In the first stage, a long-standing equilibrium in population size results from a balance between high fertility and high mortality. In a second stage, when conditions favor a decline in mortality, the population becomes unstable; it grows, resulting in a dramatic change in the age structure of society, with large numbers of young dependents relative to the aging population. But with time, and the recognition that more children will survive, a third stage takes off. Fertility declines, resulting in a more manageable ratio of dependents to working-age adults, producing a new equilibrium.

But what are the conditions that throw the system into disequilibrium, and through what mechanisms do populations adjust? Notestein saw modernization, urbanization, and industrialization as the drivers of population disequilibrium and readjustment: as family production declined in importance, education became more central to social mobility, and the cost of child rearing grew. His description was less a "theory" than a kind of overview of patterns against the backdrop of discussions of global food supply (Notestein 1945). Obviously, such a model invites elaboration in light of its congruence or incongruence with particular societies and histories. Historians and demographers collaborated under Ansley Coale's Princeton European Fertility Project to document as fully as possible the history of fertility decline in Europe, in particular testing the relationship between economic change and population decline.

What they found was surprising—namely, that economics alone could not account for the patterns found in fertility transition; there were clearly powerful cultural elements at play as well (Coale and Watkins 1986). Urbanization and industrialization did not necessarily precede decline, and fertility behavior could spread independent of socioeconomic development. Evidently, fertility decisions were not in any simple way the result of raw economic calculation. Still, certain patterns held in general: mortality always declined first, resulting in rapid population growth prior to fertility decline. As a result, there was a natural "momentum" to population growth generated by the sheer fact that there were larger numbers of women of childbearing age than in the past. Even as fertility declined, population could and often did continue to grow rapidly. On the other hand, once fertility decline set it, it rarely reversed; it too had a kind of momentum.

The search for the causes of fertility decline or its absence has always been politically fraught—after all, Malthus's original work was an antiutopian argument about the perverse incentives of the poor laws. The context for Notestein's original articulation of transition theory was the economic climate of the early postwar era and the need to ensure sufficient food for the world. Ansley Coale and Edgar Hoover took a Cold War–era interest in dependency ratios because the United States was rising relative to Europe as a force in global development (Coale and Hoover 1958). Contemporary debates about population are fundamentally debates about the cost of debt, relief, and development; about how to assign responsibility for environmental change; and about privileging individual agency over social good. It is difficult to disentangle political motives for cultural arguments and cultural motives for political arguments. Many historians and demographers have struggled to reach some kind of conclusion about the relative significance of "structural" factors (economy and rationality) and "super-structural" factors (culture, religion, values, or ideology). In this book I am alert to the political uses of arguments about culture, but that does not mean that I regard culture as unimportant. I am suspicious of efforts on any side to discount the *entanglement* of political economy and sociocultural practice, precisely because of the coincidence of biological, social, and day-to-day reproduction in the bodies and lives of women.

Whatever the debates among policy makers and theorists, women across West Africa are expected to produce children, feed families, and cultivate socially appropriate behaviors. Among the most important findings of recent work on reproduction in Africa is that, for women, the condition of being subject to a kind of ethical probation for much of their lives, as others assess their success or failure in terms of reproduction, produces enormous bodily and emotional strain. They are never quite women until they have proved themselves as mothers and their children in turn produce properly cultivated children. Success is uncertain given the unstable environment, economy, and political conditions of the region. Pamela Feldman-Savelsberg points to the anxiety women in the Cameroon grass fields region feel because of the multiple burdens that the responsibility for reproduction (producing children, reproducing societal structures, and feeding families) places on them. Women experience in an embodied manner the ambient threats to their identities, social positions, and emotional well-being, as in the case of a woman who "somatized her psychological and social difficulties as pain in the belly and interpreted them in the rubric of threats to her procreative capacity" (1999, 30; cf. Villarosa 2018; Geronimus 1994). The embodied experience of reproductive competition between co-wives conjoins fear and envy into a toxic presence that can itself cause infertility.

Women must meet these heavy expectations under conditions of structural violence that often make it impossible to meet the ideal of the good mother. Failures of development are regularly attributed instead to the "culture" of women. Not surprisingly, as Ellen Foley has recently pointed out, women experience the baby weighing of nutrition clinics as techniques to judge them as good or bad mothers, disinclining women to reveal that a child is sickly (2010, 149). Such implicit judgments depoliticize food security and economic vulnerability, making women "responsible" agents who simply need to be "made aware" of proper nutritional or reproductive practices. Failure to conform is then cast by governments, agencies, and donors as a kind of feminine irrationality. Activists then see women's resistance to external intrusion into family life as a kind of false consciousness.

The more productive approach entails a political economy of reproduction, or a "whole" demography that takes into account environmental, political, economic, cultural, and religious contexts (Greenhalgh 1995). As a historian, I see these in dynamic relationship to one another. Sometimes what appears to be a sign of continuity can disguise major shifts in meaning and experience, and what appears novel can, in fact, have deep roots in the past. Saskia Sassens emphasizes the importance of a Mande understanding of personhood that is relational rather than uniquely individual. To be fully human—neither animal nor monster—a child must acquire a name that marks survival of the dangerous liminal period after birth and that establishes legitimate paternity. But the child must then also pass through a life cycle that includes bodily modification, marriage, and the production of children and, ultimately, grandchildren. Above all, Sassens notes, "nothing is worse than 'to end' ('*ka ban*'), that is to have no descendants at all. A life is fulfilled when it ends in old age and the person is surrounded by children and grandchildren" (Sassens 2001, 17). However, to be a fully human person in this Mande context—that is to say, a freeborn person rather than the ancestor of a slave—also entails proper behavior relative to one's position, including showing shame (*maloya*). In this book, I insist that this performance of shame is not merely instrumental; it is deeply embodied, internalized, and affective.

The drama of women's lives in many ethnographic studies is experienced in the struggles to attain the stages of the life cycle and, in particular, to overcome the dangers and insecurities that thwart reproductive desires. That drama is heightened in the context of polygyny. The concept of fate, Sassens argues, provides some counterweight to the sense of failure or guilt that can accompany high child mortality or infertility. Similarly, Amal Hassan Fadlalla notes, externalizing reproductive mishaps as coming from something dangerously foreign—spirits, the evil eye, substances, contraceptives, outsiders and their influences—insulates women from a sense of failure (2007; Boddy 1989). That externalization also invites ritual countermeasures (genital surgery, spirit possession ritual, magical remedies, and protective charms) that offer a hermeneutics of blame that often targets other women.

Personhood for women is not simply a matter of producing children but of producing socially recognized children. With changes in the economy and the growing importance of women's education, women of childbearing age today face far more complex challenges to the appropriate achievement of the status positions that are marked by major life cycle events than in the past. Education, particularly where Christian mission schools took root, may be a condition necessary to achieving marriage, or to sustaining and preparing the children one produces, or of meeting the expectations of modern citizen, Christian, and mother. Catholic women in southern Cameroon, according to Jennifer Johnson-Hanks, must discipline their reproductive lives (delaying sexuality, pregnancy, or childbearing through abstinence, abortion, and fosterage) to enable them to become modern and honorable mothers. Honor here, as in the case of women of southern Sudan, rests on the capacity of women to show self-restraint. Honor—perhaps better understood as modesty and shame—requires discretion. However, rather than entailing the exclusion of the foreign as in Sudan, in southern Cameroon self-restraint calls for the embrace of a Catholic-inflected literacy and (somewhat unexpectedly) the discreet use of contraception and abortion. As a result, educated Catholic women in Cameroon no longer experience their first pregnancy, first birth, and entry into motherhood all at the same time (Johnson-Hanks 2006a).

In the industrialized world, economic and emotional considerations are often imagined to be diametrically opposed. But in a setting where there is no such thing as social security, no retirement account, no equity in a house, and no portfolio of stocks, there is one productive form of investment most people understand extremely well, and that is investment in people. Investing in people is a little like investing in livestock—once they are part of one's circle, they will go on to produce yet more wealth through their own reproduction. Not all children will become successful as farmers, or highly schooled bureaucrats, or traders. As one Hausa proverb has it, *ciki jeji ne, ba abinda ba ya haifuwa*: the womb is like virgin land, it can give birth to all manner of things. A good man may have a bad son and vice versa. But if one diversifies one's portfolio, one of those children will be successful in tapping the wealth of the state, another will be successful in attracting the wealth of the market, one will have a knack for making development projects work for the family, and another will provide cultural capital through mastery of Koranic knowledge. Parents in less developed countries don't have multitudes of children because they don't understand economics. They have multitudes of children because they understand economics all too well. There is nothing sadder or more desperate than an aging man or woman who has no kin on whom to rely.

A key argument of this book is that to understand why women and men today seek to have so many babies, one must recognize that children are not interchangeable labor units. When individuals or rulers reflect on the makeup of their families and communities, they don't see "population" in the abstract. They see children and adults who bring riches of all different kinds (*iri-iri* as one would say in Hausa—of many varieties of seed). Or they may, if they are less fortunate, see children who bring shame on the household and undermine the well-being of everyone as a result. One problem with the quantitative approach so frequently taken by policy makers, demographers, and NGOs is that in treating people as "populations" made up of abstract and homologous units, they miss the central truth that *diversity* in persons generates emotional, economic, and political value. In the enormous jump in scale from the intimacy of the body to the abstractions of the policy maker, most of what matters gets lost. This is why Nigerien civil servants may express the conviction that women should not have so many children while seeking infertility treatment themselves. In a constantly changing and uncertain world, it is hard to know which child will be the one who makes good on the intergenerational debt of entrustment. Better to have blessings in children abundant enough to weather the vagaries of drought, international commodity prices, school exams, political change, teenage pregnancy, and the unforeseeable but all too common road accident.

The term that has come to capture this approach to thinking about wealth-in-people is *compositional* (Guyer and Bellinga 1995; Johnson-Hanks 2006a, 32–34). People in West Africa have historically sought to accumulate riches of different kinds, and often those riches consist of capacities, skills, and powers. A highly skilled Hausa farmer (admired as a "king of the farmers") collected seeds of all kinds so that every conceivable environmental niche could be optimized and at least one seed crop would do well no matter what the vagaries of the rainfall. Women were skilled at recognizing the uses of leaves, fruits, barks, flowers, and seeds of the many different kinds of perennial plants that dotted the landscape of the precolonial Sahel.[5] If the harvest was poor, then wild grasses, melons, and fruits could tide a community over until the next rains. Success in gathering environmental wealth required drawing on the skills of a variety of different people of different backgrounds, families, regions, and innate ability. Such skills were highly valued by elites, who depended on their slaves, particularly slave women, to gather such foods in times of crisis and on rural communities to provide grain as a form of tax.

The Sahel as an Eco-Climate Zone

Without succumbing to environmental determinism, it helps to begin by taking the nature of Sahelian space into account in order to understand how humans have managed the resources of the Sahel in the form of people, goods, crops, and spiritual forces. One reason that the birth rates all across the Sahel are strikingly high is that the landscape itself has prompted certain strategies, limited others, and directed the flow of peoples and ideas. I will focus by and large on Niger—the limit case in the region for high fertility—but my reflections and evidence throughout this book must necessarily spill out into the territory of French West Africa as a whole and the northerly Sahelian zones within Nigeria, Ghana, Guinea, and Cameroon.

The Sahel marks the transition between the Sahara desert to the north and the better-watered savanna to the south.[6] Although for many today reference to the Sahel conjures images of a barren and impoverished region, it is in ecological terms rich in the range of desert and savanna flora and fauna it can support; historically it was the site of transregional exchange, thriving urban centers, and legendary kingdoms and empires. Before the rise of trans-Atlantic trade, the valuable products of Africa's more humid savanna and forest zones were traded toward the Sahel, which produced grain, meat,

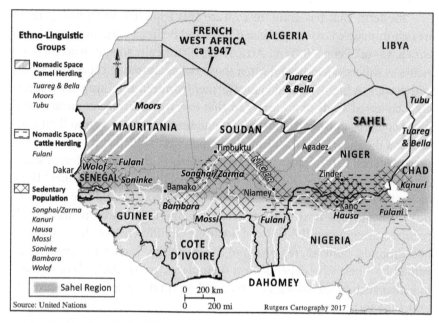

Sahel region and French West Africa, ca. 1947. Courtesy of Mike Siegel, Rutgers Cartography.

and leather. Some forestland goods, most notably gold, were then traded across the Sahara desert to the north. In exchange, Arab and Berber traders carried prestige goods such as cloth, Saharan salt, and horses. The markets of the Sahel provided the site of convergence for all these varied goods. Sahelian conditions inhospitable to the tsetse fly enable pastoralists to raise cattle. A host of edible and trade crops (some introduced through the trans-Saharan and trans-Atlantic trades) could be planted along permanent and seasonal rivers and lakes.[7]

The region is dependent on a single annual rainy season that results from the cyclical convergence of the humid winds from the south with the hot dry air mass of the Sahara. Major fluctuations in annual rainfall result in unpredictability and stress for farmers and pastoralists. This has necessarily produced long-term histories of movement as well as interdependence and borrowing between populations specializing in different lifeways. Populations developed techniques for transforming overgrown bush into pastureland, for transforming desiccated waterbeds into oases, and for generating tree cover; humans both shaped the environment and were shaped by it (Fairhead and Leach 1996).

While today we tend to speak of the Sahel, historically it was often referred to as the Sudan. As the camel made it possible to link the regional trade centers of the Sahel to those on the far side of the Sahara, Berber and Arab merchants gradually conceptualized the region as the "land of the blacks"—the *bilad al-sudan*. Ibn Battuta in the fourteenth century saw the peoples of these trade centers as different in kind, and that difference was marked as "black" (Hall 2011, 34). The *bilad al-sudan* was both the land in which black rulers, increasingly influenced by Islam from the ninth century on, controlled major centers of trade and the land in which merchants and caravan leaders could readily secure and sell slaves from both the north and the south.

Within the legal logic of enslavement in Islam, it sufficed to mark one's targets as either *kaffir* (non-Muslim infidel) or as *ahl al-bid'a* (heretical apostate) to justify their capture. Sedentary farming peoples were particularly vulnerable to capture by better-armed desert-edge warriors and raiders on horseback and camel. Over time, ideas about physical appearance (blackness) and enslaveability (non-Muslimness) tended to slip toward one another, prompting considerable debate among Muslim scholars about the relationship between race and enslaveability (Hall 2011; Hunwick and Troutt Powell 2002, xix–xxi, 35–50, 71–72; Hunwick 2000). Across the region, creative genealogical reckoning served as a means for Muslim rulers and circulating traders to stake a claim to nobility, "whiteness," or simply nonblackness (Hall 2011, 38, 58).

In the nineteenth century, slaves provided nomadic and merchant populations with a secure foothold within the zone of cultivation. Paul Lovejoy and Stephen Baier (1975) have detailed how slave and servile settlements in the Sahelian zone provided desert nomads with access to grain, secure points of water, and an emergency haven in the rain-fed zone in times of drought and famine. The labor of female slaves who gathered wild seed and grew grain supported the concentrations of populations at staging posts and trade centers. In the many European travel narratives of the nineteenth century, the Sahel was most immediately a landscape of food (Bivens 2007, 49).

Among Songhai and Tuareg, agricultural production was relegated to one servile segment of society, forever replenished through the raids of warrior classes and their slave armies on sedentary populations. Wolof, Mande, and Songhai elites, like the Moors and the Tuaregs, practiced caste endogamy. They depended on a division of labor between an extractive warrior class and a body of nominally free cultivators, second-generation slave-clients, and recently captured slaves (Olivier de Sardan 1984; Barry 1998, 29–30). Elites denigrated agricultural production as shameful and elevated the capacity to raid others—and in particular to acquire captives for exchange and for labor—as the sign of nobility. While centralized societies a bit farther east (Hausaland and Bornu) offered longer-term social mobility to captives, their absorption entailed the regular replacement of slave labor through purchase or capture. The logic of depredation produced cascading violence as societies of the Sahel preyed on sedentary "infidel" *kaffir* populations or turned accusations of apostasy into a pretext to attack.

Fulani society, like Tuareg society, comprised a mobile livestock-owning nobility, a relatively sedentary and often clerical population, a warrior elite, an artisanal caste, and a settled slave class (*rimaiBe*) whose agricultural production was taxed by their masters. Drifting gradually from west to east over many centuries, Fulani herders and mixed farmers were often dependent on cooperative arrangements with relatively secure militarized sedentary populations for access to water holes and forage. Free sedentary farmers might entrust some of their own livestock to these herders to migrate north with their herds during the rainy season. Fulbe pastoralists gained seasonal access to forage and grain after the harvest by parking their herds on the lands of sedentary farmers, while agriculturalists gained access to manure, milk, and meat in the exchange.

Nevertheless, in the eighteenth and nineteenth centuries, Fulani clerics led numerous jihads that were successful in part because of the growing resentment of herders at "un-Islamic" taxation of their cattle and the sale of Muslims into the trans-Atlantic or trans-Saharan trade (Ware 2014). In the territorial states that emerged (Futa Toro, Futa Jallon, Masina, and eventually Sokoto), slaves were a source of both labor and revenue. Slaves could be traded for guns and horses, feeding a cycle of violence. In the wake of the Haitian revolution and the passage of the British Slave Trade Act of 1807, the market for slaves at the Atlantic coast was gradually undermined. Warring states were constrained to absorb captives internally rather than export them. The Fulfulde elite of the post-jihad Sokoto and Gwandu caliphates significantly altered agricultural and slave-use patterns; the aggregation of large numbers of captive farm laborers and artisans fed the economic explosion of the region in the later nineteenth century, replicating and expanding in some ways on the settlement pattern of locating captives in oases and servile villages that had previously been more common farther to the west (Lovejoy 1978; Salau 2011). By the nineteenth century, it was clear that slave labor had become the cornerstone of Sudanic societies (Klein 1998, 12; Lovejoy 2011).

Clearly, this zone already had a coherence resulting from the environmental, racial, ethnic, and religious patterns that had emerged out of interactions among Africans dating from well before colonial rule. The scramble for Africa was played out within the context of those patterns. France, with the appearance of René Caillié's travel narrative of his voyage to Timbuktu in 1830, fixed on the Sahel as the heart of its interests in West Africa (Kanya-Forstner 1969, 263). French commercial interests imagined that linking the upper Senegal River to the Niger Bend region and then to Lake Chad would generate a vast terrain of agricultural richness. By 1854, Timbuktu was seen as the lynchpin to bridge the valuable French territories of Algeria and Senegal (Kanya-Forstner 1969, 27). Once the city of Say had been secured along the Niger, the next major interior water body was Lake Chad—the potential meeting point of French expansion south from Aïr, north from the Congo, and east from the Niger River.

The military scientists of the Mission Tilho, tasked from 1906 to 1909 with collecting scientific data pertaining to the territory between Niger and Lake Chad while demarcating the boundary between Niger and Nigeria, were disappointed to find how shallow the immense lake actually was and to discover the possibility that it was shrinking (Tilho 1910, 1928). The landscape could vary substantially depending on the timing and force of the rainfall and the depth of the underground water resources. Heavy rainfall could alter the watercourses or create pools of water that unexpectedly made it possible to plant. Poor accumulation in other sites could significantly alter the vegetation or render a well unusable (Lefebvre 2011). Human movements and settlements in the Sahel had a fluidity that was out of keeping with the fixity envisioned by the mapping of European nation-states.

The pronounced east-west orientation of France's imperial drive superimposed the new colonial order on the existing dynamics of human appropriation in the agropastoral meeting ground of the desert edge. This east-west orientation inadvertently weakened the far more commercially viable north-south links between the forested zone and the interior, the control of which had always been crucial to the success of states and markets in the region. France's landlocked territories of the Sahel were particularly poorly situated as the regional economy shifted away from northbound routes in favor of routes giving out on the Atlantic coast.

The Abolition of Slavery

European colonization of Africa was justified through an abolitionist discourse that cast "Arabs" as slave traders and Europeans as civilizing saviors. In 1905, France abolished all transactions in persons in its territories: it would no longer be possible to make a legal claim involving the sale, inheritance, exchange, or gift of a human being. This approach to the ending of slavery, known as "legal status abolition," did not abolish slavery per se. However, it did make it possible for many slaves to leave their owners without fear of legal reprisal. Between 1905 and 1908, somewhere between two hundred thousand and five hundred thousand slaves simply picked up and left their masters to return to their homelands or to settle in new villages (Roberts and Klein 1980; Klein 1998, 159–67; Rodet 2015). Tuareg groups, already weakened by the depletion of their wealth in livestock during French conquest, now lost whatever capital they had invested in anyone who chose to leave.

Not all captive populations left; some remained where they were for a host of complex reasons, giving rise to servile classes of "captives" and "domestics" of ambiguous status with ongoing linkages to the societies into which they had become, in a sense, integral (Clark 1999). The ending of the slave trade threatened to disrupt political and economic stability; France quite quickly found that the labor requirements of the region made the wholesale erasure of servitude incompatible with the maintenance of order and the raising of revenue to fund the emerging colonial order (Klein 1998, 16). The renegotiation of descent, marriage, social legitimacy, and fertility were central to the complex social revolution to which French occupation and the abolition of slavery gave rise.

One of the most striking features of colonial rule in Africa in general was the acceleration of Islamization during that period (Levtzion and Pouwels 2000). In attempting to render its new territories legible and governable, French colonial thinkers consistently drew on a schematic version of Islamic law and made reference to the racialized assumptions that subtended the slave economy of the earlier era. To do so, they also relied on the very aristocratic and scholarly elites that had an interest in sustaining relations of dominance and servitude. Colonial administrator and thinker Maurice Delafosse traced the beginnings of a binary understanding of difference even as he struggled to sidestep an overly physiological approach to "race." Whiteness for him adhered particularly well to Islamic societies.

The highly Islamicized Wolof, Hausa, Songhai, northern Mande, and Toucouleurs considerably muddied the clarity of his model (Delafosse 1912, Vol. I, 350–51). The northerly "white" peoples, although permitted by Islam to take up to four wives, tended toward monogamy. Their women had greater social influence, and their fidelity was purportedly highly prized (Vol. I, 311). In "black" societies, polygyny was purportedly functionally necessary because of the near universal taboo on sexual relations during menstruation, pregnancy, and nursing (Vol. III, 62–63). The high labor demands within desert and desert-edge agropastoral economies that had for so long fueled the demand for slaves were entirely occluded within Delafosse's division of "white" and "black" societies. The cultural dimensions of race simultaneously undercut and reinforced the very notion of racial difference.

This colonial-era distinction between white and black was superimposed on the preexisting logic of religion and racial difference that had informed enslavement in the region. Blackness was associated with marginal Muslim credentials and whiteness with adherence to the rigid orthodoxy of "pure" Islam. It would be important to French dominance to protect the black populations from contamination by the fanaticism of "Arab" Islam. The "black Islam" (*Islam noir*) both invented and cultivated under French rule was further reinforced by the bureaucratic logic of the French empire in Africa, through which North Africa and most importantly Algeria fell to one ministry and French West Africa to an entirely different one. Two separate cultures of administration and scholarship emerged, one of which functioned in French and Arabic, was driven by the logic of settler colonialism, and enjoyed the prestige of belonging to France proper; the other, clearly the poorer cousin, functioned in French and a motley array of African languages, was driven by the logic of minimal expenditure, and fell under the Colonial Ministry (Triaud 2014).

The extractive demands of the colonial economy pushed the agriculturalists of the desert edge to plant ever-greater areas of land with cash crops. At the outset, cotton production was promoted, but later peanut production for export took pride of place in the colonial economy, resulting in an increasing need for farm labor at the very moment that servile labor had become less available. The struggle to produce sufficient peanuts to meet tax requirements also prompted agriculturalists to plant seed in the northerly fringe of the rain-fed region, where in years of high rainfall it was possible to produce a crop. However, in years of poor rains serious cash and food shortages could result. The colonial period was marked by major famines in

1913–14 and again in 1930–31. Food shortages were aggravated by high taxes, requisitions of animals, and in general the erosion of the capacity to store wealth in livestock that could be sold where food was more plentiful and livestock prices high (Gado 1993).

The rise of cash cropping combined with the growing autonomy of formerly enslaved populations considerably altered the social landscape of the region. Some slave settlements established themselves as independent villages. Former slaves of Tuareg pastoralists, clerics, and merchants were among the most eager to establish their freedom and to stake a claim to sedentary status. Tuareg refer to themselves as Kel Tamasheq ("Speakers of Tamasheq"); their slaves also spoke Tamasheq and might also engage in livestock rearing; in a sense they too were Kel Tamasheq. Yet Tamasheq-speaking slaves, often referred to as Bella or Buzu, were particularly likely to mimic Hausa farming practices in an effort to make a permanent shift to sedentary mixed farming (Bernus 1981, 275–76). The colonialists found these newly independent and highly mobile populations exceedingly difficult to manage, for without masters the former slaves of the nomads effectively had no recognized chief at all.

Other agropastoral settlements were populated by Fulfulde speakers who had begun to deploy a variety of strategies for combining livestock raising with farming. Some focused largely on raising livestock near wells, others farmed long narrow strips of land through which the livestock could be rotated, while yet others opened up new farmland in the relatively marginal land to the north of the higher-concentration settlements near the seasonal watercourses (Diarra 1979; Boutrais 1994). Like the Bella, these agriculturalists were often of slave origin or ancestry, although some freeborn Fulfulde speakers also practiced a broader mix of agricultural and pastoral practices (Riesman 1992; Dupire 1962).

So long as the rainfall in the region remained unusually high, as was the case for much of the first half of the century, the vulnerability produced by these shifts did not necessarily come into evidence. The rainfall in the Sahel, we now know, is subject to great long-term variability, which was as true of the colonial period as it had been in the past (Joint Institute 2016). The unpredictable rainfall of the 1930s and 1940s pushed access to water and pasture further afield during the Global Depression and early years of World War II. Greater distances traveled with herds called for either the labor of more herdsmen or a greater burden on those already at hand. In the past, the freeborn Tuareg and Fulani had eased their own labor demands by claiming the labor of the children of their agricultural slaves. Captive boys had been enlisted to take over the task of herding, and captive girls had been charged with domestic tasks including the arduous task of finding and drawing water for animals as well as humans and finding wild grain or processing millet for consumption. Where clientage relations persisted into the twentieth century, or where coercion was still possible because of the distance from colonial structures, that labor might still be available. Nevertheless, increasingly Bella and RimaiBe populations contested the seizure of their children and laid claim to the land they worked (Bernus 1981, 61; Klein 2005).

Because colonial rule was carried out in large part through the vehicle of "traditional" rulers of both sedentary and pastoral populations, chiefs designated by the colonialists could recast former slave relations into "traditional" labor tribute for themselves, for the military, or for French major public works projects. Those who succeeded in making use of the coercive apparatus of the state to stake a claim to labor (or to the product of that labor) as part of their due as "customary" chiefs might continue to flourish. In local perceptions, slavery and the era of colonial forced labor often blurred into one another (and still do), for the coercion of labor persisted and was extracted through the hegemony of the same figures—noble chiefs and their sons—as had extracted it in the past. The suppression of summary punishments available to administrators under the *indigénat* code effectively ended forced labor in the spring of 1946 (Mann 2009).

Colonial rule and the abolition of slavery in the Sahel gradually stripped away many of the defining characteristics of nobility—military prowess; privileged access to the intimidating trappings of warfare, such as guns, horses, and camels; and perhaps most importantly the recognized capacity to redistribute seized labor, women, livestock, and grain. These shifts had complex implications for reproductive concerns. With the decline in open enslavement, virtually all that remained to mark status difference was the size of one's entourage and an exaggerated concern for the behaviors associated with free status. For Arab, Tuareg, Hausa, Kanuri, Songhai, and Fulani elites, it would no longer be possible to simply assert control over resources through violence; hegemony would now have to be sustained through visible performances of superior status.

Like other colonial powers, France found it a great deal easier to celebrate the ideal of the abolition of slavery than to actually operationalize it, given the priority of the maintenance of order and the extraction of sufficient revenues to render the colonial territories self-financing (Klein 1998; Lovejoy and Hogendorn 1993; Miers and Roberts 1988). By tacitly approving the persistence of servile relations and subtly reinforcing them through the army, courts, and schooling, France hoped to set off a very gradual shift from slavery to other kinds of labor patterns without altogether disrupting the social hierarchy. Nevertheless, the institutions that reproduced power relations could also introduce spaces through which the existing order could be contested: slaves sent to school in the place of the "sons and nephews" of chiefs could eventually become more powerful than their former masters; former slave soldiers became quite articulate about their enhanced rights as veterans, while former farm slaves could attempt to argue in court that any land they had cleared themselves belonged to them as first-comers. Eventually, through both schooling and courts, women could attempt to renegotiate the terms of marriage and their access to inheritance under Islamic law (B. Cooper 1997).

As it grew increasingly difficult to reproduce captive labor through raids, warfare, or the market, it became necessary to control servile labor through some other means. One approach was to retain female slaves as "concubines," who the French conveniently understood to be "like family" and therefore not really enslaved. As a result, there was increasing slippage between the tasks of the female slave and the tasks of the junior wife. Concubines could be treated as junior wives, and the hierarchy among and between wives was accentuated with particular emphasis placed on distinguishing between those wives who had produced children for the household and those who had not. Effectively, childbearing and leisure time were to become the most important means of distinguishing free women from servile (B. Cooper 1994).

In the numerous societies in which the children of elite men by their female slaves had been set off in a category distinct from that of the elite, the logic of endogamy in marriage played an important role in maintaining social distinctions. Rigid adherence to status or caste endogamy could serve to maintain firewalls between the freeborn "noble" stratum, freed castes with artisanal skills, and the captive slave lines subjected to strenuous labor demands. Maintaining the leisure of a freeborn wife entailed the presence of female servants, generally from the formerly captive populations. Social boundaries between status groups were (and often still are) carefully policed and performed. Across the Sahel, differences in respectability, comportment, and labor are bound up with free versus captive origin

(Pelckmans 2015). Casted men whose families are understood to have been "born" into servile relations vis-à-vis the free would never be permitted to marry women of noble background, but, by the same token, casted men would not deign to marry women from families of recent slave heritage (Olivier de Sardan 1984, 44, 120).

A History of Institutional Absence

A history of reproductive health in Niger over the long twentieth century is necessarily a history of colonial medicine, mission medicine, and global health. The case of Niger complicates many of the assumptions of the historiography of health in Africa. A conventional narrative of colonial medicine would begin by noting that imperialism in Africa was made possible with the development of treatments for malaria, a disease that decimated European adventurers in West Africa. Colonial medicine served both as the justification for and a necessary condition of colonization. At first, colonial medicine strove to improve the survival rates of soldiers stationed in West Africa and protecting colonial administrators. Early efforts at public health consisted of segregating Europeans spatially from Africans, particularly in the growing colonial urban centers. This was done in part to protect Europeans from the dangerous "ill humors" that were seen in the late nineteenth century to be the cause of illness. But such segregation also promoted a sense that African bodies were the source of contagion, an association that became even more pronounced with advances in germ theory (Greene et al. 2013).

This much of the narrative would hold more or less for Niger. However, much of the work on colonial medicine focuses on British and American colonial settings, not French West Africa. This Anglo-centric literature has generated a number of assumptions about colonial medicine that simply do not hold for most of the Sahel. If Darwinian evolutionary theory dominated the logic of eugenics in Britain and the United States, French eugenics held to Lamarkian evolutionary theory. That is, it was imagined that an individual could acquire traits through training and habit, which would then be passed on to his or her offspring biologically. A key medical concern was whether individuals or "races" could be acclimatized to new settings. French subjects were envisioned, through careful cultivation, as being amenable to evolving—hence the use of the term *évolué* to characterize the educated African.

But for this to happen, French citizens would need to bestow on the indigenous populations French language and civilization, which might or might not be seen to include Catholicism. The French approach eschewed the interventions of outsiders in the interests of turning subjects, eventually, into evolved French citizens. This important work could not be handed over to missionaries, many of whom were neither French nor Catholic. With the notable exceptions of the work of the White Fathers (limited to North and East Africa) and the Spiritans (limited primarily to Senegal), Catholic missionaries were discouraged by the French from working in Muslim regions. By contrast, in British, Belgian, and Portuguese colonies in Africa, the task of meeting the medical and educational needs of the African population was deliberately left to Christian missions, largely Protestant. Missionaries focused on saving individuals, not populations as a whole, and as a result most Africans encountered biomedicine in the intimate, moralizing, and "civilizing" context of mission medicine (Vaughan 1991; Hunt 1999; Comaroff and Comaroff 1991, 1997; Landau 1995). Mission medicine often took up maternal and infant health as part of an effort to reform African family life and sexuality, particularly polygyny. Historically, missionaries and the Africans they attempted to convert often shared a deep commitment to reproduction (Smythe 2006).

This book is as much a history of the *absence of infrastructure* as it is of childbirth. I attempt to account for why Niger's maternal health system today is so poor, its progress in improving maternal and infant health so slow, and its ability to serve the needs of women in general so limited. One reason I emphasize is that Niger was a military territory up until 1920 and a "colony" only from 1922; it was managed bureaucratically through the military for over two decades. Well after other territories of French West Africa were under civilian rule, Niger was governed by ranking military officers. Trained civilian judges arrived in Niger only on the eve of decolonization; prior to that time, military administrators had handled the tribunals (David 2007). Unlike the colonies that are the subject of most histories of medicine in Africa, Christian missions had very little impact in the medical domain here. In Niger, at the margins of the French West African empire, colonial medicine remained primarily military medicine until the time of independence. This had significant implications for the development of reproductive health services. Until independence, military doctors—whose priorities lay with ensuring the health of male soldiers and laborers—dominated the formal medical infrastructure. To the degree that

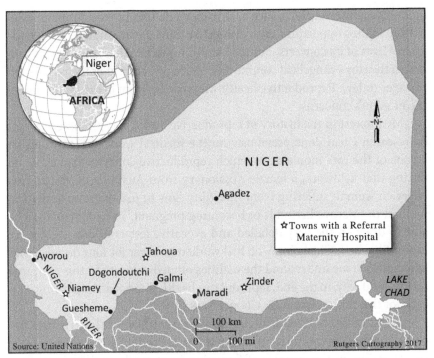

Contemporary Niger with major maternity hospitals. Courtesy of Mike Siegel, Rutgers Cartography.

military medical officers were interested in reproductive health issues, it was to prevent the exposure of soldiers to STDs. By the time nutrition and infant health were more central, during and after World War II, the accumulated effects of Niger's marginality had already left it far behind.

Furthermore, the modest missionary presence that did manage to make itself felt in Niger was limited to the Anglophone "faith" missionaries of the Sudan Interior Mission (SIM). Unlike mainstream missions concentrated along the African coastline whose vocation was to civilize Africans and thereby bring them into the fold of Christendom, the faith missions targeting the peoples of the "interior" rejected the social Gospel emphasis on civilizational uplift through hospitals and schools. Instead, the SIM strove above all to plant vernacular evangelical churches so that indigenous Christians would be called on by God to continue the work of evangelization themselves (B. Cooper 2006). SIM had no significant impact on schooling in Niger. The emphasis of its limited medical work prior to independence in

1960 was on interventions, such as leprosy work, that provided missionaries with sustained opportunities to evangelize. SIM did attempt to reshape the family lives of its converts, but the overall impact of these efforts was limited to the tiny evangelical community (perhaps 1 percent of the population of Niger today). Reproductive health was very far from being at the core of the mission's concerns.

My interest in the history of reproductive health was prompted in part by research I had done previously on the medical work of SIM in Niger. In one of the rare moments in which reproductive concerns had come up during that fieldwork, a female missionary from Australia explained to a Nigerien woman suffering from infertility how to use the reverse rhythm method to improve her odds of becoming pregnant. I was fortunate to be able to draw on the very detailed and evocative letters of one missionary nurse, Elizabeth Chisholm, who had worked in Niger for four decades. Her letters helped me understand the realities of medical work in this marginal setting, and why, in the end, reproductive health was not an overriding concern for this faith mission (B. Cooper 2018a).

It was really only with decolonization that heath infrastructure became a central preoccupation under the independent government of Niger. Drawing on the promise of financing from newly exploited uranium wealth and the income from the expansion of peanut cropping, Niger initiated ambitious plans to build schools, hire doctors and teachers, and develop maternal and infant care. The internal dynamics of nation building were to become rapidly entangled with the external logics of the Cold War, the rise of international institutions such as the World Bank and the International Monetary Fund, and the externally driven discourse of development. The first independent government under Hamani Diori encountered the tensions between addressing local political concerns and cultivating international prominence and financial support. The Great Sahel Drought of 1968–1974 altered the lenses through which the region was seen by the international community; "desertification" and "overpopulation" became ever more salient as ways to understand the difficulties of the region, entailing a push for population control on the one hand and for externally driven development on the other.

Shortly after Niger's first official coup, Seyni Kountché entertained major reforms to women's participation in public life against the backdrop of International Women's Year in 1975. At the global scale, the optimism of the African leaders at the Alma Ata conference of 1978 seemed to signal a general consensus that major investment in primary health care should be the way forward. However, without funding and against the backdrop of the gathering debt crisis in Latin America, that broad-based initiative withered. Instead, a seemingly more cost-effective and "selective" primary health approach emerged targeting maternal and infant health through inexpensive interventions including growth monitoring, teaching oral rehydration therapy, encouraging breastfeeding, and promoting immunizations (Basilico et al. 2013). Rather than a robust network of general health clinics, Niger established localized centers devoted to "the protection of mothers and infants" (PMI). This was health care on the cheap, not a national health system, and it pitted the interests of pregnant women and infants against those of male adults and older children. Still, it was a beginning, and for a brief moment Niger's schooling and health systems appeared to be coming into fruition. Civil service jobs for teachers and medical personnel helped anchor the economy, and uranium mining and peanut expansion looked like the beginnings of a viable economy.

The growing fixation of Western institutions on women's reproductive lives and population control fueled the counterdiscourses of Islamists and Islamic reformers. By the early 1980s, loans to developing countries were increasingly subject to conditions requiring the liberalization of markets: government subsidies were discouraged, civil servants were laid off, salaries were frozen, and parastatal enterprises that had provided employment were "sold" only to wither away almost immediately. Resentment at the intrusions of external powers in Niger's sovereign decision making came to a slow boil (B. Cooper 2003). The confrontation of different ideas about health care, gender, family, and reproduction initiated during the Decade for Women was increasingly expressed in an idiom of Islamic reform versus elite feminism, rendering issues surrounding childbirth—particularly contraception—extremely volatile. With the democratic transition of 1990, these tensions exploded, generating a host of competing civil society groups. Rather than improving women's capacity to push for safeguards to reproductive health, "democracy" sometimes appeared to women's rights activists to simply empower reactionary Islamic groups.

The Ambiguous Legacy of Islam

One of the ironies of French colonial rule was that its bureaucratic, military, and judicial imperatives had the effect of privileging Islamic leadership and the outlines of the Islamic legal tradition of the region (Maliki law) over other nodes of authority and modes of moral reckoning (B. Cooper 1997). Because so much of the resistance to colonial rule in the Sahara and Sahel had been couched in the idiom of Islamic jihad, administrators worked to appease the perceived sensibilities of rebellious groups, in part by discouraging Christian missions. The net effect was that practices related to marriage, inheritance, burial, child custody, sexuality, and so on were profoundly influenced by an Islamicized colonial governmentality over the six decades of French rule. By the time of independence, few Nigeriens openly rejected Islam. Nevertheless, both urban and rural populations held strongly to beliefs through which spirit veneration and occult practices endured. Such practices were not simply vestiges of an animist past; they flourished in the same urban centers and trade routes along which Islamic knowledge traveled. They were part and parcel of the fabric of Sahelian Islamic religious practice.

The perception that "we have always been Muslim" encourages Nigeriens today to interpret beliefs, practices, and sentiments that often have deeper roots as being Islamic in origin and essence. Proper comportment is therefore believed to be specifically Muslim, and improper comportment is that of the heretic or infidel. A great deal of tension and debate exists between Muslims in West Africa about what precisely are the permissible practices of a committed Muslim. Such debate had motivated the Islamic jihads of the eighteenth and nineteenth centuries in West Africa as well; they are not altogether new (B. Cooper 2006). Contemporary debates over Islamic orthodoxy and Sufism overlay but do not eliminate the deeper origins of social hierarchies in the region. Aristocratic privilege, prior to French conquest, was based on supremacy through force—the horse or camel, the gun, and the sword. French colonial rule did not in and of itself generate the profound inequities in Niger today; it amplified and at times reified differences that had in the past been more fluid. It sometimes inverted them (Pettigrew 2017). By drawing on the legitimacy of existing elites to administer its territory, France ratified the continuing privilege of the freeborn aristocracy relative to commoners, the descendants of slaves, and those of ambiguous ancestry. On the other hand, new access to privilege through the military or schooling could favor those of slave background.

In reality, the majority of the population at the time of French conquest was not Muslim, although Muslim scholars were common throughout the Sahel, and many authority figures and military leaders in centralized states were, at least outwardly, committed to Islam. However nonelite farming and pastoralist populations well into the 1950s sustained a proper relationship with the spirits of the landscape through ritual practices to placate, attract, or restrain spirits that inhabited land, waterways, and the unfarmed land where wild animals dwelled. Some spirits, known in Hausa as *bori*, were mobile, taking on the qualities and pretensions of the inhabitants of the urban centers: the prince, the pilgrim, the harlot Maria. *Bori* was essentially urban and Muslim while rural Arna spirit veneration was indifferent to Islam. In less urban areas, spiritual presences animated the landscape.

The rich visual documentation of the 1924 *croisière noire* expedition sponsored by Citroën provides a record of spiritual practices, the performance of status, and social and sexual hierarchies across the farming belt of the newly conquered military territory of Niger. In addition to advertising the engineering of Citroën, the mission was calculated to demonstrate French military mobility to restive nomadic Saharan subjects and to ignite popular interest in France's African empire. The expedition also had a mandate to collect images and objects for museums and the Geographic Society. The impulse to document the trip to render Africa visible in the metropole yielded a famous film, *La Croisière Noire* (roughly "The Black Voyage"), by cinematographer Léon Poirier; thousands of photographs (taken largely by Georges-Marie Haardt); and paintings and drawings (by Alexandre Iacovleff). Set alongside the later written accounts of the voyage, the photographs by Haardt as the mission skirted the southern edge of Niger reveal the predominance of non-Islamic practices even in unexpected settings. The still shots and paintings capture a great deal of social texture. The images and text reveal the tensions and competition between women emerging as a result of the abolishment of slavery and the growing presence of male French administrators.

Above all, the images remind us of the significance of indigenous cosmologies as the French administration began to gather administrative force in urban centers. The extraordinary flexibility of spirit practices such as *bori* meant that they could assist populations in making sense of the continually changing circumstances enriching or imperilling their well-being. The *bori* spirit possession cult was the logical extension of rural spirit beliefs in urban settings in which rural social organization and ties to the land had become less relevant. Once the shift from clan spirits fixed in the farming landscape to mobile *bori* had been made, there was really nothing to prevent the proliferation of new *bori* spirits reflecting the growing complexity of urban life (see Leroux 1948, 678; Faulkingham 1975). Many spirits were pooled by urban dwellers of various origins. *Bori* was more than an ideology or therapeutic system; it was (and continues to be) a poetic mode through which meaning could be both discerned and created (Masquelier 2001a). With the advent of colonial rule, rather than being eclipsed altogether, the spirit pantheon simply embraced new figures, such as the monsieur and the soldier.

Prior to abolition, across the Sahel the right to take captives in warfare, raids, or through purchase rested on the logic of enslaveability in Islam. Free status, therefore, was de facto Muslim status, and the misfortune of falling into captivity became proof of one's fundamental baseness, slavishness, and unorthodoxy. Only someone who was not honorable would suffer himself to be enslaved; as the adage ubiquitous throughout the region goes, "death is better than shame." It would be better to die in battle than to endure the shame of enslavement. The significance of slave holding varied to some degree between societies in the region, as did the rigidity with which social positions were kept distinct. Tuareg, Fulani, and Songhai elites did little hard manual labor themselves, depending on the labor of captives for farming and livestock management. Rigid caste endogamy ensured that social lines were not blurred. Hausa and Kanuri speakers, by contrast, did not necessarily associate heavy farm labor with slavery and were more open to an exogamy that made possible the absorption of defeated populations.[8] Preferential cousin marriage had less to do with status differences than with retaining control of resources within the family. French domination was to disrupt and recast the organization of labor and the social and affective bases on which slavery rested.

The archival traces generated by the court system established under French rule have provided me with some glimpses of how a system that linked military administrators to male indigenous authorities affected women. I draw on such judicial records to illustrate how indigenous ethical and legal approaches to pregnancy, birth, and infanticide clashed with the nascent French sense of "repugnancy" and the rising ethical positioning of orthodox Muslims. These debates among and between men were to have profound consequences for the definition of propriety and for the range of sexual and reproductive options available to women. Encounters with the courts inevitably pushed Nigeriens toward ethical arguments based on Islam, even when the desired outcome had not previously been dictated by Islam.

A History of Affect

The abolition of slavery and its very gradual enforcement in the early decades of the twentieth century under French rule profoundly disrupted the monopoly on violence of elites who owned guns, horses, and camels. It also heightened the need for labor, for colonialists placed heavy demands on the freeborn to produce laborers, taxes, and pack animals. Elites needed ever more labor at the very moment that the French began to dismantle slavery. Previously, it had been possible to assemble a following by seizing children at will from captive populations for servants, concubines, field labor, and herders. With the abolition of slavery, it became crucial to elites to maintain relations of dominance over formerly enslaved populations. In the absence of the monopoly on force, only the comportments associated with elite status remained—restraint, modesty, and respect. The performance of restraint became the signal distinction between masters and their potential clients. In the languages of the region, only the dishonorable—slaves, djinns, unruly women—lack this capacity for restraint (*kunya* in Hausa, *pulaaku* in Fulfulde, *takarakit* in Tamaschek, *hààwì* in Zarma, *nongy* in Kanuri, *maloya* in Bamanankan). These semantically rich terms, often translated as *shame* or *modesty*, encapsulate much more than a behavioral ideal. Shame is internalized as the visceral experience of status and identity, humanity and personhood. "Shame" is frequently invoked as the reason for action or inaction; it is a sensation that has the power to act on the person and thereby to situate him or her within society. However, emotions are human processes. As Julie Livingston notes, "We must contemplate them within socially complex and dynamic historical worlds. These worlds are linked and at times densely connected through movements of people, goods, ideas, and of course the prevention of movement such that some found themselves trapped in increasingly untenable worlds" (Eustace et al. 2012, 1520).

This book, in addition to being a history of institutions, is a history of the emotions of shame, fear, and envy. It takes up the existential experiences of fertility and infertility, personhood and monstrosity. Shame defines who is fully human and who is not. Hausa, Zarma, and Fulani culture have long discouraged women from seeking assistance while in labor, and this is explained in today's terms of propriety and modesty, which entail both "shame" and "respect." It is only when the newborn cries that a woman should call for the help of an older woman whose primary task is to cut the umbilical cord and assemble the placenta for burial behind the hut.

Is it "natural" for a woman to give birth alone in silence? Choosing *not* to do what is "natural" for humans-as-animals may be the most powerful mark of human culture. This is why adhering to such norms distinguishes the "civilized" from the "slave" and human from beast. The emphasis on propriety may serve to deflect attention from another significant reason why women even today do not want to draw attention to birth: fear that such a public announcement of the dangerous moment of birth would render the mother and baby more vulnerable to sorcery or to the involuntary violence of the evil eye produced by envy. In many ways, *kunya* (shame) and *'kishiya* (envy) are opposite sides of the same coin. More than anything else, given the inherent risks of childbirth, women in the region have always done all they could to avoid what they perceive to be predictable dangers, even as those dangers shift. This notion of shame or modesty enjoins them to protect their pregnancy and their newborn from the dangers of exposure to jealousy and other risks. Today, those dangers are acute in public places like hospitals where privacy is impossible, where taboo subjects are discussed openly, and where doctors and nurses insist on touching the vulnerable body.[9]

Very little literature on the demography of the region addresses what I have come to think of as the *affective* determinants of fertility. The "proximate determinants" of fertility directly shape the biological context of fecundability (the capacity to become pregnant at any given moment) and pregnancy outcomes.[10] But emotion, or to be more precise *affect*, subtends the beliefs and behaviors that produce those "proximate determinants."[11] Shame, envy, and fear together act in powerful ways on men and women; indeed, they are often understood to be forces in their own rights that, once released, can enhance or destroy fertility, success, and well-being. One's identity as a Muslim, as freeborn, as male or female, as senior or junior, as a "real" Fulani or a "proper" Hausa—all are *felt* as much as performed.

It is a tremendous challenge for the historian to find evidence that can serve to reconstitute emotions in the past, particularly in a setting where written evidence is hard to come by and in which showing emotion inappropriately is seen as dishonorable. Essays written by secondary school students across the territories of French West Africa (archived in the Fonds École William Ponty at the Institut Fondamental d'Afrique Noire in Dakar) offer a particularly rich source for exploring how a sense of proper comportment was cultivated by societies in the Sahel under French rule.[12] Because French West Africa was a federated territory, the most promising "sons and nephews" of notables throughout the federation were sent to secondary schools (*lycée*) in Senegal for their final training. At the end of their studies, the boys were given an essay assignment to do as a *"mémoire de fin d'études."*[13] Essay assignments varied, but all had an ethnographic dimension: the boys were to describe in detail some aspect of life in their home communities in an effort to prepare them to become schoolteachers and other functionaries exhibiting a high degree of competence in the French language.[14] These autoethnographic exercises, in this case written between 1935 and 1949, shed a great deal of light on how the children who were destined to enter the educated elite understood the socialization of children in their ethnic groups. They are a wonderful source of information about practices and beliefs but also about which feelings were deemed admissible and which were not. Recognition as a full person, as a proper member of the human community, came with proper comportment, and that comportment was ambiguously related to Islamic religious practice.

Colonial Accounting

Most documents produced during the colonial period were written by French administrators and were pitched at the register of the "people group" or population in the abstract. In order to govern, the thinking went, it would be necessary to know as much as possible about the customs, laws, practices, and population size of each ethnic group. An irony of colonial rule is that in order to make good on the imperialist claim to be devoted to improving life for the backward African, France would have needed to invest a great deal of manpower and financial resources to make it happen. Neither was forthcoming. Arguably, the demographic crisis of colonial rule was that there was never sufficient personnel to execute the grand vision of "valorizing" the colonies. There were not enough doctors, and what doctors there were had their hands full in urban centers where soldiers were encamped. But neither were there enough teachers, engineers, or veterinarians. The most basic administrative tasks were impossible to conduct for lack of personnel. This is why so much of the day-to-day management of civilian life (ranging from tax collection to managing family disputes to recruiting labor to build roads) was left to indigenous figures of authority.

In spite of the paucity of human and financial resources, administrators had to account for how much tax revenue they could produce, why embarrassing famines occurred, and why colonial subjects migrated from one colony to another. Reports of all kinds were produced in triplicate to be sent to the capital of each colony, to the French West Africa federation capital in Dakar, and then on to Paris. Very useful materials for reconstructing the history of medical infrastructure, staffing, training, and nutrition research are to be found in the French military medical archives in Marseille (IMTSSA).[15] Other health and law materials are held at the Archives Nationales du Sénégal. Colonial political reports for Niger and French West Africa in general are available at the French Archives Nationales d'Outre-mer in Aix-en-Provence; these helped me to understand in particular what the population figures were, how and why they were collected and interpreted, and the performative dimension entailed in their production. Those documents include an invaluable report by Denise Savineau in 1937–1938 on the state of families, prisons, schools, and medical facilities across the Sahel, which provides something of a snapshot of the entire region at a particular moment of French rule. More fine-grained materials on Niger (health reports, police reports, administrative rounds, studies related to the impact of the abolition of slavery as well as a few particularly useful student memoirs) are available in the Archives Nationales du Niger (ANN) for both the colonial period and the independence era. The Centre des Archives Économiques et Financières in Paris provided me with invaluable materials on population during the transition from colonial rule into the early independence period.

Generations of Women

From the outset, when I conceived of this book I wanted to try to bridge the enormous chasm between the intimate scale of individual women's experiences of motherhood and childbirth over time and the quantitative abstraction of the population bounded by the administrative and political units of the state. Archival materials tend heavily toward the latter. To learn something of the embodied experience, it was necessary to spend time with women, interview them, and simply observe what they actually do. The final two chapters of this book draw very heavily on oral interviews and participant observation and may appear to the historian to be dismayingly ethnographic. They address the burdens that fall to women as a result of the history I recount in the preceding chapters. They also take up how women of different generations have experienced their sexuality, fertility, and life options.

While my initial interest in the topic was sparked by my work with women in the Maradi region (where fertility rates are the highest in Niger), by the time I was ready to do fieldwork both my conception of the project and the political context had changed. I had come to feel that the study had to take the context of the state head on and that it could not focus on one ethnicity or region. In any case, because of political instability, Maradi was no longer practical as a site for this research. I decided to focus my energies on the capital, Niamey, in the awareness that populations constantly move between the capital and rural districts, between urban centers and farm villages, between international sites of labor migration and Niamey. I reconciled myself to becoming an urbanite, and I learned a great deal about Niger that I had not previously understood as a result.

To complement that fieldwork, I have also drawn shamelessly from the ethnographic work of others because there have been so many exceptionally rich studies done on the Sahel of late. In particular, I take up the central concerns traced in the work of the late Hadiza Moussa—the all-consuming problem that infertility presents for women in Niger and the secrecy surrounding contraception (2012). I would like to acknowledge how heavily I have depended on her observations and those of other scholars of the region—particularly anthropologists and sociologists—and how grateful I am for their insights.

The initial spadework for this book was conducted over three years on visits of varying duration during winter and summer breaks between 2011 and 2013. I began by interviewing key women who had emerged as leaders in the transition to democracy from 1990. I wanted to understand their thoughts on Niger's frustratingly slow progress toward longer and better lives for everyone. I learned my way around the various NGOs and government offices devoted to women's issues, human rights, legal affairs, and development. In all this, I received wise and warm assistance from Zainabou Hadari, the founder of the Centre Reines Daura. In time, I contacted members of Coordination des Organisations Non Gouvernementales et Associations Féminines Nigérienne (CONGAFEN), the major umbrella organization coordinating the activities of the plethora of NGOs that have emerged dedicated to women's interests. I made my historical project known to them so that in the course of my work my name would become familiar and snowball networking would be facilitated. I was encouraged by how supportive they were of a historical study of this kind and by their genuine curiosity about the relationship between the past and the present in the intimate domain of childbirth. Unlike my previous work in Maradi, almost all the interviews I conducted in Niamey were in French, a reminder to me that my familiarity with the history and experiences of Hausa-speaking women far to the east did not necessarily mean that I would be able to anticipate the experiences and preferences of women in the capital.

A sabbatical in 2014 enabled me to make an extended trip to Niger for the most substantive portion of the fieldwork. Thanks to Aissata Sidikou and CONGAFEN, I was introduced to Hawa Képine, a trained social worker working for the Association des Femmes Juristes du Niger. I was delighted to discover in her a kindred spirit who envisioned with little difficulty the purposive sample of women I would need to interview. We initially interviewed women in multiple households across twelve neighborhoods of Niamey. The different histories of settlement of these neighborhoods had yielded quite different housing patterns, economic activities, economic profiles, and ethnic makeups. We then narrowed our contacts down to two or three particularly interesting households in each part of the city. The households she introduced me to were known to her as a result of her work with widows, adolescents, and poor women in general. Such women often need help getting government services, finding microcredit opportunities, and accessing legal assistance. Our goal was to find settings where I could discuss and observe the reproductive experiences of women of two to three different generations from many different backgrounds. I have drawn from these interviews and observations throughout the book; all the women gave oral consent and have been assigned pseudonyms.[16]

Hawa facilitated my access to a sample of households across the neighborhoods of Niamey, she helped me gain interviews with major informants in the reproductive rights milieu, and she accompanied me during interviews with some of the Islamist women whose activism ran counter to that of the feminist NGOs with which I was already familiar. Her contacts enabled me to observe the goings and comings in one of Niger's major maternity centers (Maternité Poudrière) and to interview staff. Her authoritative presence during my interviews with dozens of high school girls and young women training to become *sage-femmes* taught me a tremendous amount about sex education and professional training in Niger. Rather than disguise the ways in which Hawa's presence, words, and silences shaped this research, I have included some of our interactions in the text to reveal her contributions to my own thinking. I commented only half-humorously to

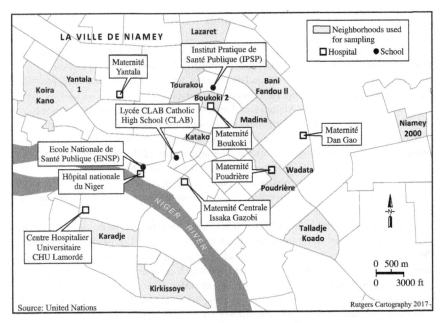

Niamey field sites. Courtesy of Mike Siegel, Rutgers Cartography.

her that if she had wanted to, she could have sat down and written the contemporary portion of this book herself, since there was little I could learn that she didn't already know.

Nevertheless, we did not agree about everything. I fear I often disappointed her when my language skills proved inadequate or fatigue left me incapable of continuing. Still, Hawa's occasional enthusiastic exclamation, "This is why we do fieldwork!" when we uncovered something unexpected, disturbing, or delightful reassured me of the mutually beneficial nature of the work. She used our visits across Niamey to seek out girls in trouble, to exhort mothers to consider contraception for their errant teenage daughters, to ferry women to administrative sites to fill out paperwork, to chide trainees about the importance of good communication with clients, to correct officials about developments they knew little about, and to seek medical advice and therapies of various kinds for herself while we were on the road. In some ways, I was simply traversing her own rich and productive networks while watching her do her work, profoundly grateful for the chance to tag along.

Notes

1. These estimates are based on the admittedly imperfect data of the United Nations Department of Economic and Social Affairs, Population Division, *World Population Prospects: The 2015 Revision*. One can quibble over the details of past estimates and question their projections, but the broader patterns are indisputable.

2. In a 2015 address to the African Development Conference, President Mahamadou Issoufou noted the challenge that a population growth rate of 3.9 percent presents and stated that to encourage a demographic transition, Niger is committed to a reduction in infant mortality and that "the best birth control is economic and social development" (2015, 7).

3. For a classic discussion of the complexities of analysis of the various senses of *reproduction*, see Moore (1988). Meillassoux (1991) insists on the importance of this broader sense of reproduction to the anthropology of slavery. For observations on actual procreative processes, see Thomas (2007).

4. For a useful overview of the history of demographic transition theory, see Kirk (1996).

5. There are at least thirty indigenous trees, bushes, and vines that produce edible seed, flowers, fruit, or internal pulp across the Sahel; these propagate naturally. But to use them one needs to know which parts are poisonous and which are edible and tasty. Some are particularly good fodder for livestock. With the expansion of monocropping of annuals, both the plants and this knowledge base is disappearing; see von Maydell (1990). For a study of the significance of these skills in twentieth-century Mali, see Twagira (2013).

6. For a much fuller exposition of the history of this eco-zone, see B. Cooper (2018b).

7. African rice, wheat, sesame, beans, cowpeas, eggplant, cabbage, cucumber, melon, pomegranate, fig, lime, lemon, mango, sugarcane, avocado, onions, garlic, tobacco, cotton, and indigo (Alpern 2008).

8. Ethnonyms are notoriously slippery and unstable despite the ways in which naming reifies ethnic groups. It suffices to speak Hausa and to live as a Hausa person to "become" Hausa. This is less true of endogamous ethnic groups in which the maternal line determines status background.

9. For the cultural contexts of risk in reproduction, see Fordyce and Maraesa (2012).

10. Bongaarts, Frank, and Lesthaeghe (1984). Any contemporary list of the relevant determinants would include percentage of women in sexual union, frequency of sexual intercourse, postpartum abstinence, lactational amenorrhea, contraceptive use, induced abortion, spontaneous intrauterine mortality, natural sterility, and pathological sterility.

11. For a concise discussion of the distinctions between feeling, emotion, and affect, see Shouse (2005). The study of what French scholars refer to as the history of *sentiments* began with the work of Lucien Febvre, one of the founders of the Annales school (1973). Debates about terminology abound. In this book, I use the word *affect* because of its reference to both feeling and motivation to action.

12. The École Normale William Ponty was founded in 1903, becoming the official teacher training college of French West Africa in 1933. Eventually, a second school was established, the École Normale Fréderic Assomption de Katibougou. Students produced assignments in bound notebooks known as *cahiers* during their vacations; most are now held in the fonds École Normale William Ponty at IFAN in Dakar. IFAN references begin with a C (for *cahier*) followed by a number indicating the class set in which the thesis is to be found. Students wrote on twenty-eight different topics. Not all memoirs made it into the IFAN set. I found

a number of fascinating memoirs among the theses in the Archives Nationales du Niger. The references for these are ANN followed by 1 G 4. All the memoirs I draw on here were produced between 1933 and 1949. Some were not dated but were found in sets of papers that enable me to make a reasonable guess as to the year in which they were submitted.

13. A great many of the students were very clearly from the families of chiefs and other notables and almost none from casted groups. For interesting reflections on the difference in schooling for the rare son of a griot, see C 14 Couyate Karamoko n.d. For the reflections on how a young man is socialized to become a chief, see C 14 Caba Sory 1949 and C14 Barry Mamadou Aliou 1949. Very few students came from Niger's rudimentary school system.

14. Two assignments have produced particularly useful material for my purposes: one in which the student was to discuss the training of children in *le milieu familial* and another on how education contributes to the shaping of society. While these topics were undoubtedly promising for the students in the sense that it would not be difficult for them to find something to write about, the topics were also of interest to the French administration, and occasionally one can glean from marginalia that memoirs were forwarded to other colonial offices. The fact that the memoirs were archived is, in itself, striking.

15. Institut de Médecine Tropicale du Service de Santé des Armées (antenne IRBA de Marseille) (Pharo)—in notes I refer to this as IMTSSA.

16. This research was conducted with the authorization of the government of Niger through the sponsorship of the Institut de Recherches en Sciences Humaines.

1

ENVIRONMENT, SEDUCTION, AND FERTILITY

THIS CHAPTER WILL EXPLORE HOW THE HISTORY OF power, the landscape, and reproduction were interwoven in the Sahel immediately prior to colonial rule by focusing on the case of Hausa speakers of the Maradi region. Power among sedentary Hausa speakers has historically been captured in the metaphor of marriage: a ruler is the husband of the land. The productive capacity of the landscape shapes how a population views various rulers; its productivity is a function of his (or, more rarely, her) potency. At the same time, the ability of a society to produce heirs, offspring, laborers—in short, people—has also been a central indicator of political and social success. While reproductive concerns are often seen as peculiarly feminine, the centrality of fertility (both productive and reproductive) to the understanding of well-being and success invites an excursion into how questions of human fertility have been understood in both political and environmental terms.

Focusing on ethnographic evidence from the Hausa-speaking region at the turn of the twentieth century, I will set out what we know about beliefs and practices related to fertility and well-being at a range of scales, from the body to the household to the kingdom. These ideas have not been static over the course of the long twentieth century, although there are deeply rooted elements that persist despite major change. The nineteenth-century jihads, the advent of colonial rule, the expansion of contagious disease, and the growing debates about what constitutes Islamic orthodoxy have all contributed to perceptions of reproduction, well-being, and fertility. They also altered how reproduction would be experienced.

The Paradox of the Malthusian Model

Despite the persistence of the Malthusian assumption that the fertility of land and the fertility of humans are at odds with one another, the historically more common perception among farming peoples of West Africa has, in fact, been the reverse. Places of abundance are sites of agricultural fertility, human wealth, and wealth in people; a large population is not a sign of impending calamity but the signal that a place is successful (Rain 1999). A parallel language of abundance (*gafi*) might apply equally to a woman's milk (*gafin mama gare ta*) or to a fertile farm (*k'asan nan tana da gafi*) or to a merchant lucky in his trade (*yana da gafin ciniki*).[1] By the same token, ideas about the blockages to good fortune (which include infertility but also poor rains, bad markets, weak soils, and illness) have resonances that link the body, the farm, and the kingdom.

Recovering the ways of thinking that characterized Hausa-speaking populations in this region prior to the advent of Islam in the fourteenth century is extremely difficult. Scholarly works on "animism" in the region date from well after the dominance of Islam in urban areas; this exposure to Islam has tended to shape both the attitudes expressed toward the practices of autochthonous peoples and the practices themselves. Nevertheless, it seems clear even from the imperfect sources we have that an array of spirits understood to have emotions and kinship relations just like humans occupied the landscape. Human well-being was very much a product of good relations with those spirits. One such imperfect source is a doctoral thesis by Henri Leroux (1948). Leroux collected a great deal of ethnographic data on Islam and animism in the Maradi region in the 1940s in the course of pursuing his law degree. Colonial scholar-administrators tended to focus on Islam because of its political importance and its increasing significance in colonial judicial arenas. Although the practices of the majority population of non-Muslims were clearly under siege even then, Leroux was able to gain a sense of the spiritual landscape as seen by rural populations, known as Arna, that had not converted to Islam.

According to him, the most senior spirit of the Arna, Baba Maza ("great old man") occupied a tree that was also the site of sacrifices; general well-being or *arziki* (health, abundance, fertility, and safety) was attributed to him. His wife Uwar Gona ("mother of the field") was associated with fields, granaries, seed, and rains—in short, with agricultural plenty. She could secure health, abundance, and fertility for women who hoped to have numerous children. She gave birth to the fruits of the fields. Like Baba Maza, she could be destructive when her wrath was aroused; for example, she protected fields from theft by causing the belly of the crop thief to swell (Leroux 1948).

If human fertility and agricultural fertility were in a sense equated and personified in the figure of Uwar Gona, the opposite was personified in the figure of Uwar Dawa Baka ("the mother of the dark wilds"). This spirit was cruel and untamed, occupying the dark spaces of the uncleared bush. Women's failure in childbirth could be attributed to her. In her benevolent guise, however, she protected hunters and gave them good fortune in the hunt. The daughters of the hunters' clan had an unusually close relationship with her, for at the moment of their weddings they might become possessed by this spirit (J. Nicolas 1967, 21). Many classic Hausa binaries reflecting the tempo of the year and the division of space are captured in the differences between Uwar Gona and Uwar Dawa Baka: cultivated/uncultivated, human/animal, wet/dry, light/dark, tame/wild, female (farmer)/male (hunter).

Anthropologist Guy Nicolas expanded on many of Leroux's findings in the 1960s and 1970s, focusing once again on the coexistence of practices of the Hausa-speaking Arna population with the Muslim practices of more urban Hausa. Careful not to tag one world as purely Islamic and the other as purely "fetishist," Nicolas nevertheless somewhat artificially segregated his analysis of the world of the rural Arna clan from his analysis of the urban Hausa dynasty. His extraordinarily rich ethnography of rural life of the Maradi valley exposed the dual masculine and feminine principles structuring Arna practice at every turn: in the construction of a home, in the planting of a field, in the celebration of childbirth (G. Nicolas 1975, 84, 254–61). Arna saw themselves as embedded in a universe that was oriented in space and time in a matrix balancing and uniting masculine and feminine principles, a universe in which "human coupling [was] the prototype, the model, a trigger of sorts for fertility in general" (G. Nicolas 1975, 91). The world humans occupied was shot through with the spiritual forces inhabiting every object; any successful endeavor had to be oriented within that matrix. The complementary balance of male and female principles was etched into the temporal and spatial practices of farming from the orientation of the furrows, to the planting of "male" millet in one direction and "female" sorghum in the other, to the days of the week during which a woman worked her husband's fields, to the tools understood to be essentially feminine or essentially masculine (223–31).

The marked attention to the sexual coupling mirrored in spatial orientation was also adopted by urban dwellers whenever they situated a new town or built a new market. From at least the twelfth century, Hausa-speaking peoples had a penchant for dense urban settings in which trade could be conducted, and by the fourteenth century, that setting was increasingly understood to fall within the dar al-Islam—the safe haven of

Islam. Highly mobile urban populations brought with them many other beliefs and modes of orientation; cities were never entirely cut off from the countryside.

The Arna spirits, rooted in the spaces occupied by Hausa speakers in the Maradi region (hills, trees, termite mounds, wells, forests), were complemented over time by a host of other spirits that were more mobile and more labile (the merchant, the pilgrim, the scholar, the queen, the prince). One effect of the advent of Islam in the region may have been the adoption of a notion of spirits as less rooted in space: the *jinns* (genies) of Islam. The local understanding of spirits was not altogether incompatible with the spirits of the Muslim urban centers and their spirit mediums. The complex pantheon of chthonic spirits was enriched by the birth or arrival of others that reflected a complex flow of peoples, ideas, diseases, and economies. These mobile and portable spirits (known as *bori*) could have Muslim names, attributes, and origins. The spirit world reflected an environment that was populated by peoples, animals, and diseases that were in motion.

Beyond simply influencing the well-being of communities and individuals, these newer spirits could actually inhabit the body of someone who either inherited that spirit or had been chosen as a host. The relation of spirit to human medium was understood to be that of a rider and a female horse. The relation between the two could be regulated through initiation into a community of spirit possession practitioners. The ability to negotiate well with particular spirits as an adept and eventually a medium conferred on the *bori* practitioner the ability to serve as a therapeutic specialist in the kinds of distress caused by those spirits. The increasing complexity of spirit beliefs was thus matched by a growing complexity in therapeutic options and a growing range of kinds of distress requiring treatment. Attaining well-being, or *arziki*, had become more complex and required the intermediation of many more invisible forces than in the past.

One sees the many-layered quality of spirit practice in the Hausa-speaking region unfolding over time in the Kano Chronicle, a treasured but complex source for the reconstruction of Hausa social and cultural life. The document, a kings' list of sorts, appears to have been constructed from bits of memory attached to the urban landscape, material culture, epithets of objects and people, and praise songs. It bears traces of stories and genealogies dating from far earlier than the moment at which it was written down in the nineteenth century. The Chronicle records the Kano analogues of the kinds of rooted spirits of the Arna recorded by Leroux; it relates the coming of Muslim traders, missionaries, and scholars; and it presents epic contests between powerful spiritual forces of various kinds. The outcome of these contests is never fixed in advance. Success results from skill in coopting the potency of different autochthonous and itinerant spiritual beings. The Chronicle declines to privilege Islam within the narrative, providing a hint of the ambivalence felt by the local scholar who compiled the history toward the successful jihadists.[2]

Drawing on the architecture of the Kano Palace and aerial photographs, geographer Heidi Nast suggests that in urban nodes within broader agricultural and pastoral economies, the power of the throne rested on the skills and knowledge assembled through the heavy concentrations of wives, concubines, and servants within the palace (Nast 2005). Wealth in people was then measurable in the grain stored within the central treasury, and it was through the redistribution of that grain that a ruler secured political ties. The productivity of the countryside and the fertility of the female concubines linking the palace to its many tributary territories were profoundly intertwined. One could literally map the linkages of the rural areas to the central space of the concubines' quarters in the palace. Furthermore, urban artisanal production, in particular cloth dying, required the assemblage of the skills and labor of women from throughout Kanoland. Human fertility, agricultural production, and wealth through trade in luxury goods were increasingly interwoven.

The assemblage of multiple kinds of power to master a complex and variegated environment was not terribly difficult to reconcile with the binary couplings of the Arna universe because Arna farmers were adept at collecting such assemblages themselves. A successful farmer matched the qualities of the soils and rains in any of his or her numerous small plots to the qualities of particular crop varieties and seeds. The metaphor—indeed, template—for multiplicity and plenty was *iri* (seed)—a word that signaled the origin of something, its essential nature, and also the way in which each thing is a thing of a certain kind with a certain temperament. The word *iri*, then, means *seed, kind,* or *type.* Just as there are many kinds of seeds suited to a host of different circumstances, so also are there many kinds of people and spirits, each useful in its own way when well understood and carefully nurtured (G. Nicolas 1975, 288–89). The true master cultivator was one who had a profound knowledge of the many different kinds of things and who had managed to assemble them to serve his or her many diverse needs.

By the late nineteenth century, multiple ways of speaking and thinking about the invisible spirit world coexisted, seemingly synonymous but only ambiguously identical: *iska* (wind, spirit), *bori* (spirit capable of occupying a human host medium), *aljani* (genie). And, of course, the notion of a single all-powerful god, Allah, was increasingly part of the repertoire. The cultivation of a mutually beneficial relationship with one spiritual force did not necessarily exclude a relationship with others; indeed, it was the assemblage of so many different forces that made for the strength of a farm, a city, a market, and so on. The development of urban centers gave rise to spirit possession cult activities that simultaneously competed with and complemented the practices rooted in farming, hunting, and pastoral pursuits. The specialists who gave sacrifices to spirits of the landscape found themselves in an uneasy collaboration with titled figures in the court hierarchy overseeing the spirit possession cult of the urban population. The linkage between agricultural fertility and human fertility remained, but it became more complex as other "kinds" of spirits intruded into the success and failure of humans in the many domains of life typical of long-distance commerce, urban trade, and artisanal centers.

Shifting notions of Islamic orthodoxy, as well, could impinge on the degree to which urban spirit possession practitioners found common cause with rural guardians of local spirits, particularly when the key seasonal hunting and farming rituals of the spirit world fell out of synch with the lunar calendar of the increasingly Muslim urban population. While the local Arna elders attuned to local spirits sometimes competed with the Muslim spirit cult leaders of the town, these spirit worlds resonated with one another and shared both figurative and literal ties of kinship. Rural practitioners and urban mediums might share a reluctance to see all spirits as *shetani* or devils despite the currency of such ideas among those who could not see any merit in the mediating capacity of the spirits. Muslims could reconcile themselves to the idea of a single god, Allah, and multiple spirits in part because the spirit world had never been understood to be transcendent or all-powerful. Spirits occupied *this* earthly world in tandem with humans; they were immanent, not transcendent. One had to negotiate good relations with these spirit neighbors; they could not simply be ignored. Thus, multiple spiritualities overlapped and coexisted uneasily: rural spirit veneration, urban possession cults, and an array of modes of Islamic practice in varying degrees of sympathy with spirit veneration. The legitimacy of urban aristocracies from about the fifteenth century increasingly depended on their ability to navigate this complex spiritual terrain.

One mark of a successful political leader was therefore his (or, more rarely, her) ability to attract good fortune to the kingdom through any and all avenues possible. Like a good husband, he would ensure the well-being of his land by providing food, safety, and, of course, abundant offspring. Thus, the chief, known as the Sarki, was understood to be the "husband of the land" or *mijin 'kasa*. Each new chief chosen by the powerful electoral college of the court from among the eligible princes of the courtly class was, through a ceremony of accession to the throne, in effect married to his territory: "Henceforth, his kingdom is bound to him as a wife to her husband. He will rule her and direct her future, and his good fortune will be her own" (G. Nicolas 1975, 338). It was, of course, essential to the kingdom that the Sarki have the qualities that attract prosperity, fertility, health, and good fortune.

However, as Polly Hill observed in her works on prosperity and poverty in Kano in the 1970s, scholars from Guy Nicolas to M. G. Smith have struggled to make sense of the key term at the heart of all this, namely *arziki* (Hill 1977, 185–87). A good ruler brings it, a woman with children has it, and a merchant needs it to do well in trade—but what is this quality, and where does it come from? Is this providential good fortune imparted by Allah to the devout (from Arabic *rizq*, meaning *provision, livelihood, wealth*; also see Pettigrew 2014, 47). Is it something particular family lines inherit through their bloodlines? Or is it something one can only reckon after the fact, just as the wise Athenian Solon suggested we call no man happy until he is dead?

One of Hill's most important insights was that success requires a great deal more than simply access to fertile land. Success, as it emerges in her work, requires a social network, tools, capital, family labor; success is highly situated (Hill 1977, 160). And yet in some ways we come up against, once again, a kind of circularity. Those who are successful have the things that lead to success. Perhaps the best way to think about *arziki* is, as Guy Nicolas observed, to see it as a kind of seductive quality—a capacity to attract and sustain those things necessary for a good life. Thinking of *arziki*—the central quality that gives rise to fertility, prosperity, abundance, and wealth—in this way helps us make sense of how Hausa speakers could find continuity in a spiritual environment that, as we have seen above, was in considerable flux. What the successful farmer, herder, merchant, or ruler had, regardless of which spiritual force dominated the landscape at any given moment, was the ability to woo, to seduce, and to placate. In other words, the metaphor of marriage signaled a great deal more than simply human coupling. The successful man had to be "charming" in both senses of the word.

The ability to captivate could come from knowing the right incantations and charms or from making proper sacrifices. It could derive from an adherence to proper ritual prayer or from assiduous Sufi remembrance of Allah. But consistent across time and space was this seductive quality, one that was not necessarily monogamous in its affections. The ambitious farmer, trader, or aristocrat might seek to attract and retain many kinds of potential. Different kinds of potential, like women, clients, or spirits, might need to be captivated in different ways.

The centrality of seduction in the success of farmers in the region is captured in a marvelous and unexpected image of nomadic millet:

> A great number of my informants [remarks Guy Nicolas] are convinced that millet walks about at night in search of food (they often use the term "pasture": kiwo). They claim often that there is much less millet today than in the past because of electrical and gas lighting; the millet, disliking the light, thus remains in the field where it perishes for lack of food. . . . This is why the Chief Farmer of Jiratawa mixes into his seed each year "medicine for the seed." The alluring scent of this magic perfume draws the spirit [*bori*] of millet to his field, causing it to abandon the one who originally planted it. (G. Nicolas 1975, 244)

By this way of thinking, the only real wealth is the capacity to attract: "The true rich man is the one who can seduce, who can subdue, who charms, who gives away without counting endless goods, who attracts the greatest number of clients through gifts, and not someone who holds on to an unused hidden treasure" (251). The competition between men of wealth and power is not a competition between productive rivals; it is, Nicolas notes, "a kind of tournament of magicians" (251). The successful Arna farmer hunts his vegetal prey in clearing new land during the dry hunting season, while the canny Muslim farmer prevents his neighbor from stealing away his growing crop by planting medicines sold by a Muslim healer to prevent the flattery of his rivals from wooing away the souls (*kurwa*) of his plants (409).

This shared understanding of prosperity and well-being as essentially a product of a successful seduction—of women, of land, of seed, of clients—produced an ethos of redistribution within both the rural and urban worlds of the Maradi region that was very much alive at the time of Nicolas's research in the 1970s. Prosperity was not something that could be stock-piled; it was transactional and required constant cultivation. It was also, therefore, quite contingent—on the success of the medicine, the precision of the incantation, the purity of the sacrificial animal, and so on. Hence, one can detect an etymological kinship between *arziki* and *risk* via a shared Mediterranean, Arabic, and Persian language of investment, provision, livelihood, and trade.[3] Circumstances far beyond the control of the husband, farmer, or merchant (such as the advent of electrical lighting) could disrupt it. Sustained success would require careful navigation and constant vigilance in the ongoing acquisition of varied kinds of potency. *Arziki* was a quality that emerged out of constant human engagement with other humans, other spirits, and potencies of all kinds.

This is not to say that *arziki*, the capacity to attract and retain the elements that make for a good life, need be understood always to be peaceful. Mawri Hausa speakers, reputed to be among the most resistant to Islamization, tell a tale that offers a glimpse of how avarice, force, and cunning figured in securing the foundational agricultural riches of the Sahelian region. The following comes from a school exercise written by the young Bakary Djibo in 1939. He later became a trade union leader and a fiery populist politician as Niger moved toward independence.

> Long ago, very long ago, Millet, Corn, Rice, Sorghum and Wheat were each a single person. The All Powerful decided to separate them. One day they came to a village seeking hospitality from the chief. He took them in willingly and found them a hut in which they could spend the night. All sorts of delicious dishes were prepared for them. But when the dishes were brought each of them wanted it for himself. Wheat thought himself superior to the others and ranted, "friends, you must really let me try these first." When he finished speaking he fell dead to the earth suddenly. Rice followed in his path in the same way. And one by one so did Corn and Sorghum. In the end Millet was the only one left standing, and he was delighted. But because he desired deeply to eat the foods all by himself he too fell to the same fate. Throughout the village the news of the tragedy struck everyone with terror. Nevertheless the villagers prepared to bury them. They carried Wheat to the shared tomb that the chief had commanded them to make. But when they readied to place him in the grave he jumped up suddenly and attempted to run away. But one of the villagers grabbed his arm and so he escaped with only one of his two arms. The remaining portion was transformed into wheat [seed]. Rice did the same and the villagers captured his two arms, which also were transformed into rice [seed]. Sorghum lost half of his body. When it was finally the turn to bury Millet, the villagers decided not to let anything escape. They transported him to the grave, and when he wanted to escape they were ready and they pressed

all around him [and buried him]. And so his entire person was transformed into millet seed. And that is why there is more millet than sorghum, more sorghum than corn, and so on. And ever since then millet has been the main staple in the region. (ANN 1 G 4 3 Djibo 1939)

The tale is fascinating, for it shows how the generosity of the villagers drew the grain-people to them but also how the asocial behavior of the guests led to their own downfall and fragmentation. By keeping their heads and working together, the villagers were able to acquire a diverse array of valuable seed and managed above all to obtain millet—resilient, adaptable, and long-living—entirely for themselves. A useful lesson for a budding populist politician.

Islamic Reform and the Persistence of Heterarchy outside the Caliphates

The seductive compositional model was very much in keeping with the Suwarian tradition of Islam in West Africa, which enabled Muslim missionaries to travel and live throughout the region. The compositional model enabled Islam to enter into the texture of West African life, while the Suwarian tradition enabled Muslims to submit to that model without seeing themselves as having been compromised. In Suwarian thinking, the role of Muslims was to present an example to unbelievers who would in God's time come to emulate them. To succeed in this important task, it was incumbent on Muslims to sustain a commitment to learning to keep their observance pure (Wilks 2000, 98). Muslims could live peacefully and profitably among non-Muslims so long as they observed a respectful relationship toward their hosts. After all, the traders, scholars, and pilgrims who entered into the region were themselves strangers, rather like our various seed grains. Chiefs and their entourages often became Muslims themselves while at the same time continuing to respect the spiritual expectations of the peoples they had drawn into their orbit.

Over time, there was growing tension between the compositional style of rule characteristic of the increasingly centralized (but nevertheless broadly representative) urban court hierarchy and the universal claims of Islamic monotheism as understood by Muslim scholars less inclined toward the Suwarian tradition. For purists inspired by the puritanical teachings of Muhammad al-Maghili (best known for his successful campaign to expel the Jews from Tlemcen), this compositional style of rule amounted to *shirk*—the association of God with other gods, in short, heretical poly-theism. The Kano Chronicle offers a vivid image for the ambiguity of Is-lamic belief in such a context. By the time of Mohamma Alwali in the late eighteenth century, Islam had been so enfolded into local practices that it was literally encased in them. Demoralized by never-ending war and fam-ine, Alwali's advisers asked, "'Why do you not sacrifice cattle to Dirki?' Alwali was very angry and sent young men to beat 'Dirki' with axes until that which was inside the skins came out. They found a beautiful Koran inside Dirki. Alwali said, 'Is this Dirki?' Dirki is nothing but the Koran. In Alwali's time the Fulani conquered the seven Hausa States on the plea of reviving the Muhammadan religion" (Palmer 1967, 127). The story sug-gests that Alwali was already inclined to reform spiritual practice, only to be toppled by the jihadists before he could complete the reforms. But one could perhaps read the story as suggesting that Kano fell because Alwali had violated the richly accreted Dirki that had successfully protected Kano from outsiders in the past.

The tension between the adaptive accretion of powers documented in the Kano Chronicle and the iconoclastic monotheism of al-Maghili came to a head in the jihad of the Fulani cleric Usman 'dan Fodio in the early nineteenth century. The successful jihadists took explicit aim at the prac-tices of the *bori* cult, attempting to expunge their representatives (the Inna, Sarkin Bori, Sarkin Arna) from political power and to erase any medicinal practices that they saw as competing with Islam's emphasis on the singu-larity of Allah's power. The assault on the Hausa kingdoms was not simply an attempt to replace one political power with another; it was an effort to replace the compositional Suwarian approach with a monopolistic under-standing (Abdalla 1981). The jihadists strove to replace the remedies (known as *magani*) associated with local spirits and *bori* with the "medicine of the Prophet."

The autochthonous populations that had previously held important of-fices and conducted key rituals became vassals within a purportedly Islamic mode of governance. The complex layering of Arna clans was gradually re-duced to a homogenous and despised ethnic group within the post-jihad caliphate (Last 1993; Greenberg 1946, 13 note 7). Urban *bori* adepts either went underground or paid tax that implied that they were not, in fact, Mus-lim. Urban Hausa Muslims now answered to a clerical hierarchy dominated by Fulani families that, ironically, became culturally Hausa over time with intermarriage. Today, the elites of the region defeated in the jihad are often Fulani in name but Hausa in culture and language.

Nevertheless, outside the territory conquered by the jihadists, the rump kingdoms of Gobir, Kano, and Katsina (in what was eventually to become Niger) carried on many of the earlier traditions of the indigenous Hausa kingdoms (M. G. Smith 1967). Arna clans of the region retained their status as autochthonous masters whose ritual expertise and mastery of local spirits contributed to the well-being and strength of the kingdoms. The *bori* spirit cult continued much as before, integrating ever more spirits into the pantheon, many of them Fulani and Muslim, as if to tame the violent reformists.

Embodiment and the Spirit Domain

The following is my attempt to pull together a host of fragmentary ethnographic observations into a more or less coherent picture of some of the key understandings of the body characteristic of the region among populations that, even at the time ethnographers began collecting data in the early twentieth century, did not regard themselves as Muslim.[4] One gleans from such ethnographic sources that in the Arna conception, each living thing in the world, whether human or animal, had an essential being, a *kurwa* or a kind of soul. This was its central living self. Only by protecting one's own *kurwa* and attracting that of others could an individual, family, market, hunt, or harvest thrive. Of course, this also meant that humans needed to safeguard their own *kurwa*, primarily by ingesting only those substances that would sustain it appropriately (given their clan, gender, and age) and through protective sacrifices to appropriate spirits.

Although the *kurwa*, like most spiritual beings, was generally invisible, it had a kind of materiality. The substance most closely associated with *kurwa* was the hailstone (*k'ank'ara*)—dangerous, hard, cold, and unforgiving, but also liable to dissolve and disappear once exposed and unprotected. But the *kurwa* was also in some sense immaterial; another quite different image of the *kurwa* is that of the shadow or double. The central bodily organs of the *kurwa* were what we might think of as the digestive system; they linked the mouth to the anus, enabling solids to both enter and leave the body. When one's *kurwa* was disrupted or troubled, it might mean that some inappropriate substance needed to be expelled through bloodletting or purgatives to cause diarrhea or vomiting. With death, the inner self melted away, a bit like the way ice melts, evaporates, and goes into the heavens (although the unsettled soul could become a ghost). During sleep, the *kurwa* might wander, becoming vulnerable to witchcraft. A sorcerer could steal the hailstone-like *kurwa*, and only when that stone was recovered (by another skilled sorcerer) would the afflicted person recover.

Each person or thing also had an outer self, or *jiki*—what we might translate loosely in English as a "body." The outer self and the inner self mirrored one another like a body and its shadow. The outward self was the site of sensory perception, social interaction, and bodily pleasure; it was substantial. The outer self was like a container, but it was also far more exposed to the world than the inner self; it was permeable. In quality it was like a fluid or vapor—breath, blood, semen, saliva. The outer self or body could be entered and acted on in a host of ways through the skin (through lotions), through openings such as the mouth (breath), nose (smoke and smells), ears (sounds), eyes (visions), anus (medicines), and, of course, through the site of vulnerability par excellence, the vagina (troublesome spirits). Most disruptions of well-being were understood to have been caused by some violation of the permeable *jiki*.

Human conception was understood to result from the conjoining of male and female *maniyi*, fluid that the body produces in the moment of orgasm. Pregnancy was fundamentally an internal experience, and the word for it is the same as the word for "inside" (*ciki*) and "stomach." However, other expressions still used to convey pregnancy are revealing. For example, *tana da juna biyu*, which is difficult to translate since *juna* normally describes a reciprocal act people do to one another, such as slap one another or meet one another, becomes something like *she has two one anothers*. The pregnant woman and the fetus are mutually constitutive beings.

The relationship between the *kurwa* of the newborn child and the broader spirit world populated by spirits and the ghosts of deceased kin was ambiguous, for a child that died shortly after birth would be said to have had no *kurwa*. But the *kurwa* of a deceased relative could enter the pregnant woman, with the result that the child would "look like" that relative. More tragically, if the intrusive *kurwa* was that of an unhappy kinswoman, the child might die. Sometimes the mother suffered because the spirit of the child was restless and easily recalled to the spirit world by other spirits, so that although she repeatedly became pregnant, each time the child was born it escaped back to its disembodied form. Such a child was known as a *wabi*, and parents would go to great lengths to persuade the spirit-child to remain: they would affect not to care about it so that other spirits would not be attracted to it. At other times someone might steal the *kurwa* of the child, and it would die. The *kurwa* was the substantial and concrete form of a kind of fluid spirit essence that only crystalized as the child became more fully human and socially recognized through ritual.

Persuading the *kurwa* of a newborn to stay and become fully human required skillful balancing of the forces of humans and spirits, in much the same way that gathering *arziki* required farmers and herders to engage in a kind of seduction of the landscape. Protecting fields, animals, and wombs required attention to male and female elements, spatial orientation, and a care to respect seasons and temporalities. As is so often the case with this kind of deeply embedded understanding of complementarity and spatio-temporal balance, it is difficult to know whether human relations and structures were ordered to be like those of the seasons and the fields or whether the fields and agricultural norms were patterned on the family compound.

Very much in keeping with this entanglement of humans in the land-scape is a lovely image recorded by Nicolas that links marriage, home, womb, and vegetal fecundity in ways that render the marriage bed the axis mundi:

> When a young woman marries she holds in her hand during the ceremony a kind of charm made of a fruit of the doum palm wrapped in cloth with a thin cord: the *kodago* [doum palm nut] or *diya* (doll) [the word also means "daughter," "offspring," or "fruit"]. People say that the fertility of the doum palm, which produces a great number of fruits, is thus communicated to the young woman. She keeps her *kodago* until the women of her family come to tamp down the soil of her new hut (*daben daki*), as is customary. They bury the *kodago* in the center of the room with other "medicines." When the wife has sexual relations with her husband, it was explained to me, she looks at the center of the roof of her hut: it is from that point, following the vertical axis linking the roof to the buried objects in the floor that will come the impregnating powers emanating from this magical pole. (G. Nicolas 1975, 256–57)

Among the distinctive features of the doum palm tree, beyond its fecundity, is that it grows in such a manner that it creates a fork, much prized in the building of huts and erection of tents, for it can serve as a critical center pole. Even in the absence of a "real" pole, the seed in the floor gave rise to a potential central axis that would support her hut, her married life, and her ability to produce children.

When a baby was born in the bride's hut, the woman who assisted the mother cut the umbilical cord (three finger lengths if the child was a boy, four if a girl) and then placed the placenta and remaining cord in a pottery shard. She placed some cotton seeds in the vessel and buried it on the eastern side of the mother's hut. When a person returned to his or her maternal home, he or she literally returned to the umbilicus, the link to the womb (Luxereau 1991, 9). The birth assistant later placed the ashes left from heating the wash water of the mother and child generated in the course of seven days in a geometric pattern at a crossroads—three points for a boy (who, like the stable triangle and hearth, could be counted on to remain with the lineage), four for a girl (who left the natal home to marry but guaranteed the fertility of her new household by working the quadrilateral fields) (G. Nicolas 1975, 84–85, 540). This process was repeated for all subsequent births.

Of course, this benign image reflects what was *meant* to be. Childbirth only rightly occurred in the context of marriage, and premarital childbearing would lead to painful public ridicule. The new bride was to be a virgin; her failure to prove to be such on her first encounter with her husband could lead to public humiliation as he placed a calabash with a hole in it over the doorway to her hut. The calabash is a highly resonant symbol in a region where most containers are made from gourds of one kind or another; the woman's womb, her procreative capacity, her capacity to contain the soul of a clan baby in pregnancy, all were called into question in such an image. Various clan-specific ordeals and tests purported to ensure that all children born to the clan were legitimate (G. Nicolas 1975, 67, 74, 84, 110, 241, 275).

A woman who proved incapable of providing children could suffer tremendously, given that her own fecundity was a measure of the good fortune of her husband and his lineage. Misfortune in reproduction could be understood in a variety of ways—weak "medicine" to protect the woman and her home, the violation of a taboo such as eating the meat of the clan totem or *kan gida*, or insufficient attention to the needs of clan spirits during annual sacrifices. Women's reproductive well-being was interpreted to be a matter of successfully seeking protection from the appropriate spirits in advance; it was not curative but rather preventative. Furthermore, the important preventative measures were collective and offered at the level of the farmstead rather than the individual (Last 1976, 130). Each homestead would have had a specific site within it for sacrifice to relevant clan spirits, often a tree planted near the opening in the compound fence facing either east or south. The tree was known as the *jigo*, or axis pole, which also became the word for an altar (Greenberg 1946, 15, Figure 2, 43–46). Spirits of the wild might be honored at a tree far from the compound in a sacred grove.

Each woman's hut would have been accompanied by her own granary, which materially represented her productivity as a farmer and her ability to provide for her children. The collective granary, overseen by the compound head (the most senior man of the *gida*) would have been used to provide for the entire household as a whole during the rainy farming season. Thus, the productivity and reproductive capacity of the household was marked spatially by huts and granaries and protected through sacrifices at the sacred tree. In many compounds, there would also have been a miniature "house" for Inna, the mother of all the spirits and protector of the harvest (Greenberg 1946, 31, 40).

Birth in an Urban Milieu: *Bori* Is Woman's War

Even today, with the lapse of significance of clans and the near invisibility of non-Muslims, *kurwa* continues to be spoken of as an essential core of being without which a baby, market, or harvest will shrivel and die (Souley 2003). The term continues to have currency despite the competition of the Arabic term *ruhu*, which also refers to the fundamental spirit or soul of a person. Most people, if pushed, would have difficulty articulating the relationship between the two (Luxereau 1991). Disruptions to well-being today are also frequently attributed to the evil eye and maleficent medicines purchased from Muslim specialists and traditional healers. Women go to great lengths to protect their babies from any potential harm by acquiring preventative charms, by respecting taboos on eating particular foods, and by using strengthening medicines.

In the more urbanized and tightly settled zones characteristic of Muslims, contact with outsiders exposed them more regularly to contagious diseases. Baba of Karo told Mary Smith that, of her scholarly father's seventeen children, only three lived to adulthood. She reported that he said in puzzled sorrow to his brother, "We are always having children, but they keep dying," to which his brother replied, "Allah grant they may live" (M. F. Smith 1954, 79). Her father's scholarly and commercial activities took him regularly to the urban areas of what was soon to become northern Nigeria, and Baba herself moved frequently from one relatively urban household to the next. His family background was rural, and he had evidently not grown up accustomed to such high infant mortality. Certainly, the disruptions of colonial rule increased the mobility of peoples and diseases (Iliffe 1995, 208–11).

So far as I can tell from the scant evidence, prior to the mid-twentieth century, rural marriages occurred much later than urban marriages; eighteen seems to be a benchmark age for women (Greenberg 1946, 24). Young brides may have been more fully developed and stronger at the time of their first childbirth. The age difference between men and women may have been small in a rural precolonial economy in which the impediments to setting up a new household were modest and many marriages were between cousins. As a result, while Arna seem to have cared deeply about the legitimacy of clan members, the punishment for pregnancy prior to marriage does not appear to have been particularly harsh; the girl was expected to identify her lover, and they would marry—the issue was identifying the appropriate clan for the child (*Coutumiers juridiques* Vol. II 1939, 293; Greenberg 1946, 24). Youthful sexuality was not only tolerated but was encouraged in the practice of *tsarance*, the sleeping together and cuddling of boys and girls from different families in a hut apart from their parents (Salamone 1974, 112). Actual sexual intercourse was forbidden, while sexual restraint was learned from a young age.

By contrast, in increasingly Islamized urban milieus, childbirth by an unmarried girl occasioned great opprobrium; she could not identify her lover (to do so would be an accusation of *zina*, a serious sin), nor could the child be legitimated. As a result, parents appear to have married their daughters off at younger ages than had been typical in Arna settings, which in turn could mean that they were not as physically mature at the time of their first pregnancies, with lifelong consequences for their fertility. Urban centers on trade routes were also more likely to harbor the many contagions that travel those corridors, including an array of sexually transmitted diseases that could be expected to inhibit reproductive success. Whereas in rural areas women were often married to cousins and therefore had the support of their kin nearby, urban life and virilocal marriage often cut women off from protective networks of kin.

Concentrated population centers, then, were spaces in which women battled to achieve their reproductive goals. It has been in relatively concentrated urban and Muslim settings that *bori* has tended to flourish. As the adage goes, "*bori* is woman's war" (Masquelier 2001b, 92). Women often had recourse to *bori* specialists to remedy reproductive problems. Unlike the preventive clan and family rituals of the rural setting devoted to appeasing clan spirits, *bori* tended to figure prominently in women's reproductive lives only after something had already gone wrong. When jealousy and competition led someone to use charms to "tie up" a woman's womb, or when the children a woman gave birth to died one after another, or when a husband lost interest in his wife—that was when *bori* came into play in the reproductive domain. In the Maradi valley, where Guy Nicolas collected his data on the Arna and where Jacqueline Nicolas and Henri Leroux conducted studies of spirit possession, only women took part: "men say, 'the gods [*bori* spirits] don't want us' but don't seem dismayed about it—it's simply not their affair" (J. Nicolas 1967, 2).

Susceptibility to spirits could be inherited, much as Arna clan spirits belonged to particular bloodlines. However, spirits could also choose to take up residence in an individual at will, violating the permeable boundary of the body. This differed a great deal from the conception of spirits as inherited in rural clan ritual. Greenberg noted that among the Arna the term *bori* seemed to refer specifically to spirit possession; some spirits engage in *bori*; others do not (1946, 28). Unlike the Arna clan spirits, any woman could become afflicted or favored by any of the *bori* spirits; the linkage to a specific inheritance was gone. Women were initiated into the cult when they faced a problem: illness, infertility, children who die (J. Nicolas 1967, 6, 25). Rural women did not seem to take part in the cult, while Muslim men were not moved to do so. Greenberg found that rural populations did engage in spirit possession; however, their possession was more serious in tone and generally therapeutic in intent, unlike the occasionally entertaining possession spectacles in more urban settings (Greenberg 1946, 50–61). On the whole, however, *bori* was a feminine affair among women who inhabited the Muslim social sphere. It was handled as an individual response to an individual problem (Last 1976, 129).

Generally, the remedy sought was not the elimination of a disease so much as release from an impediment to success in childbirth. Jacqueline Nicolas saw *bori* as complementary to the Islamic religious practice of men, from which women were largely excluded despite their status as Muslims. However, some men did participate in *bori* and still do. The resonance of *bori* with the earlier Arna clan spirits becomes evident when one examines the spirits that seem to have most commonly "ridden" the "mares" within the Maradi cult in the mid-1960s: Kure ("Hyena," harvest spirit, who causes impotence), Masharuwa ("Water Drinker" spirit of the wells and springs, who prevents women from having children), Masasao (protector of well diggers, who causes miscarriage), Sarkin Rafi ("king of the streams," associated with depression). Although these "white" *bori* spirits could cause disruption, they were not seen as bad or evil; the woman stricken by such spirits needed to assuage their anger through appropriate animal sacrifices and might eventually learn how to be ridden. Once she had become a skilled "mare," she could in turn help others through her acquired knowledge of divination and of the kinds of sacrifices and *magani* useful to remedy women's complaints.

A few other common spirits of the time reflect some of the newer stresses, preoccupations, and disturbances of urban life. Some of the figures may have been particularly pleasurable to mimic (the prince from Bornu, a spendthrift and gambler; Malam Alhaji, a pious pilgrim), and, indeed, some did not even cause any illness. Still, like epidemic disease, the truly malevolent "black" spirits came from elsewhere, bringing with them incurable illnesses and madness (Duna, Barbarbara, Bagwari); these foreign spirits had to be expelled permanently.

A diagnosis of spirit disruption to be cured through initiation and possession was a woman's last resort. Possession may not have had a particularly impressive success rate in actually reversing whatever physiological problem a woman faced (such as infertility or repeated miscarriage) (Last 1976). Still, in the past as well as today, it did surely provide women with a sense of community, a kind of imaginative and performative safe haven. It offered a mode through which to come to terms with their distress (social and psychological). And once initiated, a woman, generally at this point relatively senior and often divorced, could become a potential healer herself, for she could offer her skills and services to others for a fee. What a *bori* specialist could do was employ divination to read the past to understand the cause of a woman's distress; she might find that the problem was the unsettled soul of a dead kinswoman, a spell placed by a jealous co-wife intended to reduce her strength or her husband's ardor, or the affections of a spirit. The *bori* healer might also prescribe a variety of herbal remedies, including love potions. If the problems were intractable, she might encourage her client to undergo possession herself, enabling a spirit to voice the suffering woman's concerns in ways that could not be contradicted—in effect enabling her to temporarily take on another persona and thus find a way to become less trapped in "unquestioned yet resented social ties" (Last 1991, 55; see also Luxereau 1984, 9).

The Sterility of the Medicine of the Prophet

Rulers of both non-Muslim and Muslim societies in West Africa attempted to attract literate Muslim scribes and teachers who could provide esoteric protective remedies (*magani*). Such charms tended to take two forms. They might be inscriptions of Koranic texts or numerological esoterica that were folded into a leather or metal amulet to be worn (*layya*). But Islamic writing itself contained the blessings of the sacred word and the *baraka* (spiritual force or blessings) of the sheik (often understood to be a descendant of the Prophet Mohammed) who wrote it. One could consume that blessing by drinking the wash water with which a writing board was cleansed. Thus "drinking the word" became an essential part of protective and therapeutic practice in the region; different powers were attributed to different texts on the basis of the linkages of ideas, sounds, and images. The inks themselves, produced with plants that may have had therapeutic purposes, rendered the charms more meaningful in local terms to both men and women.

In practice, Hausa populations did not choose between occult Islamic medicine and other therapeutic traditions. They absorbed this medical tradition in much the same way they absorbed other *magani*—they took what they found useful without discarding their existing array of protective and curative techniques derived from the already highly textured Arna and *bori* traditions. The power of literacy combined with the knowledge of astrology and numerology that traveled with Muslims became much valued in the Sudanic region. Just as protective medicines were worn by hunters and blacksmiths, by women in labor and men digging wells, the written texts worn and reproduced by Muslim scholars and pilgrims entered the protective armory even of Arna populations who did not necessarily see in this cause to become Muslim. Urban dwellers did in time often convert to Islam, in part out of respect for the scholarly literate tradition with which it was associated, and they too made ample use of these kinds of protective devices. Specialists in Islamic esoteric medicine offered services that bridged the spirit possession traditions of the region and the therapeutic riches of Islamic protective sciences.[5]

By the same token, even committed Muslims continued to draw on the medical knowledge of their more rural neighbors because they seemed to work and inspired confidence. Who would know better than a hunter which barks could heal a snake bite? Wouldn't a specialist in spirit possession know how to handle a man who seems to have become another person?

When one's cattle fall ill, why not seek assistance from the previously nomadic clan that would have poultices suited to preventing the disease from
spreading? The remedies of other clans and ritual specialists drew on spirits and forces peculiar to each specialist's unique niche in the region. The
leader of any major Hausa-speaking city-state had to be adept at drawing
on and commanding the allegiance of a host of such specialists while continuing to nurture the *bori* cult, which by the late eighteenth century was
understood to be critical to founding new towns, establishing markets, and
promoting good rains (Masquelier 2001b, 49–76, 192–226). Islam, argues
Ismail Abdalla, did not alter the attitudes of the Islamized Hausa toward
magic; "it simply introduced new techniques and formulae to replace or
supplement existing practice" (Abdalla 1981, 128).

The leaders of the nineteenth-century jihads in the Hausa-speaking
region objected strenuously to the cohabitation of these local spiritual
practices with Islamic beliefs, and they rejected the compatibility of *bori*
with Islam. Usman 'dan Fodio taught that a number of prevalent practices
within the kingdoms of the Hausa were not merely sinful but were evidence
of fundamental unbelief (*kafirci*). Murray Last and M. A. Al-Hajj summa-
rize the critical distinction: "The dividing line in some cases is fine: for example, numerology, astrology, the observation of lucky and unlucky days,
the use of dust and water from tombs to anoint oneself—all these are sins.
On the other hand, among polytheistic customs he included the following:
(i) veneration of trees or rocks by making sacrifices or pouring libations . . .
(iv) divination by sand, stars, spirits, the sounds or movements of birds;
(v) consultation of soothsayers; (vi) the placing of cotton (?) [*sic*] on rocks, trees
or paths" (Last and Al-Hajj 1965, 234). Jihadists argued that if the ruler of
a kingdom was guilty of *shirk* (polytheism), the entire kingdom was to be
designated as *kafir* (heathen), regardless of the range of degrees of adherence to Islam among its subjects. Using this logic to justify war against the
unrepentant rulers of the Hausa states, who as we have seen had assembled
a host of kinds of *magani*, the jihadists toppled each of the major kingdoms
one by one (Hiskett 1994; Last 1967).

Whatever the views of the jihadists, it is unlikely that esoteric Islamic
medicine had much to offer women by comparison with the longer spirit
veneration traditions of the region (cf. Ullmann 1978). Certainly in the regions of Niger that were never conquered by the jihadists, Islamic therapeutic traditions seem to have far more salience for men than for women.
Ethnobotanist Anne Luxereau observed in the 1980s in the same region

studied by Guy Nicolas that "women have available to them other networks and resources that enter into competition with the Muslim expert" (Luxereau 1984, 5). Since the *bori* specialist, likely to be a woman herself, could be consulted on a broad array of issues ranging from behavioral problems ("nightmares, fear, vertigo, kleptomania, aggressiveness, various kinds of madness") to social problems ("women who hope to find a husband, have success in business, do violence to another") to sexual problems, it is perhaps not surprising that a male religious specialist would not be women's exclusive or even first resort (Luxereau 1984, 9).

Furthermore, in the wake of the reforms of the jihadists, women's concerns were little in evidence in the therapeutic tradition, "the medicine of the Prophet," that they espoused. Abdalla remarked that "no one who reads the many medical treatises extant in Nigeria will fail to observe the special emphasis the authors have placed . . . on matters such as male sexual virility" rather than on the diseases and problems of women (1981, 133). He argued that even with the growing emphasis on *materia medica*, the ensuing medical scholarship was of little relevance to women: "Women's complaints connected usually with pregnancy, birth, nursing or menstruation have attracted but the slightest attention on the part of these compilers. As to women's sexual pleasure in these medical writings, it is viewed as accidental, often irrelevant to the more central and more legitimate sexual enjoyment of men. Men's domination of the medicine of the book was perhaps the most important reason why Hausa Muslim women were attracted to the cult of bori in spite of men's objection" (Abdalla 1981, 133).

The striking exception that proves this rule is the poem *Tabshir al-Ikhwan*, generally known as "Medicine of the Prophet," by Usman 'dan Fodio's scholarly daughter Nana Asma'u. Nana Asma'u faced the daunting challenge of attempting to acculturate the conquered female populations who would be critical to the future socialization of children into the reformists' vision of a new Islamic caliphate. Her writings include a number of suggestions to Arabic-speaking scholars about particular texts that could be included in *layya* and *rubutu* charms to enhance the well-being of women during pregnancy and delivery or to relieve their anxiety about their fertility, the sex of their offspring, or the health of their children (Boyd and Mack 1997, 99):

Sura 56: "If written and worn by a woman undergoing child-birth, she will safely deliver the child by the grace of God the Exalted one. It is effective on everything to which it is attached." (Boyd and Mack 1997, 106)[6]

Sura 69: "If it is worn by a pregnant woman, then she will be protected from all ailments." (Boyd and Mack 1997, 108)[7]

Sura 85: "If it is read for a child, he will be guarded from all harmful things." (Boyd and Mack 1997, 111)[8]

Sura 89: "Whoever reads it a hundred times during the night and then has sexual relations with his wife will be blessed with a boy who will be a delight to his heart." (Boyd and Mack 1997, 112)[9]

Sura 90: "If hung on a child at birth, the child will be protected from any evils and from colic pain. And if the child is made to take a sniff of its water, he will have sound nostrils, be free from colds and grow up in good health." (Boyd and Mack 1997, 113)[10]

The suras favored by Nana Asma'u regularly invoked the perils of hell for the unbeliever (who engaged in illicit acts) and paradise as a reward for the patience of the true believer.

She addressed this poem (in Arabic) to the scholarly class who would presumably be called on to treat women by writing such charms. Rudolph Ware argues that Islamic education and knowledge in West Africa was not so much syncretic as deeply (and classically) embodied; he rejects the binary of masculine textuality and feminine enthusiasm that has cast Islam as the domain of men and spirit possession the domain of women in much of the literature (Ware 2014). Certainly the recitation of *dhikr*, the writing, washing, and drinking of Koranic texts, and the kinds of local pilgrimage and recitation that Nana Asma'u's female followers engaged in belie the notion of a disembodied or unlettered practice of Islam. Such remedies presupposed a deep knowledge of and confidence in the Koran as a whole; for the suras referenced to be meaningful in the absence of any broader ritual and performative frame, women would need to be literate in Arabic and conversant with the Koran.

In reality, the overwhelming majority of women did not achieve the kind of richly saturated experience of Islamic medicine that would have heightened the potency of Nana Asma'u's remedies. Certainly, in the territories that eventually fell within Niger, very few women achieved a high degree of Islamic training until very recently. Unlike *bori* ritual, these charms were not embedded in a thickly experienced context. *Bori* practices engaged the numerous sensory elements so key to the traversing of the *jiki* with perfumes, colorful clothing, pulsing music, and links to a known landscape and pharmacopeia. These charms could not counter women's fears about the *source* of their distress, which often was understood to have originated in some sort of violation of the *kurwa* by other forces, such as spirits or witches, whose existence could not simply be wished away by Muslims, however devout.

To obtain such a charm, a distressed woman would have had to seek out an Islamic scholar and reveal her physical status, potentially humiliating her husband. These remedies appear less driven by the concerns of a woman than by the preferences of her husband. Rather than reinforce a woman's bodily experience and assist her in interpreting it, these charms required her to shed the particularity of her feminine experience and submit to a series of practices (reading, writing, Koranic recitation) that were largely the province of men. Certainly, women did and still do seek out such charms, but it is easy enough to understand why Nana Asma'u's enthusiasm for the *exclusive* use of such charms would not appeal to women accustomed to a far richer symbolic field and a greater degree of participation and recognition as actors themselves.

A poignant folktale reported by Arthur Tremearne in 1913 captures the misgivings women may have had in bringing their reproductive concerns to *any* male specialist, whether a Muslim scholar or a male healer. In folktales women are often represented as hens precisely because of their reproductive function. A hen, evidently suffering from infertility, went to a wildcat (a male animal, representing a *boka* or traditional male diviner and healer) in one version of the tale and to a *malam* (a male Muslim scholar) in another. Otherwise the stories are the same. Hen said she wanted a charm for childbirth. The wildcat/*malam* told her, "Go and pluck the feathers from your head, and put on salt and pepper, and then come back and I will give you the charm for childbirth." So she went off and plucked feathers and rubbed her body with salt and pepper. Meanwhile the wildcat/*malam* had gathered wood for a fire, which had by now burned down to hot embers. "Very well," says he, "let us go close to this fire, you go in front, and I will go behind . . . " and of course he threw her on the fire, roasted her, and ate her (Tremearne 1913, 224–25). The tale hints at women's skepticism about *all* ritual specialists' claims and is suggestive of how vulnerable women felt when their fertility fell into question. A hen that no longer lays eggs is, so to speak, cooked. While not all *bori* healers were or are women, the highly feminine environment of *bori* and the likely sympathy women would find in other participants had deep significance for troubled women.

No matter how stridently Islamic reformers in the region have decried *bori*, it has proven difficult to eliminate. In one of the most engaging passages in Baba of Karo's autobiographical narrative of life in Hausa-speaking northern Nigeria, Baba reports what happened when the recognized local authority (the Fagaci) attempted to forbid *bori* in the town of Giwa in 1949:

> Tanko's wife went to Fagaci's compound to greet his wives, and as she came out from the women's quarters she had to pass through the room where he was sitting . . . As she was kneeling down [to greet him] the bori came and possessed her—it was Baturen Gwari, the European from Gwari country. "Imprison me, bind me, call the police and lock me up!". . . When the spirit was quiet for a little the women pushed her out and took her home . . . She sang this "praise-song" right before Fagaci. We are the end, we are meningitis, we are all the other illness [sic], we own the bit of earth behind the hut. (M. F. Smith 1981, 223)

One can't help but enjoy Fagaci's impotence in the face of a "European" spirit who taunted him, declaring that illness and childbirth were none of his affair. Various scholars have entertained the question of whether *bori* serves as a mode of resistance to Islam or as a counterdiscourse to patriarchy (see, e.g., Echard 1978, Onwuejeogwu 1969, Lewis 1971). At the very least, it is clear that Hausa women sustained *bori* as a specifically feminine way to seek *magani* for what rendered women's lives perplexing in particularly unsettling times.

Many *bori* practitioners today do regard themselves as Muslims; they certainly believe in the unity of Allah and adhere to the five pillars of Islam. Yet, when calamity strikes, the spirits can be difficult to ignore. The disapproval of devout Muslims toward the use of charms and spirit mediation today is, if anything, more acute and restrictive than at the time of the jihad. Not only are *bori* and Arna remedies rejected but also today the written charms proposed by Nana Asma'u are often proclaimed to be un-Islamic as well. Nigeriens sometimes find the incompatibility of Salafi reformists' version of perfect Islamic practice with the realities of their lives profoundly troubling (Masquelier 2001b, 85, 150). Undoubtedly, the fear of hell purveyed by strident reformers does shape the imaginings of many Muslims in the region, feeding the anguish they feel when they can't live up to the ideals reformists insist on. However, the fear of hell may not be as powerful as the fear of infertility. Reformist agitation can create a heightened sense of vulnerability and uncertainty rather than a sensation of well-being (Masquelier 2008, 2009).

Islamic medicine has had surprisingly little purchase on the practices of women throughout Hausa-speaking regions, regardless of their degree of commitment to the orthodoxy of various reformists. Historically, Hausa-speaking women in Niger have had relatively poor access to education, whether Islamic or Western in orientation, which has made them all the more likely to hold tight to therapeutic practices they find meaningful. Some of those practices, including *bori*, are not merely residues of a pre-Islamic past; they show the traces of a shifting reproductive landscape as populations moved increasingly into Islamicized urban settings where mobility, disease, and new forms of wealth and consumption could threaten women's fertility. Colonial rule heightened the sense of uncertainty and vulnerability women experienced, as we shall see in the next chapter.

Notes

1. George Percy Bargery's *A Hausa-English Dictionary and English-Hausa Vocabulary* published by Oxford University Press in 1934 has long been a rich resource for scholars of the Hausa-speaking region. This resource can be found online in a searchable form at http://maguzawa.dyndns.ws. My citations in this text are from the web version, which does not include page numbers. In this case, the entries are found under *gafi*.

2. The scholarly literature on the Kano Chronicle is rich and rather contentious. See Palmer (1967), M. G. Smith (1984), Last (1980), Hunwick (1993).

3. OED Online. March 2018. "Risk, n." Oxford University Press. Accessed May 4, 2018. http://www.oed.com.proxy.libraries.rutgers.edu/view/Entry/166306.

4. I am grateful to Murray Last for sharing so much of his work on these issues (among others see 1976, 142, and 2004). See also M. Smith (1967), Tremearne (1914, 131–36), Leroux (1948, 643), G. Nicolas (1975, 236–40), Masquelier (2001b, 87–91, 285), Greenberg (1946), and Luxereau (1991, 15–16, 20–21).

5. For the political complexity of "affiliations of enchantment" in contemporary Mauritania, see Pettigrew (2017).

6. Presumably the passing reference to semen in Sura 56 as part of God's intention to ordain reproduction made the Sura particularly appropriate.

7. Sura 69 "Incontestable" assures the Muslim that judgment day is inevitable with hell for the unbelievers, but for believers the fruits of their previous labors will be assured.

8. Sura 85 "The Galaxies" doesn't have any direct reference to children but does once again promise the protection of God for those who believe and hell for those who harm them.

9. The reason for linking this sura with successful procreation is obscure, although the reference to times of day and the opening of the sura with a powerful oath may be relevant.

10. Sura 90 "The Town" enjoins the believer to protect the innocent and weak, in particular orphans.

2

TENSIONS IN THE WAKE OF CONQUEST

Gender and Reproduction after Abolition

A Visual Inventory of Niger in 1924

Photographs taken by the celebrated *croisière noire* mission capture the complex social field of the populations of the Sahel just as French colonial rule was being consolidated after two decades of struggle to subdue the Tuareg. They reveal that social tensions were heightened rather than erased, and they convey the textured quality of spiritual practices in the interwar years despite the growing hegemony of Islamic law. Sponsored by automobile company Citroën, the "mission" featured a caravan of eight specially designed caterpillar vehicles (antecedents to the military tank) built to traverse the difficult and variable terrain of the central Sudanic zone. The caravan began in Algeria and traversed the desert to Niamey, where it then followed the southern shore of the Sahara, circled around Lake Chad, and eventually plunged south into the Belgian and British colonies of East and Central Africa. This adventure-cum-publicity stunt carried forward both an exploratory and a military tradition. The "penetration" of the continent through the superior technology of Europe would contribute to taming the landscape and the people within it. Beyond advertising the engineering of Citroën, the mission was calculated to display French military mobility to Tuareg subjects and to attract commercial interest in France's African empire. The expedition also had a mandate to collect images and objects for museums and the Geographic Society. Fortunately for the historian, the impulse to document the trip yielded a famous film, *La Croisière Noire* (by cinematographer Léon Poirier), a multitude of photographs (taken largely by Georges-Marie Haardt), paintings and drawings (by Alexandre Iacovleff), and published travelogues.

The first major stop within Niger was Niamey, which was not at that time a major urban center (the capital being in Zinder). All children there under about thirteen years old were entirely naked, whether girls or boys. Only adult men had the privilege of wearing the embroidered *riga* gown and *hula* cap associated with Islam.[1] Once a young woman was married, she too would begin to dress more modestly, in locally woven cloth, and in town she might drape another cloth across her head (MQB Vol. 2, 162, November 27, 1924, PA000115.211). During the entirety of the mission's time in Niger, while it traversed the length of its southern edge from Niamey to N'Guigmi, every "chief" the mission encountered wore the turban associated with power and authority in Islam, and at each stop the mission was greeted with an intimidating military display of mounted Zarma, Hausa, or Tuareg on horseback and camel. Power was unambiguously marked in this colonial display as masculine, Islamic, and based on the superior capacity to do violence.

And yet, at each stop the mission was also fêted with local drumming and dancing and with the cultural curiosities particular to the region. Many of the photographs capture the diverse and delighted audience and not simply the performers. A familiar pattern emerges: women sat and stood separately from men, older women separately from younger, sedentary separately from nomadic, and powerful people sat higher and weaker sat lower. Older women regularly wove their wealth in coins into their hair. Generally infants were not in evidence; women did not expose their vulnerable babies to the eyes of others. The performances varied slightly from one region to the next; however, we see women dancers, male drummers, and young men engaged in spectacles that have little relationship to Islam and are suggestive of the enduring importance of the skills of hunters to tame the dangerous world of the bush. In Niamey,

> Toufounis [the hunter] wears on his forehead a piece of wood curiously wrought and representing the head of a *kalao*, the wading secretary-bird, whose long crooked beak surmounted with a hollow horn gives it the appearance of a bird from the Apocalypse . . . The fact is that this strange bird scents danger from a great distance. It is the protector of the heavy flying bustard and the wingless ostrich . . . These two great birds have need of warning at the approach of danger; and so they seek out the neighborhood of the *kalao*, which gives them due notice. (Haardt and Audouin-Dubreuil 1927b, 42–43)

Hunters, although often belonging to subordinate groups absorbed into larger and more powerful polities in the region, remained feared and respected figures whose prowess drew from protective magic and knowledge of the wild spaces outside the zone of cultivation. Hunters had an important role in ritually "opening up" the hunting season during the dry season after the crops had come in.[2] Toufounis has to seduce his prey in order to conquer it; this kind of wily deception with a view to literally "eating" one's opponent was deeply respected in folklore of the region.

The members of the expedition were also treated to a dance by two women in Niamey. Accompanied by drumming, the "priestess" Songo danced an intimidating knife dance, threatening suggestively to cut off the sexual organs and breasts of her beautiful dance partner, Kadi. "None of you [in the crowd] dare come near me," she taunted in song, "because you feel shame that there is one among you who always surpasses you in beauty and the pleasures of the flesh, who is always chosen by the Conquering Warrior or the passing lover. It will always be thus, so long as she is present, because her beauty will forever crush you. . . . Therefore if you hope to find love, I must kill her. *Diaram, diaram, diaram!*" (Audouin-Dubreuil 2004, 42–44, my translation).

The dance is reminiscent of *holey* or *bori* spirit cult initiation ceremonies, which would also have been common in the dry season. Here the priestess Songo was possessed by a fearsome warrior spirit from the south. The sexual and reproductive violence intimated by the dance hints at the anxiety peoples in the region felt when their daughters and wives had been captured and taken south through slave trade networks. But by the same token, the dance gives voice to the fears of married women whose husbands would have had sexual access to captive women.[3]

The threat of violence that lay just beneath the surface in this early colonial moment emerged in other ways as well. Just three days of travel short of Niamey, as the members of the expedition were resting by firelight at Bourem, they were startled by the appearance of a young Tuareg leader named Igounana. When asked what he wanted, Igounana replied that he needed to know when the expedition would arrive in Niamey. Having been summoned by the French administrator in Niamey to welcome the expedition when it arrived at that post, Igounana and his large group of Tuareg horsemen hoped to gauge how quickly they needed to move in order to arrive in time. The expedition leaders told him proudly that their group would make it in three days thanks to their all-terrain

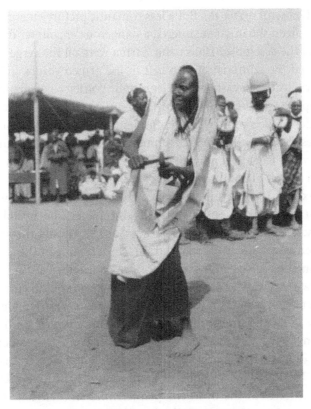

Kouli-Kouta dance in Niamey, November 1924. Courtesy of
Musée du Quai-Branly-Jacques Chirac (Art Resource, NY).

vehicles. Igounana reportedly replied, "Good, maybe now we won't be
forced to supply camels and build roads anymore," and took off into the
night with his entourage (Haardt and Audouin-Dubreuil 1927a, 29–30, my
translation).

Later in the accounts, Igounana and his men thundered into Niamey at a gallop just as the Kouli-Kouta dance was being filmed by cam-
eraman Georges Specht. In the sanitized published account, the dramatic
arrival of these galloping horsemen was cast as a colorful and stylized
spectacle between Priam and Achilles; Igounana faced off with the Hausa
chief who had killed his father in a prior moment of violence (Haardt and

Audouin-Dubreuil 1927a, 36). But a less romantic picture emerges from the diaries; in effect, the mission suffered a dangerous encounter in which the Tuareg and the assembled Hausa and Zarma were on the verge of violence that required the administrator to call in the armed *gardes civils* to reinstate order: "In the devastated battleground, Poirier has tears in his eyes, Specht appears stricken" (Audouin-Dubreuil 2004, 40). The region was barely under French control; the resentments between former masters and the peoples they had dominated simmered just beneath the surface. The spirit of rivalry went beyond verbal abuse or dance; it was both contained and fueled by colonial military power.

The expedition captured some of the ways in which this extraordinary mix of populations historically interacted, both violently and pacifically. It inadvertently offers traces of the rituals through which age, gender, and status were marked. In Zinder—one of the strongholds of Islam in the region—the expedition was treated to a kind of puppet show known as Daï-Mabo, which attracted a large and diverse audience; the puppets represented nude figures both male and female.[4] Images taken in Zinder the preceding day of the same or very similar figures label them rather as "fetishes" (MQB Vol. 2, 196, December 5, 1924, PA000115.315). Startlingly, these figures had been preserved in the Great Mosque: "In the Great Mosque of a spare and primitive architecture, ancient statuettes of the heathens [*d'anciennes statuettes de féticheurs*] are preserved. Long Islamized, the population respects these objects of worship. The Sultan invites our company to an initiation ceremony" (Audouin-Dubreuil 2004, 46). The initiation ceremony, if there was one, made the "puppets" or "statuettes" all the more striking; these naked and sexually explicit figures were probably not intended simply to entertain, as the term *puppet* would suggest. They had a deeper spiritual origin prior or parallel to Islam in the region. The sultan, as both head of the Islamic community and sovereign over the far bigger non-Muslim population, had the duty to preserve and protect them. They were not hidden; they were viewed by men, women, and children out in the open square.

The album also captures young dancing men whose age and distinctive haircut suggests that they were part of a recently initiated age group linked to the public showing of the "fetishes." Other striking photographs from the same day show Hazena women performing a dance known as the *koraya*, their faces painted an intimidating black and white (MQB Vol. 3, 201, December 6, 1924, PA000001.2). By absorbing rather than annihilating the spiritual practices of the region, Muslim-led polities such as Zinder succeeded in maintaining a relationship with the surrounding non-Muslim populations. Such populations, referred to in French as *autochthones* and in Hausa as *people of the earth* ('yan 'kasa), had a rootedness in the landscape that rendered their spiritual skills particularly important. Clearly, their significance endured after French conquest.

Children at the margins of crowds in many photographs, mostly naked, generally appeared to be healthy. But sometimes the photographs reveal the kind of distended belly typical of protein-calorie deficiency. Some of the more troubling images of such malnourished children were taken in the most agriculturally rich part of the territory, at Madaroumfa. In this region, the lake and the valley lands of the seasonal watercourse, the Goulbin Maradi, make a longer and more varied agriculture possible. Elsewhere, the sandy land of the dunes is suitable only for growing millet, cowpeas, and peanuts. The presence of such clearly malnourished children seems to have struck Haardt, who photographed more children here than in other settings. The particular vulnerability of children in the very heart of the agricultural zone where the market for food and commercial crops was strong was already in evidence as early as 1924.

Frustratingly, the images are otherwise unrevealing about food or indeed about children. The mission appears to have eaten its own food apart, prepared by its own cook, Baba. Interestingly, the one set of images in which a meal was served was taken in the palace of the Sultan Barmou of Tessawa. In them, his numerous wives huddle in a circle in such a way that the photographer can see neither their faces nor the dish itself. Clearly, modesty in the consumption of food was part of the generalized set of practices related to status, reserve, or shame. The sultan's meal was accompanied by the music of blind musicians, because, we are told, no one must ever see the sultan eat (Haardt and Audouin-Dubreuil 1927b, 48–50).

The sexual interactions between local women and administrators and soldiers were well known and evidently did not require discretion on the part of the photographer. In Niamey, an African woman dressed in a simple dress posed with her two daughters of about six and eight years old. The two mixed-race girls were dressed in Western dresses and matching white sunhats. All three wore shoes and bracelets. Around their mother's neck was a string festooned with amulets; the girls wore matching

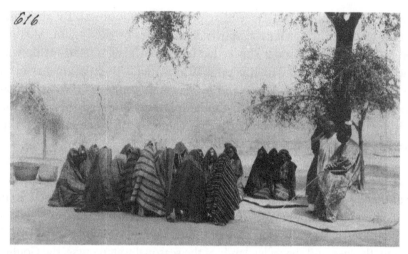

Sultan Barmou with his secluded wives in Tessawa, November 1924. Courtesy of Musée du Quai-Branly-Jacques Chirac (Art Resource, NY).

necklaces with a pendant of some kind, perhaps a religious medal. The text refers to the girls as "orphans." Clearly, although the girls knew their biological mother, as mixed-race *métisses* they were being schooled in an entirely different cultural setting.[5] In Dosso, the administrator, M. Coupe, posed unabashedly with his Fulani "wife," who was judged by the all-male team to be quite beautiful (MQB Vol. 2, 159, November 27, 1924, PA000115.202). In Madawa, Audouin-Dubreuil was disgusted to arrive in time to find the half-dressed and sleepy administrators with their mistresses; one of the men quipped that it is easy to get a good night's sleep in this region because of the "loyalty" of the populations (Audouin-Dubreuil 2004, 44).

Some of the more sensual photos (which do not appear in the published book) seem to have been staged with prostitutes, who dotted the same landscape as the soldiers and administrators. The photographer was particularly taken with three nubile Kanembu girls in N'Guigmi, who posed for him nude in numerous photos (MQB Vol. 3, 264, December 17, 1924, PA000001.220; MQB Vol. 3, 262, December 17, 1924, PA000001.214). Images of adult Kanembu women dancers performing impressively athletic leaps

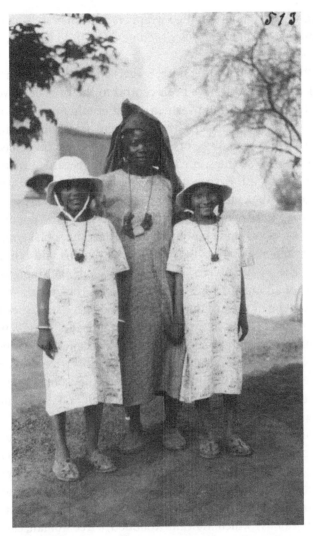

Two mixed-race girls with their mother in Niamey, November 1924. Courtesy of Musée du Quai-Branly-Jacques Chirac (Art Resource, NY).

show them wearing modest indigo wrappers and a hairstyle markedly different from that of the nude "*filles gallantes*" (MQB Vol. 3, 248, December 1924, PA000001.174).

The album as a whole, therefore, reveals an extremely diverse population in which Islam may have been central to the lives of powerful men in relatively large towns but in which a host of other practices important to women and men (especially younger men) were vibrant and openly performed. While sexuality outside of marriage may have been tightly controlled in some settings, it was evidently not regarded with the same censorious eye by all. Even within the restricted spaces of the Muslim leaders (such as the court of Sultan Barmou), we see evidence of a wide variety of practices in keeping with the diversity of the population. The numerous "wives" of these powerful men reflect the social landscape, for they were taken systematically from diverse regions and ethnicities. To refer to these women as "wives" is surely to occlude the ambiguously captive origins of all but the four legitimate wives. Integrating "wives" into the court reiterated the accumulative and seductive strategies necessary to the assertion of power in the region. A great deal of slavery and concubinage continued openly in such courts three decades into French rule in southern Niger. Barmou's sexual monopoly over his wives and concubines was ensured by the use of eunuchs to oversee the women's quarters and of blind musicians to entertain the court (Haardt and Audouin-Dubreuil 1927a, 41–42).

The complex tensions generated by this mix of nomadic subjects and sedentary chiefs, concubines and wives, and white men and their African mistresses, emerged in yet another form in an incident in N'Guigmi. As the painter Iacovleff decided which of the women assembled at the administrator's residence he wanted to paint, Haardt and Audouin-Dubreuil noticed "the look of jealousy which Mairam-Kouddou, a free woman, cast upon the beautiful captive Ayagana whose portrait Iacovleff [was] painting" (Haardt and Audouin-Dubreuil 1927a, 57). They report the words of the mocking song Mairam, clothed in a dark indigo cloth, sings to Ayagana:

I am named Mairam, Mairam
Mairam sister of Kondoukoye,
Mairam is more beautiful than all others;
Go ask her suitor Boukar
If that is not so.

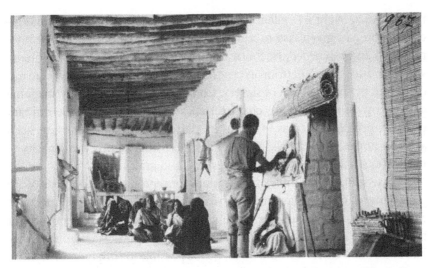

Alexander Iacovleff paints Ayagana in N'Guigmi, December 1924. Courtesy of Musée du Quai-Branly—Jacques Chirac (Art Resource, NY).

Just as the black boubou
Is different from the white boubou,
So is Mairam distinct from other women.
If the indigo boubou and the white boubou
Are the same as one another,
Then Mairam is just like the others.
Mairam, the daughter of a chief, is beyond compare.
Before her, daughter of a mosquito,
You can do nothing but flee. (Haardt and Audouin-Dubreuil 1927a, 57–58, my
    translation)

Even a woman of relatively high status such as Mairam was threatened by the sexual availability and reproductive competition of a captive woman like Ayagana.

Production and Reproduction

The visual record of the *croisière noire* offers a glimpse of a diverse zone in which Islam had a visible presence but was by no means the single most important spiritual and social dimension of people's lives. The tensions captured in the accounts reflect some of the striking ruptures of the era: warrior elites continued to have the power to intimidate but no longer had the legitimate right to violence; relations between European men and local women had given rise to a mixed-race social group that was at once marginal and privileged; freeborn women and their slaves were in intense sexual and social competition as criteria demarcating social status were undermined by the abolition of slavery. Colonial rule was gradually stripping away many of the defining characteristics of nobility—namely, military prowess; privileged access to the intimidating trappings of warfare, such as guns, horses, and camels; and perhaps most importantly the capacity to redistribute seized labor, women, livestock, and grain.

These shifts had complex implications for reproductive concerns. With the decline in open enslavement, virtually all that remained to mark status difference was the size of one's entourage and an exaggerated concern for the behaviors associated with free status. For Tuareg, Hausa, Kanuri, Songhai, and Fulani elites, it would no longer be possible to simply assert control over resources through violence; hegemony would now have to be sustained through visible performances of affect, ritual, religion, and routine. This pattern has been remarked on in studies of the implications of the decline in slavery in the region, most notably in the work of Olivier de Sardan (1984, 29–32, 201–5). However, the focus has generally been on the ways in which the performance of honor among elite males has been contrasted with the attribution of a lack of honor to former male slaves. Here I wish to direct attention more precisely to the feminine side of the story—after all, most slaves had been female.[6] In the case of women, status performance had as much to do with shame and its correlates (restraint, modesty, and reserve) as it did with honor, inviting a rather different approach to tracing the unintended consequences of colonial intrusion and abolition.

Prior to colonial rule, most captives in the Hausa-speaking region of Niger (as opposed to Nigeria) had worked alongside family members in farm units that, while sometimes large, could not really be described as slave settlements or plantations. As it grew increasingly difficult to reproduce captive labor through raids, warfare, or the market, it became necessary to retain servile labor through some other means. One approach was to retain female slaves as "concubines," who the French conveniently understood to be "like family" and therefore not really enslaved. As a result, there was increasing slippage between the tasks of the female slave and the tasks of the junior wife. Concubines could be treated as junior wives, and the hierarchy among and between wives was accentuated with particular emphasis placed on distinguishing between those wives who had produced children for the household and those who had not. Effectively, childbearing and leisure time (marked by seclusion and veiling) were to become the most important means of distinguishing free women from servile (B. Cooper 1994).[7]

Thus, the burden of reproducing the labor force, the social structure, and the family fell largely to lower-status women, who in this region continued to contribute significant labor to the agricultural economy as well as to food transformation and child rearing. This solution to the labor problem is particularly tidy when one recalls that in West Africa most slaves were women, and most female slaves were understood to be sexually available to their male owners (Olivier de Sardan 1984, 118–20). However, this solution would be most workable and plausible in a setting in which the offspring of concubines could be absorbed into the master's lineage, as was more or less the case in much of the eastern portion of Niger, the so-called Central Sudan.

By contrast, in the numerous societies in which the children of elite men by their female slaves had been set off in a category distinct from that of the elite, the logic of endogamy in marriage played an extremely important role in maintaining social distinctions. Rigid adherence to status or caste endogamy could serve to maintain firewalls between the freeborn "noble" stratum, freed castes with artisanal skills, and the captive slave lines devoted to strenuous labor. Maintaining the leisure of a freeborn wife entailed the presence of female servants, generally from the formerly captive population. Olivier de Sardan has insisted, rightly, that the depiction of servitude as a continuum of relations from slave to free misses the ways in which social boundaries between status groups were (and often still are) carefully policed and obscures the qualitative differences in comportment and labor associated with different statuses. Casted men whose families are understood to have been "born" into servile relations vis-à-vis the free would never be permitted to marry women of noble background, but by the same token, they would not deign to marry those of captive slave heritage (Olivier de Sardan 1984, 44, 120).

In the regions to the north and west, "freed" but not "free" women brought into households were likely to occupy an ambiguous status between that of the concubine and the wife. This would be particularly true where the work of nursing and caring for small children during the day was turned over to "servants" whose own children would thereby become "milk" kin rather than blood kin to those of the master. The words of one elite Seryanke son of such a household, written in the late 1940s, convey the ambiguity well: "[The child] spends most of the day on the back of the servant girl that his father has assigned to him. The child comes to feel a deep affection for the one who calms him with flattering lullabies and this emotional attachment from a young age may explain the large number of 'taras' (a servant woman married by her master) that appear in the headcount of the families of chiefs" (IFAN C 14 Barry Mamadou Aliou 1949).

In both absorptive and endogamous societies, the most important means of distinguishing those lower orders susceptible to "recruitment" for involuntary labor from those leisured classes above them was, from the 1920s on, through an almost obsessive attention to what generally is glossed inadequately in English as *shame* or in French as *honte* (*kunya* in Hausa, *maloya* in Bamanankan, *haawi* in Zarma/Songhai, *tekaraqit* in Tamasheq, *semteende* in Fulfulde, *nongu* in Kanuri). These terms are all difficult to convey in English or French, since they refer to the capacity to *feel* shame, not simply to shame itself, and they encompass a far greater semantic field than the words generally used to translate them imply. The capacity to feel shame is laudable; it is a sign of good breeding in a rather literal way. Someone "without shame" lacks a sensibility associated with nobility, humanity, and freedom. This sense of shame and the self-mastery that results from it marks freeborn adults as fully socialized humans, distinct from animals and small children. The capacity to feel shame sustains the honor of an individual, a family, and a social group.

The multiplicity of local terms and their lack of a shared Arabic root suggest strongly that the emphasis on shame across the region was neither introduced by Islam nor was it a mere by-product of the trans-Saharan slave trade. Some of the most pronounced behaviors designated through such terms are to be found in Sahelian societies resistant to Islam, such as the Bambara, whose expression "death is preferable to shame" (*saya ka fisa ni maloya ye*) finds echo in virtually every other language in the region (Barreteau 1995, 264). A willingness to die rather than be enslaved was the mark of the freeborn nobility; enslavement in itself was therefore understood to result from an inborn inferiority, an incapacity to feel shame (for the Zarma context, see Bornand 2017).

Understanding Shame and Honor

Shame is not quite identical to honor; one inheres in the individual and is felt as a sensation, while the other is a quality attributed to him or her by others as a result of comportment. Someone who is seen as being honorable deserves to be treated with respect. Proper behavior with regard to others is the most important dimension of the capacity to feel shame, and so to "have" shame is also to be respectful. Honor, shame, modesty, and respect are entangled and all are the mark of humanity and proper upbringing and breeding. The visible evidence of someone who has this capacity to feel shame is his or her modesty in the presence of others to whom deference is due: in dress, in speech, in bearing. Those who have shame also have the ability to discern those members of society to whom deference is due: those who are of a higher caste, those who are older (particularly in-laws), men over women, free over slave. A woman must be modest before all freeborn men and must defer to her husband; a man must be modest before his in-laws and show respect to elders in general. The self-restraint that gives a man the alluring capacity to *distribute* (food, wealth, wives, slaves, livestock, land) rather than consume is the behavior that most invites respect toward men. For women, the self-restraint that gives a woman the capacity to remain *modest*, patient, and hardworking brings honor. To varying degrees, these qualities, particularly generosity, are admired in both men and women.

This capacity to feel shame means that one must also demonstrate a *public* response to any circumstance that could provoke shame. "Having" shame is not simply experienced; it is also performed. Womanly modesty is demonstrated through restraint in speech, sound, and visibility. A bride will ostentatiously flee the presence of her father-in-law, for example—such avoidance relations can make every waking moment an exercise in the performance of reserve, modesty, and shame. A man's demonstration of shame occurs through the distribution of food, clothing, and gifts to his wives, extended family, and clients. To ignore the sensation of shame would be a mark of baseness; a man who had no gifts would refuse to return home from a trip until he could provide them.

Proper comportment is a sign of good breeding in a literal way. Failures of comportment give evidence of a kind of bastardization of the free or noble bloodline. Thus, nobility must respond aggressively to anything that threatens the honor of the group, and individuals are expected to take specific action to redress any shame they bring on their household, family, or society. To fail to do so would be to reveal one's fundamental baseness, one's lack of capacity to feel shame, and by implication the baseness of one's lineal relatives.[8] Where hierarchy became overlaid with Islamic practice and an accentuation of patrilineal descent, shame and honor came to be seen as attributes of a good Muslim. Fittingly, the performance of Muslim piety could become a mark of self-restraint and good breeding.

The lack of shame is regularly associated with casted groups (whose sometimes distant origins were linked to defeat or captivity) and in particular with griots, whose task it is to speak openly about precisely those things about which those with shame would never speak.[9] The spirits who occupy the Sahelian zone are also frequently shameless; consequently, their mediums (often women) appear to act in ways that are immodest and even un-Islamic when possessed. Very young children cannot yet be held accountable for their actions, for they have not yet begun to "feel" or "have" shame. Across the entire region, one of the most common claims is that slaves (and their descendants) have no shame (Meillassoux 1991, 128). In fact, in the absence of actual captivity, what most marks slave origins is shamelessness—the incapacity to provide wealth, protect feminine modesty, or act with restraint. This is not to say that slaves and former slaves never articulated their own alternative views and practices contesting, reestablishing, or redefining honor (Stilwell 2000).

Of Livestock and Slaves

Recalling that historically most slaves were women, scrutiny of the close association of slaves with shamelessness is in order. Women taken captive in warfare or raids were distributed as booty to soldiers and raped. Their bodies were sexually available to their masters and, until they found a place in a stable domestic space, to any men of the elite classes. Klein rightly emphasizes that "for the freeborn woman, one of the horrors of enslavement was to be suddenly removed from a situation where her sexuality was carefully controlled and her virginity valued to one where her body was someone else's property and subject to that other's will" (Klein 1998, 247). As a result, female sexual vulnerability was central to distinguishing the genuinely free from the freeborn and the emancipated: "ending the right of the master to command female sexual behavior was undoubtedly one of the most important concerns of the emancipated slave" (Klein 2005, 844).

More than anything else, it was the involuntary sexual vulnerability of the female slave to rape that marked her as different from the free woman. Women protected by free families were sexually available exclusively in marriage (at least in principle) and only on the consent of their fathers or other male kin, particularly in their first marriages. If a woman was to voluntarily deviate from such norms, shame/respect required that she successfully hide her behavior. Freeborn Tuareg women, for example, had greater license than women of other societies in the region, in part because their children belonged to them and their tent, not to their husbands. One outcome of this pattern is that, in Niger at least, many of the children of French soldiers were born to Tuareg women in Bilma and Agadez, whose families simply absorbed them. By contrast, the children of liaisons between European men and women of other ethnicities, like the "orphan girls" photographed by Georges-Marie Haardt, might be assembled in an orphanage managed by Catholic nuns to receive a European education once they were of school age (2 H 1 37 Court 1937).

Formal marriage throughout the region was marked by the transfer of gifts from the groom's family to the bride's, often in the form of livestock. Among Hausa in Niger, when a bride went to her new home, her father also sent her with a milk cow or a sheep so that she and her children would have milk and so that she could prove to be the kind of wife who prepares rich and varied food. Eating well and having good marital relations were linked to one another and were in turn linked to the prospect of producing children. This wedding cow would be said to bring *arziki* and *albarka* to the household: fertility, wealth, and marital happiness.[10] Women and milk cows belong together, linked by their production of food, milk, and offspring, all signs of wealth. Shame and *arziki* were related—to lack shame (*rashin kunya*) was also to lack prosperousness (*rashin arziki*).

The *absence* of these transactions—not simply of the "bride wealth" but also of such symbolically important gifts as grain and milk-producing animals—marked the slave woman as a slave and therefore as sexually available without her consent. Gift exchange was and is profoundly bound up with the demonstration of women's worth, marital status, and respectability. The absence of abundant wedding gifts to a woman marked her as unmarried and her children as illegitimate. For a woman to be sexually available outside the context of marriage was to be shameless, servile, animal-like. The captive was sexually available, and so by a kind of logic of inversion, that woman was therefore shameless. In a final turn, it was that shamelessness that marked her as non-Muslim and suitably enslaved. To sustain her claim to freeborn Muslim status, a woman had to remain, or at least appear to remain, sexually unavailable. A woman who had sexual relations outside of marriage revealed herself to be base; such a woman undermined the humanity, nobility, and honor of her family, and in particular of her mother. The daughter who proved to be shameless was imagined to be herself the product of an illicit coupling on the part of her mother, tarnishing the legitimacy of her paternal line and therefore of all her full siblings.

In many ways, slaves were regarded as equivalent to livestock (Meillassoux 1991, 76, 109). The slave woman, like the female cow, had no right to her offspring; her offspring belonged not to the genitor but to her owner. A Tuareg expression captures the logic and resonances of the association of slaves and livestock:

> *Celui [qui] possède captive, possède captif*
>   He who possesses the female slave possesses the male slave
> *Celui [qui] possède vache, possède bœuf*
>   He who possesses the cow possesses the ox
> (Bernus 1981, 92)

Female slaves would have been sexually vulnerable to men of free status in general. Yet a slave woman's progeny in effect had no lineage; they only had *appartenance* in the sense of "belonging to" a specific master. Slaves might breed, but they could not give birth; their offspring were not really recognized free persons (Meillassoux 1991, 107). Rules for the transfer of slaves regularly followed the same logic as rules for the handling of livestock. In this regard, slaves were the product of a specific womb, whereas the freeborn Muslim belonged unambiguously to a particular patriline or matriline.

In the end, the female slave and her womb always belonged to someone, and her offspring belonged to that master. Paul Riesman noted in the mid-1970s that both "noble" and "servile" Fulani used the same analogy between slaves and cattle to explain the continued hierarchy in status between them long after the abolition of slavery. He cited the explanation of one person of hereditary captive status as an example: "It is like stray cows . . . if a cow goes astray and wanders into someone else's herd, everyone knows that the cow does not belong to the herdsman—but it does belong to somebody. Even if the cow has calves and those calves have calves, they do not belong to the herdsman; they belong to whoever is the cow's rightful owner" (Riesman 1992, 28). The memorable title of Riesman's book on the reproduction of this hierarchy is *First Find Your Child a Good Mother*. This advice is not, Riesman insists, an exhortation to seek out a woman with good child-rearing skills; it marks the Fulani perception that parents do not shape their children—breeding in a more literal sense does. If a man wants to have honorable children, he will have to seek out a marriage to a woman from an honorable lineage. Among Tuareg, a similar conviction is expressed in the adage "*le ventre teint l'enfant*"—the child derives his color from the womb. The status of the child follows that of the mother (ANN 3 ECOL 115 5 Guemas 1953).

The notion, then, is that the sensitivity to shame is inherited, not learned, and that it adheres to those whose ancestors had always been free. For a man to have permitted himself to become a captive rather than to die in battle was, in a sense, the original moment of shamelessness, the echo of which we can hear in the 1930s exhortation to a young Zarma man to "prefer death to shame" (C 71 Jean-Louis Méon n.d.). The children of such a captive, born into slavery, have shameless parentage. Women of servile heritage have no shame, and accordingly, their sexuality is always suspect; their offspring are, in a sense, illegitimate in advance.

Controlling access to women in both sexual and reproductive terms was the means to control the labor of other men. In the Tuareg proverb cited above, the control over the female slave secured control over the male slave, because in order to gain access to her, the male slave must follow her wherever her master sends her. The slave armies of the region (including the French armies of conquest) were assembled the same way: the continued loyalty of such men was bought through the redistribution of sexual access to female captives. But sexual access is not the same thing as marriage or paternal rights; the male slave in the proverb is not like a bull but instead like an ox used to draw a cart—not a genitor, but a beast of burden (Bernus 1981, 92). The way for a male slave to acquire a "wife" over whom he had more control was either to capture her or to purchase her for himself. His master, however, would nevertheless inherit her and other accumulated wealth when the male slave died.

Patriliny and Shame in Niger

Despite the fact that Islam insists that religion is not inherited, the capacity to feel shame in Niger came to be seen as the attribute of the observant Muslim, something that accompanied a woman or man's membership in a Muslim community and household. By the same token, honor was associated with whiteness, which is one reason why Maurice Delafosse had a hard time delineating whiteness as a strictly racial category; those lineages that could project honorableness and Muslimness were by definition "not black." Thus, in the complex and inconsistent overlay of associations at play, being susceptible to enslavement called to mind blackness, non-Muslimness, femaleness, and shamelessness.

One effect of this entanglement, importantly, was that one could attempt to bypass the genealogical dimensions of nobility by emphasizing Muslimness and deemphasizing one's maternal origins, which was easier to do in some societies than in others. Among Hausa-speaking communities, the son of a nobleman and a slave woman could enjoy the same prerogatives as his half-brothers from the womb of a legal wife. This absorptive dynamic could considerably enhance the position of the nobleman's slave mother. With the abolition of slavery, taking on the identity of a Muslim head of household became another way freed men could emphasize their free status. In effect, they could assert themselves as the head of a new patriline. In the starkest of terms, what had most distinguished the free man from the slave man was the capacity to form legitimate marriages producing recognized children belonging to the presumptive biological father. Without such progeny to embody the history, memory, and afterlife of a man, particularly in settings in which patrilineal descent had grown in importance with the expansion of Islam, a man was nobody.

For the freed man, then, having a wife and children in a male-headed household had become tantamount to being free. The corollary, however, was that the purity of all men's bloodlines—not simply those of the nobility—increasingly became the signal marker of their claim to free status. The more patrilineal the society, the more likely it would be that men would mark their own free status through control of the sexuality of their wives and daughters and find status in producing a substantial line of male heirs through which to be remembered.

Patrilineal descent among regional elites had become the norm by the nineteenth century across much of the Sahel, even in societies that had previously tended toward matriliny. This shift accelerated very rapidly under colonial rule as all segments of society jockeyed to establish free status. This process was facilitated under French rule because local justice within Niger was handled largely on the cheap through recognized Muslim scholars. By 1946, the commandant of Agadez reported that the legal practice of the region had become so imbued with Maliki legal approaches ("*malikisé*") that "the only time custom is observed is when the maternal line of descent is relevant in the context of inheritance or property, and even then it is only in certain regions. In just a few regions inheritance or property may follow the mother's family line. With such vestiges it is hard to make out the previous social fabric" (ANN 5 E 2 5 Chapelle n.d.). In the nomadic and pastoral zone, free noblewomen among the Tuareg could continue to enjoy some status and sexual license as a result of bilateral and sometimes frankly matrilineal kinship norms. Tuareg women inherited livestock and other property through their maternal line. This property was known as "living milk" and could sometimes include slaves or houses.[11]

By contrast, former captives who settled in the sedentary zone were likely to be drawn to the prevailing patrilineal norms in which offspring of a woman belong to the male genitor—the husband. By purchasing the freedom of a female slave (in Hausa *fansa*), a man of captive descent could gain rights over the children she produced (Rossi 2010, 101–2). The colonial administration struggled to find ways to encourage the emancipation of the slaves of nomads without upending the authority of masters. One element of this effort was to attempt to persuade masters to let female slaves go in exchange for a traditional marriage payment to be paid either by a male representative or the woman herself (ANN 5 E 2 5 Chevet 1949). The redemption fee paid to acquire the slave bride was treated euphemistically as a bride wealth payment, but it went to the master rather than the bride or her male representative (as would occur in a legal marriage transaction), effectively compensating the nobility for the loss of female slave labor on emancipation.

This patrilineal tendency was reinforced by French efforts to impose some kind of order on the movements of the former slave populations and of the Bella in particular. The governor of neighboring French Sudan in 1949 proposed that Bella households should be counted in the census as being "under the tent" of the male head of family along with his wife and children and any property (ANN 5 E 2 5 Louveau 1949). In free Tuareg households, the tent always belonged to the woman; clearly, these new households were to be modeled not on noble Tuareg patterns but on sedentary norms. In setting up such a male-headed household and by being recorded in the tax rolls, a man could in a rather literal way "count"; by paying his own tax, he would achieve "official consecration" of his status as independent from and equivalent to his former master (ANN 5 E 2 5 Urfer 1949). Consequently, the freed captive men initiating such family lines were likely to value female virginity and to embrace the prospect of polygyny, in contrast with the lesser importance placed on virginity among Tuareg nobility and the strong preference for monogamy enforced by Tuareg noblewomen (ANN 5 E 2 5 Reeb 1947).

Still, masters endeavored to reinforce their status through rituals of submission well after abolition. For example, one means of controlling former captive populations was to refuse to accept bride wealth for such marriages or to decline to provide meat for the naming ceremony of a child born to former slaves so that it would, by implication, be seen as a bastard.[12] Former slaves and their lineages often chose to maintain a deferential or "loyal" attitude to their former masters in the interests of retaining access to land through membership in recognized social relationships (Iliffe 2005; Klein 2005; Kelley 2008; Pelckmans 2015). Shamelessness could therefore have its uses as a means to claim rights as dependents. By the same token, without slaves, the nobility would have no way to mark themselves as such, for the antithesis of nobility is enslavement. The performance of nobility required female leisure, the paternalist redistribution of wealth, and the presence of slaves. For example, noble Tuareg girls, as Sara Randall explains, were gorged with milk to render them fat before marriage: "force-feeding both demonstrated wealth and was a means of storing excess production; wealth in cows who produced a surplus of milk used for the feeding, and wealth in Bella. A family could only initiate force-feeding if there was a Bella woman to supervise it, and once the woman was married she could only maintain her weight if she had Bella women to do all the daily work" (Randall 2011, 50).[13] The immobility and obesity of the Tuareg noblewoman also revealed the nobility of her husband and kin; that bodily abundance rendered her sexually alluring. Male status was profoundly bound up with the performance of nobility of their wives, mothers, and daughters. The significance of sheltered and leisured wives to male status accounts for a Tuareg chief's indignant declaration to the French commandant of Dori in 1933: "If our Bellas are taken from us we would rather die than have our wives pound grain and our children take up the hoe" (ANN 5 E 2 5 Bourgine 1933).[14]

Gender and sexuality were, as colonial rule progressed, far more central than in the past to the structuring of honor and shame, both of which were becoming ever more closely associated with Muslim status. Because of the profound importance of the sexual vulnerability of women in defining the slave condition for both women and men, and because of the urgency of securing offspring for freeborn and freed men in the sedentary zone, women's bodily comportment rapidly became a major battleground in the postabolition struggle to mark slave from free, dishonorable from honorable. As we shall see in the next chapter, this meant that women's performance of shame could become the site of complex struggles within the family and in the legal domain.

Notes

1. Musée Quai Branly médiathèque, "Mission Citroën Centre-Afrique (1924–1925)," Territoire du Niger (hereafter MQB). Photographie de l'album "Expédition centre Afrique," 1924–1925, Vol. 2, 148, November 25, 1924, PA000115.157.

2. The bird mask the hunter wears is reminiscent of the bird mask seen by Ibn Battuta in medieval Mali (King 1995, 53–54).

3. Erin Pettigrew's work on Mauritania shows that sorcery accusations could derive from the resentments and fears freeborn wives felt toward the slave concubines of their husbands (2016). For a song expressing a similar sentiment collected in the Hoggar of southeast Algeria, see Haardt and Audouin-Dubreul (1924, 228–29).

4. Haardt refers to it as a *guignol* in French in the labels to the photographs. MQB Vol. 2, 197, December 6, 1924, PA000115.321.

5. On orphans as by definition fatherless rather than motherless, see Guillermet (2009).

6. The broad literature on gender ratios among enslaved populations confirms this finding across the continent. See Robertson and Klein (1983). For this region, see Olivier de Sardan (1984, 118–20).

7. Similar patterns probably exist elsewhere, for example in 1949 Fanne Fode opined that Peuls in Kolda, Senegal, were prolific because the Muslim men there often had up to five wives, which suggests that at least one was in fact a concubine. IFAN C 3 Fanne Fode 1949.

8. Catherine Baroin (1985) explores the implications of such avoidance in a context in which the absence of a marked centralized hierarchy renders shame/avoidance behavior of this kind the most significant shared idiom through which social cohesion is generated.

9. It is not uncommon to be told, in response to a sensitive question, to ask the griot, whose capacity for gossip and innuendo is likely to be as impressive as his or her knowledge of local social relations. Part of being shameless is insisting on being compensated for such information.

10. Throughout the Maradi valley, marriages contracted prior to the 1950s were almost invariably contracted with livestock for the bride wealth or *sadaki* entrusted to the bride's male kin and a gift of a dairy animal for the bride from her father (Université de Bordeaux, Maison des Suds, Collection Claude Raynaut, Carton "Enquête 100 Villages").

11. Tuareg attitudes about mingling between men and women, female sexuality, and extramarital sex have varied but have generally been more relaxed than among the sedentary societies to their south, except among the clans that self-identify as Islamic that have adopted highly patrilineal norms. On "living milk," see Walentowitz (2011).

12. ANN 5 E 2 5 Questions des Bellas, "Les Iklan ou les Touareg Noirs," Mémoire du Capitaine Reeb, Chef de Subdivision Nomade de Tahoua, 1947 pour l'admission au Centre des Hautes Études Musulmanes.

13. Caillié also noted the role of slave women in enforcing the force-feeding of girls among the Moors (1830a, Vol. 2, 67).

14. Interviews in the Sahel in the late 1980s echo the profound adjustments Bambara and Tuareg nobility had to make when they could no longer count on slaves to do all the female labor (Cross and Barker 1992, 75, 79, 91).

3

PERSONHOOD, SOCIALIZATION, AND SHAME

Social Personhood, Legitimacy, and Infanticide

In this chapter, I argue that the shifting meanings of *shame*, long an element in maintaining social hierarchy throughout the region, also crucially contributed to shaping the reproductive landscape. I am here interested in the period from the early 1930s to about 1945, as the implications of abolition were already being felt and as status reckoning became one of the most important ways in which individuals and families could lay claim to the resources of the state, to the labor of subordinate groups, and to the produce of herding and farming. In the same period, colonial institutions prompted the extremely rapid expansion of Islamic practices. Saba Mahmood's revealing exploration of the moral attribute of "modesty" illustrates why we should reflect seriously on the terms women use to account for their actions (Mahmood 2005). We know surprisingly little about "shame" or its history in this setting, despite its ubiquity. I will show that among non-Muslim societies in the early decades of French rule, shame could entail a moral obligation to eliminate an infant conceived before a girl was properly transformed into a woman through ritual and marriage. With the rapid advance of Islam, the moral focus shifted from the monstrous and dangerous infant to the disruptive sexuality of the mother. Yet, despite the emerging rejection of infanticide, there was no corresponding accommodation to bring the child into full humanity. The illegitimate child continued to be, in a sense, monstrous. Like a slave, such a child had no lineage and no shame.

What can we tease from the available evidence about how a new social order was generated and about how the behavior of women in particular was disciplined in the reproductive realm? How were men and women socialized to feel and to behave in particular ways with regard to their reproductive behavior? I will draw on three remarkable sources of different kinds that speak to several different registers of history: the legal, the practical, and the normative. Colonial-era judicial correspondence touching on women and legal texts recording local custom provide a glimpse of the kinds of social and moral constraints women experienced in the context of infanticide cases. Such documents provide a rather atomized depiction of particular individuals, cases, and social norms. Fortunately, we also have the 1937 study of family life conducted by Denise Savineau across the entire French West African territory. Her observations give us a sense for the broad patterns that resulted from these kinds of cases at a time when the presence of the colonial state was increasingly being felt even in more rural settings. The practical social implications of the unresolved problem of pregnancy outside of marriage troubled Savineau a great deal. Finally, we have the very rich body of simultaneously normative and anecdotal evidence that emerges in the many student memoirs produced by the young men who attended the École Ponty in the 1930s and 1940s.

Such sources present a signal challenge for exploring the history of affect—they are all written in French, whereas practices and feelings were expressed in a host of different Sahelian languages. Because the texts were written in French, it is not possible to know the specific local terms for which the terms *la honte* (shame) and *l'honneur* (honor) often did service in translation. When the judicial record presents *la honte* as the reason a woman offered for killing her newborn, what is lost? Similarly, in the student essays, one senses that the French vocabulary available to the boys was ill suited to conveying the complexity of their thoughts. The French term the boys used was more often *honor* (*l'honneur*) than *shame* (*la honte*). This makes sense. While in English or French these are different terms, this is not generally the case in the Sahel. For example, the Hausa term 'kunya' can be translated, depending on the context, as many different terms in English (*shame, honor, respectfulness, embarrassment, restraint, dignity, forbearance, timidity, reserve*). No single French term comes close to being adequate to capture all these nuances. The colonialist teachers, for their part, complained in their comments to the students that their writing was incoherent, inconsistent, or contradictory—which one readily understands when a student might start an essay by referring to "honor" and end lamenting young men's "timidity" with no clear transition.

Bearing in mind the broad meanings of the indigenous terms today makes it easier to make sense of the sources available to us. Despite their limitations, these sources provide invaluable historical insights into the gendering of adulthood and the training of the girl child, about which it is difficult to obtain evidence through other sources. The disciplining effects of the judicial realm are clear enough, and the confusions, struggles, and inconsistencies in the judicial record bespeak profound shifts occurring in the ethical domain in the first half of the twentieth century. While the claims of schoolboys about how girls were trained must be taken with some reservations, these were the observations of young men about their own societies, surely derived from their awareness of how the training of their sisters differed from their own. The memoirs give us evidence of how French education in a handful of urban centers was destabilizing some of the gender assumptions of the prewar era; they offer as well glimpses of how these young men felt about those changes. Despite the limitations of the sources, the general familial and social dynamics through which moral conditioning of girls was instilled come through clearly.

The Uneven Geography and Evolution of the Colonial Judicial System

Senegal had the longest experience of French judicial intervention of all the Sahelian colonies. There, urban families intermarried with Europeans, resulting in populations whose complex and ambiguous adoption of French language and custom accorded them special legal status as *originaires* including some of the privileges of French citizens. Among the *originaires* were influential Muslims who insisted on the continuation of Islamic courts to handle civil matters. Military considerations also shaped the development of law in Senegal. Beyond the exceptional spaces of the *originaires*, local disputes continued to be mediated in many informal settings in which prominent figures (referred to as *notables*) and Muslim scholars negotiated between parties to broker mutually satisfactory resolutions to conflict. It was not until *le décret du 10 novembre 1903* that something resembling civilian legal structures crystalized in French West Africa (FWA) to serve the needs of the general population of French colonial subjects.[1]

These early courts, known as *tribunaux de province* (provincial courts) were regulated by African chiefs appointed by the administration who were to make their decisions on the basis of local customary practice. Richard

Roberts has traced the shifting ways African populations made use of the courts in French Sudan from 1905, when slave condition could no longer in principle be recognized, to 1912, a moment of major reorganization of the courts (Roberts 2005). Roberts found that with the abolition of slave status, struggles over control of land and labor between former masters and former slaves became intense. Masters used litigation over debt and land to reduce the mobility of former slaves. At the same time, the decline in access to slave labor caused husbands to pressure wives to perform tasks previously relegated to servile members of the household. Women therefore went to court to seek divorce, and they used income derived from the increasingly monetized economy to repay the marriage expenses claimed by their husbands' families. In this relatively early period, women found the courts preferable to informal dispute mediation fora in which reconciliation between spouses was a priority. The *tribunaux* briefly offered women a way to circumvent the increasing labor demands of their marital relations.

However, the appeal of such courts to women declined significantly in later decades, as French priorities shifted to privilege order, access to labor, and patriarchal hierarchy over the interests of women and slaves. After the *décret du 16 août 1912*, the provincial courts headed by local chiefs were replaced by *tribunaux de subdivision* headed by the French administrator overseeing that subdivision (Mangin 1997). The court could, as in the past, seek advice from two local African judicial advisers (*assesseurs*) knowledgeable about local practices and morals. In principle, courts were to respect local customary practice wherever it did not conflict with civilization or public order. In the interest of efficiency, the French administration increasingly sought to textualize local custom. French ethnographic descriptions of the structure of family and of the authority of male household heads became a far more rigid charter than the fluidity of the early court cases seems to reflect. With the increasing bureaucratization and standardization of rule, some of the avenues available to women to cushion the impact of the abolition of slavery disappeared, and the significance of marriage as a means by which to control labor and reproduction increased.

In part to ensure that the practices in such courts were reasonably consistent and that they distinguished clearly between civil or criminal cases and the minor infractions to be handled through summary police powers (known as the *indigénat*), in 1931, the French instituted courts of review. In *le décret du 3 décembre 1931*, a system of appeals courts (*tribunaux coloniaux d'appel*) was created. Even without a formal appeal, the new system enabled the judicial hierarchy to annul prior court decisions in the *Chambre d'annulation*. From the 1930s, the decisions of lower-level courts were reviewed up the chain of command, going first to the lieutenant governor of the colony and then sent on to Dakar to be reviewed by the general prosecutor—the highest-ranking prosecutor within FWA, before whom appeals would be made. In the same period, administrators were instructed to collect information useful to understanding local practice. One of the most useful primary sources for the history of this region is the three-volume collection of texts known as the *Coutumiers juridiques de l'A.O.F.*, which assembled what administrators believed to be the relevant local custom in various jurisdictions (Coutumiers 1939).

On the whole, women as agents, as opposed to victims, are invisible in the earliest colonial-era judicial records for Niger, for by the time the region was secured in the 1920s, the openness of the courts to women's concerns had long dissipated. Unlike regions that had been colonized at the close of the nineteenth century, Niger didn't feature in the early colonial flurry of civil court cases around divorce, property claims, and slavery described by Richard Roberts for French Sudan. In part, this is because the Military Territory of Niger was treated as a special case. In principle, each people (*ethnie*) was to be governed by its own customary law. Courts were to respect the particular customs of each "category" (nomads, sedentary populations, Muslims, and non-Muslims) and each "race" (left unspecified). The designated chief of each newly delineated province would preside over the proceedings.

The sizeable nomadic population presented a particular challenge. Could the customs of mobile populations be respected in courts designed on the assumption that chiefs govern demarcated territories? Would not the sedentary populations (thought of as "black") end up sitting in judgment of the nomadic populations (read "white")? And what of the ambiguous import of Islam in the customary practices of all the various permutations of categories and races? Would the solution be to introduce more provinces and increase the number of *assesseurs* significantly?[2] Would it be best to leave the management of the courts largely to the discretion of the European military command? In the end, the solution was to rely on the presumed fairness of European administrators rather than the "chiefs" while leaving room for administrators to call on a very large number of *assesseurs* where needed. Niger was not to share the same tribunal system as French Sudan and Senegal until the 1930s.

As a result, in general, commercial agents kept their disputes outside of the formal commercial court system unless the conflict involved one of the European trading houses. Women tended to prefer to handle civil matters related to marital, property, and custody disputes in assorted sites invisible to the colonial archival record: the courts of the local qadi, the palace of a local chief from a noble family, or in the compound of a respected family elder (Cooper 1997, 20–39). Among the rare early civil cases in Niger was a dispute in 1906 between two African soldiers over the status of the property of a woman named Zeini Diarra. The woman, having been determined by the appeals court to be "a source of trouble" in Niamey because of her "extremely erratic behavior" was forced to return to her village. This would have been a sobering outcome from the vantage point of a woman in the growing urban center trying to get her property back.[3]

In another case, a Niamey woman named Mariama wanted to leave her husband, but her husband insisted that he wanted her back. Accused of the crime of "abandoning the marital home," she was, on appeal, persuaded to "reconcile" with him.[4] Such criminal cases, in which men attempted to use the courts to control the mobility and labor of women, are much more richly documented for Upper Senegal (later French Sudan) (Rodet 2007). From the scant record for Niger, it appears that courts were not particularly favorable to women even in this relatively early period. Prior to the 1930s, Niger's courts handled criminal cases almost exclusively, where women often figured as victims of the continuing slave trade. Thus, in 1906, a man in the region of Zinder was sent to prison for a year for selling one of his female "captives" for a camel and ten sheep.[5]

In the slowly evolving system after 1912, as *la justice indigène* was established across FWA, some irregularities had to be worked out through a system of review. The prosecutor general in Dakar reported to the governor general of FWA that the courts functioned reasonably well in the Military Territory of Niger. Nevertheless, he pointed out, the lower-level courts seem to have lacked a certain precision at times in distinguishing civil from criminal, and the *indigénat* (entailing summary but circumscribed punishments for specific offenses) from *justice indigène*. While a man could be punished with a year in prison in the criminal court, he could not be forcibly divorced from his wife as a form of punishment. That would require a civil case. Furthermore, Muslim chiefs, marabouts, and qadis, whose authority was threatened by the growing presence of the colonial tribunals, occasionally interfered with the workings of the court system.[6] Courts were used very differently in different settings; in Zinder, where the large numbers of soldiers and their wives and lovers were quite familiar with the workings of the judicial system, individuals occasionally formalized agreements with one another.[7] But in other settings where the courts were more alien and less useful, they seem to have left little or no record.

With the eruption of war in Europe, the court records for Niger dwindled away for lack of paper, only to reemerge in 1930, in anticipation of the revision of the court system resulting in the *décret du 3 décembre 1931*.[8] It is striking how much more prominent the use of the courts had become in a setting such as Senegal, which saw 2,553 civil cases in 1930, in comparison to Niger, which saw only 99. The 516 criminal cases in Niger paled in comparison with the 3,662 cases for Senegal.[9] The reform of 1931 was intended to make the lower-level courts, to be renamed *tribunaux du premier degré*, more appealing to Africans by permitting indigenous judges to handle all civil and commercial cases with a view to reconciling the parties. Despite the introduction of indigenous magistrates in the lower-level courts, relatively few subjects in Niger aired civil disputes before the courts.[10]

Serious criminal cases and disputes involving relatively large sums of money fell automatically to a European administrator. The definition of what constituted a crime was dictated by French law as promulgated in the colony; indigenous custom could enter in the sentencing stage. The hope was that as indigenous customs were codified, Africans would be more and more inclined to make use of the courts rather than what were deemed by the French to be extrajudicial mediation settings.[11] The overwhelming majority of the accused in the criminal cases were men. Women surface in the scant records largely as victims of rape, theft, or battery. Some cases involved "captives," whose status was ambiguous and who were therefore particularly vulnerable. A case in 1933 involved the rape of two captives of about twelve years of age (a boy and a girl), both of whom contracted syphilis as a result. One suspects that the rapes only became evident because the two children had been diagnosed with the disease.[12] In rape cases, the local courts tended to take into account the evidence of the accused male, sometimes not even troubling to interview the victim.[13]

When women were the accused, their crimes often reflected competition between women involved with or "married" to the same man. Typical of the kinds of challenges presented by indigenous disputes was a case in 1934 brought against a woman known (rather generically) as Fulani. Very likely a captive in a farming household in largely Hausa-speaking

Dogondoutchi, she was accused of poisoning the four-year-old son of her "co-wife," Soje. Fulani had fed the child, Nahalla, while the two were alone together in the fields one day, and ten days later the child's belly began to swell, a sign perceived locally to indicate that a poison (known as *gouba*) had been administered. Fulani denied the poisoning three times and then eventually "admitted" that she "had wanted to poison" the little boy. Aware that this was essentially a witchcraft accusation, the court in Niamey instructed the lower court in Dogondoutchi to release her pending a report by Pharmacien-Lieutenant Heroud on the capacity of the purportedly poisonous substance to actually cause death.[14]

This request for more "scientific" evidence appears to have been a new development; women imprisoned for "poisoning" or "murder" in the 1920s often got quite long sentences because of the presumption of premeditation in the absence of any attention to the actual presence or efficacy of charms and substances.[15] Erin Pettigrew's study of sorcery accusations in Mauritania shows that freeborn women in affective and reproductive competition with women of slave ancestry often made such accusations. The resentments, jealousies, and hunger of women of slave status were understood to have acted on women of higher status and their children; such attacks could only be remedied through the death of the accused (Pettigrew 2016). Accusations of witchcraft may therefore have been a means of intimidating and controlling former slaves.

On the Visibility and Invisibility of Infanticide as a Crime

By and large, however, when one gains a glimpse of women as agents rather than as victims in the judicial records of colonial Niger, it is in the context of infanticide cases. We see traces of the early handling of an infanticide case in eastern Niger in Zinder in 1926; the prison register notes that the woman convicted could be released in 1946 after enduring a twenty-year sentence.[16] The heavy sentence suggests that the infanticide in question in this Hausa/Kanuri region was treated as equivalent to *assassinat* or premeditated murder.[17]

However, correspondence surrounding a 1934 case, the Affaire Mata in Niamey, suggests that such long sentences may have disinclined judges to convict women. This Zarma woman was acquitted of infanticide for lack of consistent witnesses. Evaluating the handling of the case, the head of judicial affairs in Niger remarked, "Certainly the five year minimum that would have been required . . . was too high with regard to certain crimes, among them infanticide. In Zarma territory the infanticide of a bastard, far from being punished by custom, is even required by it. Given that the aforementioned MATA has already been in prison for three months and given the contradictory accounts of the witnesses, I consider the decision of the Niamey criminal court to acquit to have been sound."[18]

The early 1930s were difficult throughout West Africa, but the triple scourges of drought, high taxes, and economic depression caused particular stress on the Sahel.[19] In another case in 1934, the *procureur général* in Dakar returned comments to Niger on the puzzling outcome of an infanticide case known as Affaire Fourératou, judged by the tribunal in Dosso.[20] A young woman of apparently about nineteen had given birth to a baby girl that had been seen by more than one witness. The baby later disappeared, and the young woman confessed to having strangled it. The body was never found, but a medical practitioner provided testimony that supported the claim that Fourératou had recently given birth.[21]

The prosecutor general was troubled by the rationale through which the woman who had been convicted was then released without a sentence; this was clearly a far cry from the Zinder case from 1926. The reasoning behind the leniency in this case seems to have been twofold: that "Zarma custom" does not regard the infanticide of an illegitimate child to be a crime, and that the woman had been subject to *contrainte morale* or a kind of "moral coercion" or duress from her community in acting as she did. Infanticide was in this specific setting a kind of "ethical practice" through which women as ethical subjects could be apprehended as such; women were "docile" agents constituting themselves as moral within their communities in yielding to the "moral coercion" referenced in the case.[22] The prosecutor in distant Dakar insisted that the courts should not have had reference to custom in such a case; they should have referred only to the *décret du 3 décembre 1931*, which sets out the acts that the *justice indigène* must handle as crimes. Regardless of prior practice, "infanticide is in reality a murder, which is the first crime enunciated in the aforementioned document, and it must be punished by the same punishments as murder, whatever the custom may be."[23] He did allow for some latitude in the sentencing, when custom could be taken into account; as examples, he noted that a recent infanticide case in Niamey had resulted in a ten-year sentence, whereas in Dosso (where custom did not see this as a crime), a lighter sentence of five or six years and temporary exile might be appropriate.

Infanticide had long presented a particularly complex legal quandary even in France. The Republican code in 1791 had not treated infanticide as a specific crime; it was simply a form of premeditated murder liable to the death penalty. By contrast, an unpremeditated murder had a maximum sentence of twenty years. Debates about reforming the law were intense; some argued that the death penalty was too severe for a crime a young woman might commit "to hide her shame." Others argued against reduced sentencing or deportation; infanticide involved cold calculation, they insisted—it was not a crime of ungovernable passion. However, judges were not comfortable imposing the death penalty on women accused of infanticide and therefore tended instead to acquit (Cournot 1885). Furthermore, the problem of distinguishing miscarriage from infanticide, and a viable newborn from an unviable newborn, gave rise to tremendous debate that prompted the elaboration of forensic techniques to clarify the circumstances of the infant's birth and death (Burton 2007, 154–65).

One can readily understand, therefore, why French administrators who had not been trained in the law and who typically had few reference materials might find confusing the instruction to treat infanticide as "by definition" premeditated murder.[24] While the French law of 1901 treating infanticide as a form of premeditated murder had been promulgated in FWA, the attenuating circumstances under which it might be treated simply as manslaughter were unclear, and the potential reduction of the sentencing was exclusively to be applied to the mother, not to any eventual accomplices (Haute Commissariat de l'Afrique Française 1941). As a general rule, it was customary practice that was seen to be the appropriate benchmark for adjudication for French subjects on matters of family life. Colonial administrators relied on the expertise of indigenous *assesseurs* to serve as the brokers of local custom; such individuals were generally notables from influential families, and they were always male. Determining what constituted a marriage, when it could be broken, how divorce could or could not occur—all these kinds of civil matters were to a significant degree overseen by these men, who freely made reference to local custom on the one hand and Maliki judicial practice on the other in a selective and occasionally opportunistic manner.

Judging from the *Coutumier juridique de l'AOF*, collected in the 1930s, infanticide of illegitimate children within the cultural zone broadly surrounding Niamey was seen to be a matter of family honor, part of the internal regulation of domestic life, and an issue that was not open to public discussion or debate. A close perusal of the *Coutumiers juridiques de l'AOF* reveals a very consistent pattern throughout the region along the Niger River from Bamako to Niamey: there was, according to the local authorities surveyed on the subject, a very strong disapproval of children born of mothers who had never been married (Vol. II, 27, 98, 144, 311, 354). Throughout the region, such children were seen to have no lineage, no inheritance rights, and few prospects for marriage. They were, in effect, not recognized as social persons.

This was not generally true of regions to the south of the Sahel, where any offspring of a "wife" could be regarded as part of the wealth in persons of either her or her husband's lineage. Nor was it true of the Senegal and Gambia basins (for example, among the Wolof) and only in an attenuated fashion in the region leading to Lake Chad (as in Zinder), where bastard children were generally taken in reluctantly by their mother's family. It is, if you will, a distinctively Songhay/Zarma and Mande/Bambara pattern. In the *Coutumiers juridiques*, local practice was understood to be grounded in immutable "custom"; the administrators who drew up the texts did not suggest that the attitude toward illegitimate children had any direct relationship to Islam. Indeed, it was often among ethnic groups marked explicitly as having *rejected* Islam (such as the Bambara) that the pattern appeared to be strongest. Thus, in the compilation on local custom for the Bambara of Bougouni, we find the following remark: "any woman who puts her bastard child to death will be excused" (Vol. II, 26). In the section on the Songhai of Gao we find, "custom is extremely severe towards the illegitimate child [*l'enfant naturel*], in no case considered to be akin to or in any way comparable to a legitimate child" (Vol. II, 309).

The observations of Denise Moran Savineau confirm this pattern. Commissioned by Governor General de Coppet to conduct a systematic study of the condition of women and family life across French West Africa in 1937, she produced an extraordinarily rich body of observations of the entire region. She noted in her report on the Zarma region near Niamey, "Infanticides are common because of the public reprobation towards them [illegitimate children]."[25] Indeed, in her final overview report, Savineau specifically singled out the Zarma: "The illegitimate child [*l'enfant naturel*] may be, with the mother, the subject of such reprobation that both mother and child are exiled. Regions where girls are rigidly constrained by chastity are the same ones in which one sees abortion (often provoked by the mother of the girl), the abandonment of children, and infanticide. In the face of such crimes the administrator too often shares the perspective of the family and the assesseurs. He ought to make an effort to draw their attention to the sources of this problem" (Savineau 2007, 11). Evidently, the pressure to eliminate the unwanted child came from all sides, whether "traditional" or "colonial."

The *assesseurs*, in brokering a relatively lenient response to the death of Fourératou's child in 1934, appear to have condoned the pressure to eliminate an illegitimate infant that was recorded in the *Coutumier juridique* and was observed by Savineau in 1937. However, to be aware that an infant had either been born or had died would require intimate knowledge of a woman's menstrual cycles, her prayers or lack thereof during times of impurity, her physical appearance, the length of her absence from communal activities, and her lactation. Someone had to have brought the issue of infanticide to the attention of the colonial administration. Why do so if it was not seen to be a crime?

Men increasingly schooled in Maliki law may well have been appalled by this local practice through which women could cleanse themselves of the opprobrium of sex outside marriage and an illegitimate birth. If "custom" condemned illegitimate children, Islam condemned sex outside of marriage (*zina*). These may appear to amount to the same thing; however, there is an important difference. In the first case, the resolution to the immoral action is enacted on the child, and in the second, it is enacted on the immoral woman and only indirectly on the child. Devout Muslim men may have hoped that the courts would make it possible to circumvent local custom in the interests of a more severe punishment directed at unchaste women. As an interpretive matter, one might also note that in the first case the moral and social danger to be overcome was understood to reside in the monstrous child, and in the second in the immoral mother. The *assesseurs* in the early 1930s (as opposed to the often invisible accusers) do not appear to have been driven to modify local custom to bring it into closer accord with Maliki law. The handling of the Affaire Fourératou is suggestive of tension and disagreement within the community of Dosso about how to respond to extramarital sex, illegitimate births, and infanticide.

Details of the Affaire Kanni in 1934 are suggestive of confusion within the administration as well. In that case, the initial *notice d'arrêt* gave no age for the unmarried woman involved, named Kanni. The assumption of the general prosecutor seems initially to have been that leniency had been accorded in sentencing because she was a minor. Kanni had given birth to a girl infant that she then strangled. She confessed, and witnesses also testified that she had strangled the baby.[26] The *assesseurs*, in limiting punishments, appeared to systematically treat the typical defendant as *by definition* a minor. Judicial overseers in Dakar requested further information on how local custom defined minority and majority and craved further information on precisely how *old* Kanni might be.[27] The simple fact that she was not yet married meant, in local terms, that no one would have considered her a full adult. But when it was reported that she was twenty-one, the notion that she was a minor became somewhat less plausible in the French manner of thinking.

Chronological age was not particularly relevant to adulthood across the region. Excision was often a *prerequisite* for marriage; a young woman or girl's chronological age was not what determined her marriageability. Sarah Brett-Smith's art historical research in Bambara settings in Mali reveals the historical link between excision and acceptable childbirth. Her work underscores the profound importance placed on protecting the community from the dangers of monstrous illegitimate infants (1982, 1983). Ritual excision, controlled by older women, was the means whereby the powerful and dangerously excessive life force (*nyama*) of young women could be safely channeled by postmenopausal women through the vehicle of the excision cloth. Women who abandoned their newborns in the bush or in rivers may have regarded them as dangerously asocial beings that were not and never could be fully human. In focusing exclusively on the criminality of the *mother*, one risks losing sight of the construction of the *child* as monstrous, which contributed to the "moral coercion" to commit infanticide or abandonment.

Denise Savineau's visits to penal institutions in 1937 suggests that by the late 1930s attitudes toward women who bore illegitimate children had hardened such that *assesseurs* were less inclined to implicitly condone infanticide by mitigating sentences. Instead, they sought the maximum possible sentence for women, presumably adopting as an alternative strategy the more typically Maliki approach to controlling out-of-wedlock births. In Goundam (French Sudan), Savineau noted, "Two women who had been prisoners were condemned of infanticide; one was a young girl who abandoned the baby in the bush. The other was a married woman who strangled the child conceived before the wedding. This is the consequence of custom that is too harsh towards women who make mistakes. In these cases the *assesseurs* had demanded capital punishment and the presiding judge had quite a lot of difficulty saving them" (CAOM 17G381 Rapport 4, 13). By the late 1930s, administrators and *assesseurs* alike were perhaps disinclined to set aside such cases quite so quickly, feeling that the details were salient and that women should be held accountable for their sexual misconduct in the increasingly unruly colonial economy, since the practice of treating such cases with leniency was not seen to have a deterrent effect.

Significantly, cases often involved married women who had fallen pregnant while their husbands were in Gold Coast or Nigeria in search of the relatively high wages to be found there. Within the territory of Niger, the western region had long been known for male labor migration to coastal cities, a pattern that began before colonization and accelerated with the abolition of slavery and the increasing burden of labor, taxes, and unfavorable commodity pricing (Painter 1988). The most detailed of the cases I have studied dates from 1939, a particularly difficult moment for the region. From 1937 through the end of the decade, Niger was wracked by a succession of droughts, bad harvests, and epidemics.[28] In the midst of this crisis, a twenty-eight-year-old woman named Lobo of Tillabery was brought before the Chambre d'Accusation of Niger to determine whether she should be tried for the infanticide of which she had been accused.[29] Her husband had been gone since the harvest of 1938; she had gotten pregnant around April of the subsequent year. Everyone, according to the witnesses, knew that she was pregnant. The village chief, noting that no one had seen the baby at the termination of the pregnancy, brought the matter to the attention of the French Commandant de Cercle, thus initiating the process recorded in the documents.

Lobo claimed to have had a miscarriage and that she had placed the fetus in the river at sunset three days after the miscarriage. When asked by the judge (an administrator in Niamey), she claimed not to have seen the sex of the child. The judge expressed skepticism, noting that "the body should have been well formed"—why would the accused be so vague on this point? Typically, in infanticide cases, it was the purportedly *deceptive* nature of the crime that seemed to render it "premeditated" murder. Lobo claimed to be unaware that others knew she was pregnant in order to account for why she hadn't discussed the miscarriage with others. The administrator felt that this was a "childish argument of someone who senses themselves to be at fault and hopes to vindicate themselves" of the accusation of deception. Why, he wondered, did she hide the fetus for three days? Rather than show it to her neighbors, she threw it in the river. Indigenous custom, he opined censoriously, would have dictated that the body be buried immediately.

He discounted her claim that it was "shame" that caused her to hide the body, for if she had been so "ashamed" why did she not throw the body in the river at night when no one could see? Note the tremendous confusion over just what exactly was shameful. Was it the pregnancy? The act of childbirth itself? The fact of having miscarried? The illegitimacy of the child? The administrator assumed that it was the infanticide that was shameful to her. However, everything surrounding pregnancy and childbirth is typically treated with the greatest discretion (or shame) across the region. No one in the village, so far as we can tell from this record, would speak either for her or against her. The judge determined that there were sufficient grounds to try her, although no body was ever found.[30]

The case is striking because on the face of it there was no evidence of a crime in the absence of a body or a confession. FWA had no crime of "concealment" of pregnancy in the penal code. Her claim that the fetus miscarried had not been countered through any physical evidence, nor had any witnesses come forward to claim to have seen a child whether alive or dead. No one saw her dispose of the body. It appears, then, that the decade of the 1930s saw a transition in attitudes toward infanticide, not only among French administrators but also among the *assesseurs* who were their advisers as well as among local-level village chiefs whose intervention would have been necessary for a case to have been brought in the first place.

Several silences in the judicial records of these cases are striking. The first is that no one in a position of judicial authority ever made explicit mention of the fact that in all the cases in which the sex of the fetus or infant was established, the body was that of a girl. The sex of the babies emerges in passing, although clearly the question was asked or one would not be able to glean that detail from the scant records that exist. In other words, in the early decades of colonial rule, it may have been easier to tolerate an illegitimate boy child than an illegitimate girl. There is some suggestion in the *Coutumiers juridiques de l'A.O.F.* that in Bambara regions a gender imbalance was emerging favoring males over females.[31] The second silence is that no one in a position of judicial authority ever made explicit reference to the position of Islam on infanticide. One of the signal innovations of Islamic legal practice was the explicit condemnation of infanticide of female children in particular (Seignette 1911, xxvii Note 1). Perhaps explicitly mentioning that the logic by which the punishment for a crime was to be assessed had shifted from local *coutume* (condoning it) to Maliki religious practice (condemning it) troubled the very notion of a consistent body of "customary law."

In each instance, someone had to make public the disappearance of the pregnancy and/or the infant. Given that Christian missions were conspicuous largely in their absence, and given the initial ambivalence of the French administrators when faced with these cases, Western or Christian influence is unlikely to have prompted the change of heart. Far more probable was the tremendous expansion of Islam and Islamic education in the colonial period, which raised ethical qualms about a practice that had hitherto been regarded as not only acceptable but as morally desirable.

It is also possible that the reproduction of slave labor had become important to the kinds of elite men who were now standing in judgment of poor women. The biological reproduction of a servile labor force had replaced capture of new slaves. In rejecting out-of-wedlock births as improper and unrectifiable except through infanticide, local "custom" rejected the very notion that such children could be integrated as social persons. Like slaves, such children had no patriline, and like slaves, their options would be limited without the patronage of a "master." In the past, this rejection of certain children had been managed and enforced, it seems, largely by senior women. The shift in thinking about infanticide in the late 1930s was probably initiated by Muslims, largely those men exposed to Islamic judicial reasoning and Islamic identity in the context of colonial rule.

Such a shift *could* have led to a broader rethinking of whether and how children born outside of proper marital relations might be otherwise understood, accommodated, and integrated, or about how the circumstances leading to the production of such children could be alleviated. Certainly, Denise Savineau felt that the thinking behind the handling of the infanticide problem on the part of both administrators and local *assesseurs* needed to shift from punishment to prevention (2007, 11). It is one thing to punish a young woman for adultery by refusing to condone the cleansing act of infanticide, but it is quite another to find a way to integrate the child as a social being. The focus was not, therefore, on the welfare of the child or the fetus but on the punishment of female sexual misconduct and fertility control. Women who failed to adhere to the gender norms expected of freeborn women were effectively forced to occupy permanently the status of an unfree woman, and their illegitimate children were effectively consigned to the social status of slaves.[32]

The Autoethnography of Gender Socialization

While the ethical consequences of bearing an illegitimate child were shifting, the opprobrium attached to sex outside marriage was not. Essays written by secondary school students across the territories of French West Africa archived in the Fonds École William Ponty at IFAN in Dakar offer a particularly rich source for how proper comportment was cultivated by societies in the Sahelian region.[33] Because FWA was a federated territory, the most promising "sons and nephews" of notables throughout the federation were sent to a single secondary school or *lycée* in Senegal for their final training. At the end of their studies, the boys were given an essay assignment to do as a "*mémoire de fin d'études.*"[34] Essay assignments varied, but all had an ethnographic dimension: the boys were to describe in detail some aspect of life in their home communities to prepare them to become schoolteachers and functionaries exhibiting a high degree of competence in the French language.[35] The assignments required the student to objectify "indigenous life." These autoethnographic exercises, written between 1935 and 1949, shed light on how the boys who were destined to enter the educated elite understood the socialization of boys and girls in their ethnic groups.

Like all autoethnography, these are complex texts given the conditions of inequality under which they were produced (Pratt 1992). The essays regularly began in a nostalgic tone only to conclude by denigrating as backward everything previously described. The ethnographic present was frequently disrupted by lamentations about the decline of morals with urbanization or education. Normative accounts may have hewed closer to realities for the students' parents or grandparents than to their own times. These unruly texts also provided license for a degree of criticism of French administration—for example, in an essay on the interpretation of dreams, a student named Koke Issaka from Niger recounted a dream in which a pack of noisy and discordant hyenas were unflatteringly interpreted to be French colonial administrators whose inconsistent demands were best ignored (C 53 Koke Issaka n.d.).

Despite their contradictions, these accounts of family life across the Sahel impress on the reader the significance placed on teaching children submission to authority from a very young age. Even small children were to greet the more senior members of the family formally each morning to make visible their awareness of their "low social position" (C 30 Oumar Diouf 1949). Their speech was quite restricted; if they were to speak at all, the voice was to be soft and their words agreeable (C 30 Magatte Fall 1949). Children were to keep their heads bowed and their eyes down, and girls were to offer water to drink in a pose of genuflection (C 30 Magatte Fall 1949). But the very importance of showing respect could mean that a mother might not punish a child publicly for misbehavior, as that would only draw attention to the dishonor it has brought on her and the family (C 30 Diallo Seydou 1949, C 30 Oumar Diouf 1949). A child's shameful behavior shamed his mother as well, particularly relative to her co-wives.

Under the circumstances, then, when a parent became angry enough with a disrespectful child (usually an adolescent who had "dirtied the name of the family") to curse him or her publicly, the social rupture it entailed required that the child be exiled permanently, as if to contain a contagion (C 30 Oumar Diouf 1949, C 30 Elhadji Diouf 1949). The implications of such a curse on a child were so significant and so formalized among the Zarma that we find reference to them spelled out in judicial guidelines as late as 1952 (ANN 1 F 3 1 Author unknown 1952, 15). A student of a warrior family line lamented, "The least infraction is punished with excommunication because the son who does not respect custom is considered to be beyond all hope, someone from whom one must remain distant for fear of being corrupted" (C 3 Kane Bousra n.d.). In the Hausa-speaking region, a son who had been cursed by his mother could not be buried in the cemetery; he had to be buried at least six kilometers away, otherwise his corpse would lead to death and misfortune (1 G 4 6 Condat Georges Mahamane 1938–39). Shameful behavior threatened the very links between the living and the dead.

Such a rupture might be caused by alcohol drinking by a Muslim, or an attachment to a girl of low status, or in the case of a girl, refusal to marry the partner chosen for her or, even worse, sexual misconduct leading to pregnancy. Flagrant inappropriate sexual or romantic behavior was not to be tolerated by either unmarried sons or daughters. Girls, thought to be more flighty, were subject to even closer scrutiny than boys. In an urbanized Muslim setting, they might not be permitted to leave the house at all, and their very physical gestures would be scrutinized (C 30 Diouck Sanor 1949). The training in obedience and reserve had taught children to be extremely timid, which some of the male students felt did not serve them well once they entered the French school.

Proper behavior was performed in the context of eating. For girls, proper comportment was displayed in their manner of serving food or drink; for boys, it was particularly marked in the context of the communal dish. Boys ate with their fathers and girls with their mothers. A well-trained boy, we learn, was to wash his hands and sit or crouch properly. During mealtime, as the men were seated on the floor around the communal food platter, the boy's task as the youngest was to hold still the dish with the fingers of his left hand while eating with his right hand. He was not to cough, take large handfuls of rice, watch the others too closely, drink while the meal was being eaten, or use his left hand to eat (C 30 Amadou Badiane 1949, C 30 Seydou Cissoko 1949, C 14 Caba Sory 1949). Nor was he to touch the meat or fish but was to wait for it to be given to him (C 3 Kebe Babacar 1949). Social status was marked by how much meat went to which person at the meal. Given the significance of shared meals for marking membership in a community, the injunction to Muslim boys never to eat with Christians would have been a stark indication of the limits of social inclusion (C 14 Pascal L. Macos 1949).

Once a boy reached about eight years old, he was expected to spend little time among women. A boy's training in masculinity among the men regularly entailed deference to elders (whether male or female), sharing, fortitude in the face of suffering and pain, and a willingness to engage in physical violence to counter injury to individual or family honor. In many ethnic groups, circumcision and initiation into adulthood were collective activities bringing together boys from about nine to fifteen, after which in more Islamized settings a young man's full entry into male responsibilities in prayer and Muslim ritual would begin. Adulthood would be marked formally by a shift in clothing toward the cap and longer gown of adult men. Young men across the Sahel generally received Koranic training under a Muslim scholar for varying lengths of time, but it was always, according to the memoirists, far more significant than that given to girls.

In settings that rejected Islam altogether, major rites of male and female initiation seem to have been typical and were often parallel to one another. Rites for boys entailed the retreat of a large number of boys of roughly the same age into the forest with a ritual specialist, a healer, or sometimes a blacksmith. Boys would be "initiated into the fetishes" of their family and taught how to show reverence by making food offerings (C 14 Caba Sory 1949). Male circumcision would frequently be part of the initiation, and later stages of achievement of masculinity might also entail painful tattooing. In other words, the endurance of pain was a key marker of the stages of entry into adulthood (C 14 Caba Sory 1949, C 14 Sow Ibrahima n.d., C 14

Diakite Mamadou 1945, C 14 Sagno Mamady 1948–49). Where Koranic education was in a sense integrated into this larger system of socialization into endurance and submission to authority, training and occasional punishment by the teacher could be quite painful as well (C 14 Sow Ibrahima n.d., C 30 Elhadji Diouf 1949). As seasonal migration to coastal towns grew in importance in the Zarma region of Niger, this too entered into the repertoire of rituals marking male entry into adulthood, offering opportunities to demonstrate endurance and the willingness to defend their honor, for the Zarma, we are informed, "prefers death to any form of dishonesty or dishonor" (C 71 Jean-Louis Meon n.d.).

Where male rituals and female rituals appear to have been more or less parallel, female genital cutting was understood to be functionally parallel to male circumcision. The degree and character of such cutting for girls, generally near the age of puberty, could vary from society to society; in some cases, it entailed clitoridectomy and full infibulation, in others clitoridectomy alone, and in some the cutting of the skin above the clitoris. Obviously, the memoirs can't reveal much about these kinds of rituals for women, but they do offer some sense of how the boys understood them. Diakite Mamadou had been told that this cutting was to make women less sensitive to love and less likely to commit adultery—the *exciseuse* (a female ritual cutter) would tell the girl to work hard and obey her husband and would impress on her that infidelity would lead to hell (C 14 Diakite Mamadou 1945). Sagno Mamady remarked that, unlike boys, girls only had a single ritual leading to marriage, that of excision, whereas men might go through eight years of tattooing marking the successive stages of military and civic training (C 14 Sagno Mamady 1948–49). For him, women were formed to become wives; men were formed to become warriors. Intriguingly, the gradual and fairly recent shift among some Muslim societies toward infant circumcision of boys by the interwar years had disrupted the continuity of the older initiation rituals. Infant circumcision undercut the public endurance of pain as a mark of belonging, masculinity, and movement toward adulthood (C 71 Jean-Louis Méon n.d.).

The education of girls was the exclusive province of women, whose task it was to teach them that respectability required submission to the authority of others. A woman had no authority over her sons, reported Kebe Babacar of Cayor, Senegal, but "she has true authority over her daughter. It is she who is in charge of the girl's education. A young girl is less free than a boy in the family and in the village. One says that a woman is a slave, so she must experience early her social condition. She will never command, she must always be guided" (C 3 Kebe Babacar 1949). The one moment in which a woman could, it seems, count on commanding authority was in teaching her daughters submission. Enjoying that authority would be the exclusive province of women who had successfully raised children—once again, to be freeborn was equivalent to bearing children. Proper feminine comportment for the freeborn woman required an attitude of submissiveness toward her parents and her future husband. Sometimes preparation for feminine fortitude in the face of the pain of adulthood and the temptations of sex entailed cutting or painful tattooing, which a girl was to withstand without complaint (C 30 Diouck Sanor 1949, cf. Thomas 2003, Davison 1989).

Despite a certain tolerance for nonpenetrative sexual experimentation in the home communities of a few of the students (see, e.g., C 14 Diakite Mamadou 1945), all the essays on family life attest to a universal concern throughout the Sahel for the virginity of the girl at marriage (C 33 Samoura Sinkoun n.d.; C 14 Diakite Mamadou 1945). If, in the forested zone of West Africa, a woman might prove her worth prior to marriage by becoming pregnant, one decisive mark of the Sudanic belt was that a properly socialized girl was to protect her virginity. In effect, "shame" and virginity went hand in hand. This emphasis on virginity was not merely a projection of *male* understandings of honor on women, as Iliffe (2005, 3) suggests; rather, women as successful mothers cultivated, enforced, and benefited from upholding virginity.

Virginity gave evidence of the restraint understood to be the mark of those who have the capacity to feel shame—the characteristic of the freeborn and the noble. Virginity was not simply important because it made clear the genitor of the child, although surely that was relevant; it was important because the virgin bride thereby demonstrated her own capacity to feel shame. That restraint marked her as the bearer of the status of her family. Most of all, her own chastity was visible proof of the chastity, and therefore capacity to feel shame, of her mother. The honorable girl was evidence of the faithfulness of her mother. The cultivation of a moral sensibility entailed conditioning the child to *avoid* anything that might give rise to shame, for that too was part of how a woman revealed her proper breeding.

Thus, according to Diakite Mamadou, a mother will regularly tell her daughter before marriage, "My daughter, try to honor us when you are at your husband's house. I won't be with you to guide you in your household. Like a sheep, be submissive, it is our destiny. You are my pride. It is your task to increase my bloodline" (C14 Diakite Mamadou 1945). Every mother's honor depended on the comportment of her daughters, which in turn required the demonstration of submission, restraint, and fertility. According to Diakite, in addition to virginity, female excision was a prerequisite for marriage and for honorable childbirth and was understood to have a role in ensuring the sexual restraint of the woman and in preventing adultery. True to form, the essay closed with a lamentation that educated girls can't cook and are not as submissive as they should be; the best bride, he averred, would be one with limited French education.

A story recounted by a young man from Kaya in Upper Volta (contemporary Burkina Faso) suggests that romantic adolescent dalliances complicated the picture. This relatively defensible plateau region of the Sahel offers a rare case in which the majority of the population is today neither Muslim nor Christian. The concern in this narrative for establishing the paternity of the child suggests strongly that the emphasis on virginity and women's fidelity was *not* simply a product of Muslim mores but was part of a broader set of understandings of how to establish the full humanity of a child and membership in the human community that predated Islam in the region. Gayego Leopold related the fate of a young woman of about seventeen named Saissi who had already been promised by her father to her future husband when she fell pregnant by her boyfriend (C14 Gayego Leopold n.d.). In her marital home, her in-laws treated her badly, offering her food only in a broken calabash (a common symbol in the Sahel for a woman who has lost her virginity). Her husband attempted (through unexplained means) to abort the baby, and so she ran home to her parents.

At this point in the text, Leopold shifted from relating a past event to presenting a series of more general, perhaps hypothetical, observations. The unfaithful woman would suffer great difficulties in childbirth until she revealed to the old women assisting her "the name of the man with whom she has had bestial relations [*des relations animals*]." The woman could die if she did not tell the truth. Then, once the baby was born, the husband would thrust the baby on the boyfriend. The boyfriend might have identified someone to serve as wet nurse, or his family might provide the baby with cow's milk. The child born of such difficult labor might be said to be a devil; such children, he reported, were often abandoned under a granary. If someone were to take the baby it might live, and, if so, it would be named Moussa. Leopold observed that there were very few people named Moussa in the region.

Such abandoned children, like the Biblical Moses, were probably taken in by neighboring peoples at least occasionally. Certainly, historically in other parts of northern Upper Volta (now Burkina Faso) region, children understood to have maleficent powers discernable when their lower teeth emerged first had been abandoned and taken in by neighboring Fulani, who then raised them as household slaves (Baldus 1977). Such children entered into a separate slave caste. However, if against all odds the imagined woman's boyfriend were to succeed in keeping a girl child alive, the woman's legal husband could claim the girl's bride-price when she married. We see here how the maintenance of status groups and the hierarchy between them rested in important ways on policing "shameful" behavior of women in the context of sexuality. The rejection of the bastard child was necessary to establish the fully human characteristics of the husband's line. Fully human procreation could occur only in marriage; by extension, a child born of an illicit union could not be fully human. It was bestial or demonic, fit to become a slave.

A fully human child could come into being only through proper human constraint; consequently, when a woman suffered a difficult labor, it was assumed throughout the region that she had committed adultery. A properly human birth should occur smoothly, silently, and with restraint; it was not animal-like. Perhaps the association of a host of ills (maternal mortality, stillbirths, physical or mental defects in the child, or incontinence in the mother) with long and difficult labor contributed to a perception that the woman was being punished for something, most likely infidelity.[36] A properly cautious and restrained woman would obey all injunctions about how to avoid the many perils facing a pregnant woman: she would not go out at certain times, she would obey her husband in every particular, and she would fortify herself with charms and prayers of many different kinds. In order to preserve the integrity and humanness of the baby, she would avoid looking at ugly things, deformed people, and animals such as monkeys.[37] All of the memoirs that discussed in any way pregnancy and childbirth placed great stress on the responsibility of the pregnant woman to ensure the health of the baby through her own comportment. In Cayor, Senegal, a woman could guarantee the future happiness of her child by working hard and ensuring the happiness of her husband during her pregnancy: "whatever happens to the child, whether good or bad, people will say, 'that's the work of his mother'" (C 3 Kebe Babacar 1949). In some settings, the death of the child might be attributed to the failure of its mother to keep promises made to the ancestors or protective spirits (C 3 N'Diaye Mody Diabe Maurice 1949).

The duty of the adult man or woman within a social group was to have children; Diakite Mamadou reported that in male initiation, the adepts where exhorted to produce children: "Your duty is above all to procreate, for without that you would never have been born on this earth. Your children will continue to multiply your bloodline after your death" (C 14 Diakite Mamadou 1945). The injunction to produce children, therefore, weighed as heavily on men as it did on women. But those children could only be received into society if they met the conditions of membership; they had to have been born to men and women properly initiated into the expectations of society and publicly joined in marriage. The full humanity of a child, its suitability for integration into the family and community, had to be publicly and ritually marked.

The Importance of Naming

Throughout the Sahel, the students explained in their essays, a naming ceremony would be held on the eighth day after the birth of a child. This ceremony was (and continues to be) known by various indigenous terms that are rendered into French as *baptême* (baptism), the Christian analogue. The ceremony rendered visible the child's entry into the human community. As Barry Mamadou Aliou expressed it, "The baptism marks the triumph of the being that is coming to birth over nature, sometimes cruel to beings so small; the baptism celebrates the integration of the child into the family and into society" (C 14 Barry Mamadou Aliou 1949). Caba Sory made explicit what is normally simply implicit—that the ceremony also serves to exclude. If the father recognized the pregnancy as legitimate, the naming ceremony would go smoothly and the baby would have a surname redolent with meaning. The child would also receive a Muslim name chosen from the Koran and very likely over time an assortment of sobriquets and nicknames that would enable everyone to avoid using that spiritually potent name (C 14 Caba Sory 1949).

However, in the event that the child was illegitimate, three days after the birth, when the respected men and women of the community gathered to discuss the case, they would decide that the baby must not be given a conventional naming ceremony (C 14 Caba Sory 1949). The child would go by its mother's family name instead, excluding it from the community and from the rituals of collective life. Such a child, another student reported, might even be denied a name associated with the mother's family and instead be named for a friend (C 3 Toure Alpha n.d.). In Hausa, one of the many ways of pointing out that someone was a bastard was to say *"ubansa bai yi masa ragwan suna ba"* (his father didn't slaughter a naming day ram for him). It would be exceedingly difficult for such a child to get by in life; he or she would have no right to inheritance and few prospects for marriage. Effectively, such a child had the same status as a slave.

These passages in the memoirs give us a richer sense of the nature of the "moral constraint" women faced that led them to commit infanticide in the face of an unwanted pregnancy. To violate the norms of submission and obedience could lead to exile or ostracism. Such a woman damaged the stability of the family's claim to whatever status it had traditionally claimed: nobility, freeborn status, the renown of particular caste, a scholarly family's descent from the prophet. In a context in which claims to resources such as land and labor were no longer determined by the capacity to capture and subdue, but rather by bloodline and reputation, the birth of a child of uncertain blood could destabilize the entire system. Better to expel both the mother and the baby altogether. The mother would have no support whatsoever from her family—especially from her own mother—and the child would throughout life bear the stigma. There would be no apprenticeship into the farming, smithing, hunting, or military skills that indicate status and adulthood; there would be no initiation, no circumcision or excision, and very likely no marriage. Such a child would face a difficult life and would be resented forever by its mother and despised by its family.

Infanticide Today

If a child could not be integrated ritually, the alternative for the mother was to show publicly that she understood the gravity of what she had done and the impossibility of humanizing such a creature. The judicial records suggest that up to the late 1930s, by showing that she did in fact recognize that the child could never be embraced as fully human, a woman could show that she herself was indeed from a family of a worthy background, the kind of family made up of those who have the capacity to feel shame, unlike animals and slaves. The deepening implantation of Islam throughout the colonial period was simply grafted on top of a profound rejection of the bastard child, the origins of which were older. That rejection was enracinated in the culture women taught one another and imposed through ritual sanction. Gradually, the means by which such children were publicly rejected became ritualized and Islamicized through the refusal to "name" the child.

The conditions that led young women to commit infanticide have not disappeared. Studies have regularly shown the high proportion of imprisoned young women who have been incarcerated for infanticide in Niger. In a 1987 public health thesis during another period of tremendous economic and environmental stress, female prisoners accounted for their crime through reference to shame—the same reason offered in the 1930s (Boulel 1987). This does not mean that the material conditions of the moment—economic depression, food scarcity, poor rainfall—are irrelevant, but it does mean that if we want to understand women's own feelings and existential reality, we need to take seriously the force of this term *shame*. While much has changed—indeed, what shame means and how it is felt or imposed seems to have changed—the language and desperation with which women express the unimaginableness of a future that includes such a child has not.[38] Niger continues today to struggle with three desolate implications of the refusal to recognize the personhood of the illegitimate child: infanticide, clandestine abortions, and child abandonment.

January 9, 2014

Lazaret: I ask a woman from near Tillabery what happens when a girl is pregnant before she gets married. She is quiet for a moment. Then she replies, she will be rejected by her family. In fact there was a girl who had a baby and threw it down a latrine just over there, she says as she points vaguely. The girl is in prison now. Her father had died and she had no family, so she was doing what girls do and got pregnant. She has no kin. The women who had gathered around us to listen wondered who was feeding her while she was in prison. The neighborhood chief, she supposed, he visits her from time to time.

The others described a similar case of a girl whose mother was so angry with her for becoming pregnant that she rejected her daughter. So the girl "did something" to try to remedy her situation, and in the process of trying to abort the pregnancy she died, but the baby lived. So now her mother has to live with the guilt of having caused her daughter's death and with the burden of taking care of the baby.

Numerous studies confirm the long-standing pattern: young women, often from rural backgrounds and with very little education (three-quarters are illiterate), become pregnant and the impossibility—the unimaginability— of attempting to raise an illegitimate child in the face of the rejection of their families leads them to kill their newborn babies, generally by throwing them into a latrine or abandoning them on a garbage heap (Seyni 2001; Adamou 2001; Aougui 2008; Boubey 2008; Cusson, Doumbia, and Yebouet 2017). These young women's kin very likely knew that they were pregnant. Women do not by and large commit infanticide to hide a pregnancy—they do it to reconcile themselves with families that will not accept the child when they know they have no means to support the baby without help from the father or their kin. Thus, for example, in a 2001 study of infanticide in Niamey, women gave as reasons the shame of her social circle (*honte de l'entourage*) (33.3%) and family rejection (*rejet familial*) (33.3%) far more frequently than insufficient means (*manque de moyens*) (13.3%) (Adamou 2001, Tableau XI p. 29). The cause of the unimaginableness of raising a child alone is social rejection, not simply poverty, although of course the two are related.

In an interview in 2014 with a lawyer who assists women in legal trouble pro bono, I asked about infanticide cases. Magistrate A responded that when she went to the prison to do outreach, generally the younger women were being held for infanticide. She talked with a young woman who had been convicted along with her mother. It seems that the young woman's mother had abused her emotionally and physically because she was so angry about the pregnancy and that this was common knowledge in the neighborhood. When the girl gave birth at home, the neighbors heard the cry of the newborn. Two days later, the girl and her mother were claiming it had been stillborn. As is common, the neighbors called the police—generally, it is the *entourage* of the family and neighborhood that draws attention to the issue. The magistrate said that the girl appeared to be repentant and hopes eventually to get out and find work. However, unless women have legal representation, they are often held even when they are meant to get out on parole. No one keeps track of the dates (Magistrate B. A., Niamey, June 11, 2014).

At the time of my fieldwork in 2014, out of a shifting roster of forty-five to fifty women in the Niamey women's prison, there were eleven being held for allegations of or convictions for infanticide. According to Madame H. F., the social worker assigned to the women's prison, girls whose mothers abuse them verbally and physically because of the pregnancy know that they will have no support because illegitimate children are despised. Sometimes the baby is thrown in the latrine, sometimes the girl leaves it in the road, and sometimes she buries it. Divorced women whose ex-husband wouldn't recognize the child are under suspicion; they often have other children to support and can't handle another mouth to feed. Puzzled about the problem of how one distinguishes miscarriage or stillbirth from infanticide, I asked Madame H. F. how the authorities know that a woman is guilty of murder.

Any time a girl who isn't married has a child at home and it dies, the presumption is that it was infanticide, she replied indignantly. Because there is rarely the means to follow up with a gynecological exam, perform a rapid postmortem of the baby, or even interview the girl, these girls end up in "preventive detention" until an investigation can be done and the judge considers the case. Unfortunately, because the system has insufficient funds, there is often no investigation. The accused is in prison, but she can neither leave nor prove her innocence one way or the other.

BC: So you think there are girls in there that really did just have a still birth?

HF: Yes! I went to a judge because I discovered a woman who had been in the jail for four years and her case had never come up. Why? Because one document was missing, the one from the coroner's office that releases the body for inhumation. That form is what indicates how the baby died. "Why can't they let her out provisionally until the court date?" I asked the judge.

"We keep them in for two years to protect them from becoming pregnant again." That was his reply! "That way they will have time to rest before they get pregnant again. You know," he said, "if we release them they could just get pregnant all over again, so that's why we keep them whether or not the court case has come." (Madame H. F. Niamey, June 12, 2014)

Implicitly, a girl or woman who has sex outside of marriage is automatically guilty of something. The pregnancy itself is the proof.

Notes

1. For the history of law in French West Africa as it touches on the lives of women, see Cooper (2010a, 2010b), Miers and Roberts (1988), Roberts (2005), Mann and Roberts (1991), Lawrance and Roberts (2012).

2. I have Anglicized ranks and titles to ease the flow of reading throughout the body of the text but retain the original French nomenclature in citations in the notes. AS M 89 Note de service N 32A, Lieutenant-colonel Lamolle, Commandant le Territoire Militaire du Niger, September 1, 1906. AS M 89 Letter from Lieutenant-gouverneur Haut-Sénégal et Niger in Kayes to the Gouverneur Général de l'AOF, January 10, 1907. AS M 89 Letter from Procureur Général to Gouverneur Général de l'AOF, March 29, 1907. AS M 89 Letter from Lieutenant-gouverneur Haut-Sénégal et Niger in Kayes to Gouverneur Général de l'AOF, July 24, 1907.

3. One man, having compensated the other for the value of the woman's bride wealth payment, intended to marry her. She evidently preferred to return to her original husband, whereupon the "new" husband seized her belongings. The dispute under appeal was over the value of her "things" and whether they had all been returned. AS M 119 État des jugements rendus sur appel en matière civile et commercial, Tribunal de cercle de Niamey, 2ᵉ trimestre 1906, June 18 and June 26.

4. AS M 119 État des jugements rendus en matière civile et commercial pour le Tribunal de province de Niamey pendant le 2ᵉ trimestre 1906, June 11.

5. AS M 119 Région de Zinder, Cercle de Tahoua, Jugements rendus en matière criminelle 2ᵉ trimestre June 22, 1906.

6. AS M 123 Letter reporting on the functioning of la Justice Indigène in the Territoire Militaire du Niger 3ᵉ trimestre 1911 from Procureur Général de l'AOF to the Gouverneur Général de l'AOF, February 27, 1912; AS M 123 Letter reporting on the functioning of la Justice Indigène in the Territoire Militaire du Niger 1ᵉʳ trimestre 1912 from Procureur Général de l'AOF to the Gouverneur Général de l'AOF, March 27, 1912.

7. ANS M 123 Conventions entre Indigènes 1914. Agreements recorded land transfers, usufruct rights to a woman's palm trees to her daughter as dowry, terms of commercial credit, formal recognition of a civil marriage, loans of houses, and the paternity of a three-month-old girl whose mother declined to leave Zinder if the father were posted elsewhere.

8. ANS 3 M 20 Rapport sur le fonctionnement de la justice indigène pendant l'année 1934.

9. ANS 3 M 11 Rapport sur le fonctionnement de la justice indigène pendant l'année 1930.

10. ANS 3 M 20 Rapport sur le fonctionnement de la justice indigène pendant l'année 1933. That year, 112 civil cases were brought, by contrast 734 criminal cases.

11. ANS 3 M 11 Rapport sur le fonctionnement de la justice indigène pendant l'année 1932.

12. In a murder case in the same year, a woman named Coumba was murdered on the road toward Togo and her earrings stolen. ANS 3M109 Notices des arrêts 1933.

13. ANN M 6 16 Justice Indigène Relations avec le Parquet, Letter from the Officier du Ministère Publique près le Tribunal d'Appel du Niger to the Procureur Général près la Cour d'Appel de l'AOF à Dakar, October 17, 1935.

14. ANS 3 M 109 Affaires connues par le tribunal de Niamey (Niger) et expédiées au Procureur Général pour Contrôle 1933. Arrêt no.50. Men could also be accused of "eating" the souls of children, particularly if their families were thought locally to be witches.

15. ANN 2 F 1 Extrait du Registre d'Ecrou, Cercle de Niamey 1ᵉʳ trimestre 1929, cases of Tanou (assassinat 20 years) and Larba (assasinat 29 years); Niamey 1ᵉʳ trimestre 1930, Fatou (empoisonnement et assassinat 20 years) and Adiza (empoisonnement 20 years).

16. ANN M 5 15 Notices des actes d'instruction. Extrait du registre d'écrou Zinder, December 31, 1937.

17. By 1921, laws treating infanticide as murder in France had been extended to apply in FWA and should certainly have been relevant in this case; Gaston-Jean Bouvenet and Paul Hutin (1955, 698).

18. ANN M 6 16 Justice indigène. Relations avec le Parquet. Letter from the Officier du Ministère Public près le Tribunal Colonial d'Appel du Niger Segealon to the Procureur Général of the AOF, December 27, 1934.

19. ANS 3 M 20 Rapport sur le fonctionnement de la justice indigène pendant l'année 1933.

20. ANS 3 M 109 Letter from Procureur Général to Lieutenant-gouverneur du Niger, October 15,1934.

21. ANS 3 M 109 Notices des arrêts January–April, 1934. No.19.

22. On ethical practice, see Mahmood (2005, 29).

23. ANS 3 M 109 Letter from Procureur Général to Lieutenant-gouverneur du Niger, October 15,1934.

24. By 1824, in France punishment could be reduced to a life sentence under extenuating circumstances if the act had been committed by the mother. This leniency was expanded to include persons other than the mother in 1832. In an impassioned speech in 1885 encouraging members of the Cour d'Appel d'Angers to revise the law, Louis Cournot argued that infanticide by an unwed mother was not premeditated murder but rather a crime of passion (Cournot 1885, 20). Another round of reforms resulted in significant softening both toward the mother and her accomplices—after 1905, the sentence might be as low as two years (Gauban 1905). Alarm over depopulation in the wake of World War I gave rise to a particularly pronatal legal reform in which contraception, abortion, and infanticide were all subject to judicial efforts to punish the refusal of women to produce children (Ronsin 1980).

25. For background to this document, see Lydon (1997). Cited here CAOM 17 G 381 "Rapport no. 5." Savineau reported on conditions in prisons in the territories she visited. The final report is now available in a print volume edited by Claire Griffiths, to whom I am very grateful for making the text so accessible (Savineau 2007).

26. ANS 3 M 109 Notices des arrêts January–April 1934, Case 22.

27. ANS 3 M 109 Letter from Procureur Général to Lieutenant-gouverneur du Niger, Affaire Kanni, July 28, 1934.

28. Fuglestad, *History of Niger* (1983, 138–39).

29. ANS 3 M 117 184 Notice des Arrêts rendus par la Chambre d'Accusation, Réquisition 12, March 1940.

30. From there, Lobo disappears from the records as the war in Europe rendered staffing and judicial oversight more and more difficult.

31. In later decades, the reverse appears to have been the case. By 1953 in Songhai and Bambara regions, the sex ratios at 90 and 97.8 respectively seemed to indicate unusually high stillbirths among boys over girls. ANS 1 H 122 versement 163, Author unknown 1953 La répartition des sexes Table V Sex-ratios à la Naissance et Mortinatalité pour les principales races de l'AOF August 1951–July 1952.

32. For a similar shift in criminalization of the reproductive practices of poor women in the context of a postemancipation society, see Roth (2017).

33. The École Normale William Ponty in Senegal, founded in 1903, became the official teacher training college of French West Africa in 1933. Eventually a second school was established, the École Normale Fréderic Assomption de Katibougou in French Sudan. Students produced assignments in bound notebooks known as *cahiers* during their vacations; most of these are now held in the fonds École Normale William Ponty at IFAN in Dakar. Such IFAN references begin with a C (for *cahier*) followed by a number indicating the class set in which the thesis is to be found. Over the years, students wrote on some twenty-eight different topics. Quite a few of the memoirs probably never made it into the IFAN set. I found a number among theses collected by the French administration in the Archives Nationales du Niger. The references for these are ANN followed by 1 G 4. All of the memoirs I draw on here were produced between 1933 and 1949. Some were not dated but were found in sets of papers that enable me to make a reasonable guess as to the year in which they were submitted.

34. Students were not equally gifted, diligent, or honest. At least two clearly plagiarized memoirs turned up in the sets I read. Others were so poorly written that they occasioned

very stern grades and commentary. A great many of the students were very clearly from the families of chiefs and other notables and almost none from casted groups. For interesting reflections on the difference in schooling for the rare son of a griot, see C 14 Couyate Karamoko n.d. For the reflections of chiefs' sons on how a young man is socialized to become a chief, see C 14 Caba Sory 1949 and C 14 Barry Mamadou Aliou 1949. Very few of these students came from Niger, which had an extremely rudimentary school system even by 1945.

35. Two assignments have produced particularly useful material for my purposes—one in which the student was to discuss the training of children in *le milieu familial* and another on how education contributes to the shaping of society. While these topics were undoubtedly promising for the students in the sense that it would not be difficult for them to find something to write about, the topics were also of interest to the French administration, and occasionally one can glean from marginalia that memoirs were forwarded to other colonial offices. The fact that the essays were archived is, in itself, striking.

36. C 14 Pascal L. Macos 1949. This appears to be linked to notions of retribution for asocial behavior: C 3 Sarr Alioune 1949.

37. The belief that taking too great an interest in wild animals will act negatively on the child is very common, C 3 Toure Alpha n.d.

38. In 2001, 68.2 percent of female prisoners were detained for infanticide (Seyni 2001, Tableau 5, 26). In 2006, according to Niger's Ministry of Justice, 80 percent of women incarcerated nationwide were charged with infanticide. US Department of State (2007).

4

COLONIAL ACCOUNTING

GIVEN THE DEBATES ABOUT INFANTICIDE IN THE PRECEDING chapter, it is clear that Sahelian populations were not pronatalist in an unqualified sense in the first half of the twentieth century. Children had to be brought into the world in ways that did not disrupt the moral order. The revulsion toward the bastard child, despite its vaguely Islamic trimmings by the mid-twentieth century, does not appear to have derived from Islam per se or simply from the significance of patriliny among Muslims. It had a deeper origin in conceptions about the relationships between the environment, invisible beings both monstrous and benevolent, human procreation, and the possibility of a moral order. The truly freeborn gave birth to humans in the context of marriage. Only slaves and animals bred with so little restraint. In this chapter, I open by setting out the clash between two very different modes of reckoning—the moral and cosmological reckoning typical of peoples of the Sahel and the crudely quantitative accounting of the French colonial order. These fundamentally antagonistic ways of understanding "population" made it extremely difficult for the colonial administration to gain a clear sense of the demography of French West Africa (FWA).

After France's defeat in the Franco-Prussian war in 1870, French patriots turned their attention to their empire to counter the declining birthrate in France, an impulse that contributed to the drive to colonize the Sahel (Andersen 2015, 1). The French public became intrigued by its empire's potential to address metropolitan France's manpower and military needs. In the end, the concern to promote population growth in the colonies took two forms: an investment in managing colonial subjects' reproduction in a handful of places, notably Madagascar, and a push to support a prolific settler presence. Pronatalism could be inconsistent and contradictory. On the one hand, the colonies presented a space of expansion and possibility that might encourage French families to produce more children than in metropolitan France. Settler territories, notably Algeria and Tunisia, would enable the rebuilding of the French "race." Pronatalist policies were focused "almost exclusively on the French settler population" (Andersen 2015, 9). In such settings, a rapidly growing indigenous population could be experienced as a threat, triggering divergent treatment of women of different races (cf. Klausen 2015 and Kaler 2003).

On the other hand, indigenous populations could provide crucial manpower. West Africa was seen to be a promising source of soldiers to replenish France's army (Andersen 2015, 12; Mangin 1910). From the outset, soldiers figured prominently in population thinking about French West Africa. From the 1920s, it was increasingly argued that to "valorize" its colonies, France would have to promote the growth of the indigenous populations. Historians tend to assume that the postwar pronatal mission had a significant impact on women and the direction of health services in FWA. For example, Jonathan Cole has recently argued that "by virtue of their reproductive capacities, women were the central focus of this new health policy" (Cole 2012, 118). However, in reality only in Madagascar and Indochina did colonial governments invest substantially in measures aimed at decreasing mortality and increasing fertility among the subject population.[1] Despite Albert Sarraut's 1931 declaration that to make progress valorizing its African colonies it would be necessary first to make more blacks (*faire du noire*) (cited in Bonnichon, Geny, and Nemo 2012, 558), relatively little headway was made before independence in improving reproductive health in the Sahel outside Dakar and Bamako.

The conundrum of colonial rule in the Sahel was that for imperial domination to be worthwhile—both to France and to the populations under French control—there would first need to be an investment of human and economic resources. Those resources, given the political logic in metropolitan France, had to come from *within* the territories themselves, which paradoxically could not be adequately "valorized" without a staff equal to the task. Colonial administrators would need to extract wealth in order to create it. The necessary impossibility of gathering credible population data in Niger—the central concern of this chapter—encapsulated the absurdity of French colonial rule in the Sahel. Repeated commands, requests, and pleas for the collection of such data went either ignored or were fulfilled in a perfunctory manner for the simple reason that there was neither the staff nor the resources to take up the task.

For overworked administrators, demographic data tended to be reduced to information relevant to raising revenue through taxes. Rough numerical estimates to determine the tax burden on each village and household were necessary to anticipate the tax revenue to be generated within defined geographic units known as *cercles* (districts). Obviously, it was not in the interests of the indigenous populations to volunteer accurate information. These figures were subject to myriad errors of over- and underestimation and could be reckoned differently from one locale to another. Some administrators counted the names on the tax lists, some estimated village size, some counted granaries, and many turned the matter over to indigenous chiefs and hoped for the best. The figures were in effect a kind of accounting—an accounting of the populations under a particular jurisdiction, but more importantly an accounting of the potential tax resources of the colony overall. Ideally, the figures would always be going up. What mattered were the *perception* of their accuracy and the intimidating spectacle of census-taking as an assertion of French authority. This was as true at the local level as it was at the level of each colony and each federation (Gervais 1997).

Local commissioners sent their population figures to the lieutenant governor of their colony, who then packaged them to send to the governor general of FWA in Dakar. Most of the intellectual investment in this sequential exercise was devoted to accounting for any decline in numbers. The impulse to produce figures moving in the right direction was high at every level (Gervais 1997, 967). This fixation with visible declines in numbers of villages and households resulted in greater attention to dramatic population movements than to more subtle shifts in mortality and natality—losing taxable subjects to neighboring British colonies, in particular, was a matter of consistent anxiety.

In effect, France did face a serious demographic problem in its empire. But at its heart, the demographic crisis concerned not the indigenous population but the inadequate numbers of appropriately trained colonial administrators. Senegal (the best endowed of all the Sahelian colonies) had in 1908 some 4,229 French residents against an estimated indigenous population of 1,163,620 (CAOM 22 G 20 Statistiques "Senegal 1908"). Taking the whole of FWA in 1905, the total "European" population was on the order of 11,118 (including wives and children and assorted non-French expatriates) in a territory estimated at 3,913,190 square kilometers over which an indigenous population of perhaps 10,062,208 was dispersed (CAOM 22 G 20 Statistiques "Table: Colonies de l'Afrique occidental française 1905").

France never invested sufficient human or financial resources to have an appreciable positive impact on reproductive health in the Sahel.

A Cosmology of Population and Reproduction

> At first God agreed to let the children of Adama and Adam enter the new world with the promise that their children would live forever without death or illness, as in Paradise. But over time people became more and more flawed and debauched. Up until that point there had been no such thing as punishment or purgatory.
>
> Then the population became so dense that there wasn't enough space for it on earth. To solve this problem God sent down the Angel Gabriel to ask the populace what it wanted. God received from his representative all their grievances and concluded that death was a necessity for humans.
>
> God turned over to the oldest person the keys that would enable him to open up the chambers enclosing the lives of each being, as well as a silver staff, a rope and a chain. But Death complained that he was continually threatened. So to ease his task God made him invisible, tireless, and able to run through the world as swiftly as the wind. (ANN 1 G 4 6 Condat Georges Mahamane 1939)

In the Hausa tale related above, École Ponty student and future politician Georges Mahamane Condat shared a narrative in which death emerged as a gift from God necessary to resolve some of the limits of the earthly environment and of human needs and behaviors.[2] This account of human mortality was, in Condat's 1939 essay, the origin of the cycle of beings through which the death of a grandparent opens the way for the birth of a child (see also C13 Gaston Dory 1943). In demographic terms, the tale seems to be a meditation on population equilibrium: overpopulation resulting from a surfeit of births created the conditions for a corresponding rise in deaths. The peril of "overpopulation" had been permanently resolved by Death. Reproducing no longer contributed to an absolute increase in the number of "beings." With the creation of mortality, that number was fixed. Having children enabled one's virtuous ancestors to continue to circulate between the worlds of the living and the dead.

In his charming 1945 essay on dreams among the Cadot-Songhai of Niger, Mossi Adamou described a variety of invisible beings with magic powers. The Atacourma, he explained, live in termite mounds and cool sandy places and come out only at twilight. They move as fast as sound and eat our food out from under our noses, which is why sometimes a large platter will be consumed and yet people will still be hungry. Genies, on the other hand, are so gigantic that their heads touch the heavens; they are able to overhear the private conversations between God and his angels, which is how they can tell the future. The Guingi-bi, which are "black spirits," are the most fearsome to humans. Tall, naked, and dragging a long train of hair, they drink human blood and go out at night bearing an enormous cauldron into which are caught the dream-wandering souls of those who are not protected by charms: "For the Songhai, then, we [humans] are nothing but a tiny minority of the inhabitants of the earth, and we are disconcertingly feeble compared to the beings of the invisible world . . . Fortunately [good] sorcerers, magicians, the Holley spirits and Genies are all here to protect us!" (C 53 Mossi Adamou 1944–45).

Humans, it seems, coexisted and sometimes competed with the numerous invisible beings with which they shared the world, some of which were malevolent, others more benign. Survival was a matter of shoring up good relations with protective beings while warding off the dangers of those whose power derived from swallowing the dream-souls of others. Against such a perilous backdrop, a refusal to bear children altogether appears as a kind of betrayal of an intergenerational and transworldly compact. Marriage was the means through which the elders of a particular family ensured the return of their "grandparents." The appearance of an illegitimate child disturbed the social contract. The child might "look like" and reiterate the wrong family altogether; it took up space, if you will, that was not fairly obtained. Indeed, only an evil being would enter the world in such a rapacious, dishonest, and dissembling fashion. For the Songhai, women were central to the maintenance of the moral order: their wombs do not appear to have belonged to them or even to their own families.

The moral dimension of this circulation of beings made each reproductive event—a miscarriage, a stillbirth, a deformity, a set of twins, a bastard child—subject to moral appraisal. Why this "being" rather than another? How did the actions of humans and the other kinds of invisible beings (witches, sorcerers, genies, devils, angels) influence the unfolding of a particular pregnancy, the reproductive career of a particular woman, or the reproductive success or failure of a particular group? Women of reproductive age faced a multitude of dangers and responsibilities. Seydou Cissoko elaborated in his essay on childhood in Senegal: "People say that the soul [in a fetus] is in constant battle with evil forces acting all around it. Consequently it is necessary to create a protective environment around the pregnant woman through a collective effort. It is a matter of great responsibility—because the pregnant woman carries in her a gift of God:

the human-gift that only the Eternal can give" (C 30 Seydou Cissoko 1949). This collective protective labor succeeded best when the pregnancy, the birth, and the general details about a particular family or people remained hidden. There was no advantage to provoking the jealous ill will or resentment of those beings or humans with less success in attracting souls/beings into the world. Certainly, it would not be wise to presumptuously take the gifts of God for granted.

Given the intense competition between beings and the urgency of protecting every pregnancy and birth, it is not surprising that the students of the École Ponty were acutely discomfited by an assignment given to them in 1949 requiring them to produce "a demographic study of a specific locale." The students were to gather information on the numbers of births and deaths of boys and girls in their chosen locale over a given period and to indicate whether the babies had died at birth or later on. Seydou Cissoko politely explained to his teacher that people don't like to talk about demography; they worry that talking about a child will put it at risk (C 30 Seydou Cissoko 1949). Oumar Diouf made excuses for his scanty data, offering a more frank assessment of the difficulty: "First of all the natives don't have any civil registry and out of superstition they refuse to give any information about their age, whether precise or approximate. Being terrorized [sic] by the taxes that the district chiefs take from their meager crops, they try as hard as possible to hide the real size of their families to reduce the size of their tax" (C 30 Oumar Diouf 1949). With characteristic obtuseness, the teacher underlined *terrorized* as being a poor choice of words. Oumar Diouf's classmate Elhadji Diouf, who diligently attempted to extract such information from the village chief, was dismayed to find that the chief became very suspicious of him and would tell him nothing for fear that the hapless student would tell the whites and as a result taxes would go up. In any case, he noted, "to reveal the number of deaths could cause misfortune, that is, there would be more deaths" (C 30 Elhadji Diouf 1949). Amadou Badiane, evidently sidestepping the dangers of talking directly to the chief or the people in his village about the size of their families, drew on notes kept by a former soldier, who had presumably become accustomed to the idea of a civil registry because birth and marriage documents were necessary for soldiers to receive their compensation (C 30 Amadou Badiane 1949).

Clearly, the colonial context had amplified and complicated the matter of *protecting* as opposed to *counting* people. Taxes were reckoned by the number of members of a household and village. Avoiding being counted had become more than a matter of protecting one's family from invisible spirits or malevolent people—it had become a matter of economic survival. Of course, one could think of the depredations of the colonial order as being akin to, or perhaps even caused by, the agency of already familiar beings. Mossi Adamou offered a "literary translation" of a magic Songhai incantation, the powerful *Guingui Hau*, used to protect against the bad dreams that occur when one's soul is being stolen. It had clearly been adapted to confront the contemporary challenges facing any occult specialist in the colonial context:

> Not through me, but through my fathers, Gareyfarma, Boureima, Molia, Maharou, Toussounda, Kababe, Walo, Bibaga, Mahama Nkuma [all great wizards, Adamou explains]—it is with a huge iron nail that they nail down and immobilize evil genies, the souls of the dead, the evil enemies from the East, from the West, from the North, from the South, the Whites [Europeans, in particular the French], the *Tirailleurs* [colonial soldiers], the cold, stomach problems, colic, pains in the side, the evil night walkers, the evil sorcerers of the wild and the evil sorcerers of the village, the cruel poisoners of men, the Red Blacksmiths [fearsome wizards]. (C 53 Mossi Adamou 1944–45)

Whites and their soldier consorts had joined the malevolent Guingi-bi as a class of beings to be neutralized at all cost. Changing circumstances, as always, required adapting one's protective repertoire. In the early colonial period, spirit cults integrated newer spirits, often creatures conjured by the colonial regime, so that the spirit mediums might, by embodying them, tame them and master their secrets (Stoller 1995). For those that could not be tamed, this powerful incantation could serve as protection.

On the other hand, in the colonial context, new resources were available through the act of registering marriages, births, and deaths; anyone employed in the military or the colonial bureaucracy quickly became accustomed to this logic. The literate could earn a salary performing such acts of registration. The business of enumeration also offered a means of extorting labor and wealth from the population: chiefs could skim considerable sums off the top of the taxes they collected by raising amounts in excess of those to be turned over to the French. The Ponty students were being apprenticed to this new world, where counting and speaking French were rewarded with salaries and lifestyles unheard of for farming and herding populations. These positions could provide for large numbers of people while offering a hedge against the risks of an uncertain agropastoral economy and a commercial world in constant flux. The logic of attracting and celebrating publicly a large entourage conflicted with the logic of evading taxes. Still, the benefits from the new order in the form of wage employment and family allowances proportional to the size of one's family could also become part of a broader strategy for diversifying kinds of expertise. The Ponty students were caught in the middle—aware of how local populations experienced colonial intrusion but schooled to contribute to this profitable and prestigious order.

Political Arithmetic

As the experiences of the Ponty students suggest, the figures recorded as a result of this political arithmetic were at once hard-won and inevitably flawed. Administrators were aware that there was neither sufficient staff nor appropriate local cooperation to produce figures of any real value. In a draft letter in response to one of the many pleas from the Colonial Ministry for such data, Ernest Roume, the governor general of FWA at the time, attempted in 1905 to prepare the Colonial Office for disappointment: "As I informed you in my letter of 12 September, 1904, n. 1213, in the interior regions [of Senegal], which have the simplest of administrative structures, there is no civil registry; there is no useful information available to the administrator to determine with any precision the figures on births, deaths, or population movements required by the tables you have sent us" (CAOM 22 G 20 Statistiques draft letter n.d.). The absence of a consistent civil registry was to haunt the administration for decades and continues to be the source of innumerable problems across the Sahel. Tables related to births, deaths, divorces, marriages, and so on submitted by Niger beginning in 1928 annually repeated the exculpatory formula: "As a civil registry service for the native population does not yet function in a consistent fashion, it is impossible to provide even approximate figures" (CAOM FM AGEFOM 395 "Divers"). If the population of available bureaucrats (whether French or indigenous) was too small to perform such basic tasks as the recording of births, deaths, marriages, and divorces, it was *a fortiori* unlikely to be in a position to perform a serious census.

Under the circumstances, one might logically look to the military to perform such normally civilian tasks—certainly all mass "campaigns" of any kind within FWA prior to 1945 drew heavily on such labor to tax, count, vaccinate, or draft local populations. The earliest taxes in the Troisième Territoire Militaire (Niger) were in principal based on estimates of the resources of different regions determined during what were known as "police rounds." Idrissa Kimba characterizes these census operations as little more than military raids in which surprise tactics and force were used to extract information on the size of families and harvests (Kimba 1993, 99). Because Niger was a military territory up until 1920 and a "colony" only from 1922, it was managed bureaucratically through the military for over two decades. Soldiers were useful for intimidating civilian populations into producing the requirements of the administration. On the other hand, the presence of large numbers of soldiers amplified the challenge of raising resources to feed and to pay them. What subjects experienced most directly was not the French administrator but rather the soldiers, chiefs, and private cavalries of the nobility.

In 1909, Commissioner Clozel forwarded the following population figures on the Territoire Militaire du Niger to Dakar in 1909: 218 French, 1,051,657 "subjects," and another 1,500 "subjects of other colonies" (CAOM 22 G 20 Statistiques "Envoi statistiques 1908 territoire militaire du Niger"). In other words, there were considerably more Africans from other colonies than there were Frenchmen—largely soldiers from other parts of FWA. From the 1909 materials, it becomes clear that, for the administrator at the margins, there would be little short-term incentive to make a precise count of the population. Taxes were collected according to quite different criteria in the various districts. Among nomads, each tent head paid seven to ten francs and each shepherd another three to five francs. The unit of taxation was therefore tents and shepherds, except in Agadez, where the unit was the tribe.[3] In different districts, sedentary populations were charged different rates depending on a rough sense for which regions could afford more and which less—in Kayes the rate was 4.50 francs per adult, and in Koury it ranged from .25 to 2.50 francs.

Districts were ranked according to how much tax they could yield (CAOM 22 G 20 Statistiques "Envoi statistiques 1908 territoire militaire du Niger"; "Envoie statistiques 1908 Haute-Sénégal Niger"). For example, the "yield" in Zinder (369,873 francs) in 1909 was considerably lower than the "yield" in Bamako (641,326 francs). Such differences in revenue had cumulative effects: the more revenue there was to invest, the more productive the region could become and the more desirable it would become to invest in it further. Administrators on the ground had an interest in squeezing ever more taxes out of the subjects within their reach, which resulted in astonishingly high rates of increase in the tax rates in very short periods of time. Finn Fuglestad calculated that the per person poll tax rate alone tripled in

Niger between 1906 and 1916; at the same time, ethnic groups were added to tax rolls, such as the Fulbe (or to be more precise, their cattle), that had not been taxed previously (Fuglestad 1983, 83–84). In order to increase the tax yield it was, of course, necessary to "count" ever more subjects or their proxies through whatever mechanism available.

The Africans governed by this military hierarchy were subject to two sorts of law. One, handled through the judicial court system overseen by the military commandants, would in principle draw on *justice indigène* (the customary law discussed in chapter 3) and would seek counsel from local *assesseurs*. The other system, the *indigénat*, was far more intrusive to subjects on a day-to-day basis. The administrative sanctions of the *indigénat* could be applied on the spot for disrespect, reluctance, or an uncooperative attitude. These summary punishments facilitated the collection of taxes, the seizure of animals and crops as "requisitions," and, most notoriously, the imposition of forced labor on adult males. While there were limits to the punishments to be inflicted through this summary administrative law (fines could not exceed fifty francs, and imprisonment could not exceed fifteen days), Africans had little recourse if the system was abused. It was the threat of the *indigénat* that compelled indigenous populations to provide taxes, labor, and animals.

Historian Boureima Alpha Gado has documented the relentless growth of tax receipts in Niger. For example, in the *cercle* of Ouahigouya alone, taxes collected went up by an average of 13,643 francs per year between 1900 and 1914 (Gado 1993, 61). Gado notes that under this level of extraction, the least deficit in rainfall or the most minor of locust invasions could provoke disaster (Gado 1993, 63). The 1900–1903 famine provoked major population movements from north to south. Families in search of grain "sold" children, a phenomenon documented across the whole of the central Sahel (Gado 1993, 72–76).[4] Evidence for a resurgence in sales of slaves appears to be clear across the region as well (Gado 1993, 85). Famine had visibly increased the numbers of people of slave status within the better-endowed receiving regions. Individuals whose families had willingly exchanged them for food could not easily expunge the shame of their origins in subsequent generations (Gado 1993, 87).

Mothers and Laborers

In the wake of World War I, France was preoccupied with rebuilding the population in Europe and obtaining the raw materials necessary to rebuild her industrial economy. In one of the more surreal episodes of French colonial history, the subject populations of FWA were exhorted in 1921 to purchase badges, flags, metal medallions, and postcards to show their sympathy toward and recognition of patriotic French mothers reproducing the nation. In his cover letter, Governor General Merlin pronounced to the commissioner in Niger, "I have no doubt that you are as aware as I am of the benefit of this day of celebration which, in honoring large families and in rewarding the most deserving, aims to make France ever more prosperous and powerful in the future" (ANS 2 H 6 versement 26, Merlin 1921). Across FWA, the colonies raised 165,015.35 francs to send to the committee (ANS 2 H 6 versement 26, Mayet 1922).

These pronatal and mercantilist concerns also shaped the understanding of the valorization (*mise en valeur*) of FWA during the interwar years. In the conventional narrative of France's colonial engagement in West Africa, the interwar years are marked as the period in which France began to develop its *Grands travaux*—its proud accomplishments in the development of the transportation infrastructure (particularly the Dakar-Bamako rail line), the health services (the work of Eugene Jamot on sleeping sickness and the creation of the Institut Pasteur), and the school systems (the medical school in Dakar opened in 1918). In this period, Colonial Minister Albert Sarraut drew up an ambitious (and ultimately unfunded) plan to equip and develop the colonies. "The era of lazy and sterile domination is past," he declared prematurely in 1931 (Bonnichon, Geny, and Nemo 2012, 558). It was in this context that the infamous phrase *faire du noir* (make blacks) emerged to capture the concern to improve the human capital in the colonies "in quantity and quality." African human capital was, in effect, the only capital available.

In 1920, Governor General Merlin created a commission to study how the medical services for subjects, known as the Indigenous Medical Assistance (Assistance Médicale aux Indigènes, AMI), could be reorganized and improved. The report revealed a striking paucity of medical staff of all kinds as a result of the war; the number of *sage-femmes* was so small that it was "practically negligible" (ANS 2 H 6 versement 26, "Situation Actuel" 1920). There was nothing in place to reduce infant mortality beyond the smallpox vaccine, and the only assistance women were receiving in childbirth was that of the traditional birth attendants. The first of the students trained in the medical school would not graduate until 1921. The report uncovered other problems related to the persistence of the military medical system alongside the newer civilian system: the military doctors were paid better than civilian doctors, had more mobility, and had access to the highest positions. There was not much, in short, to entice a civilian doctor to come to FWA.

Increasingly, the medical services targeting the African civilian population would need to draw on what were known as "auxiliary" health workers: African doctors, *sage-femmes*, and pharmacists who had been trained at the École de Médecine de l'AOF in Dakar. The medical school not only trained African doctors to augment the small pool available but perhaps more importantly for this story, it trained educated women from within FWA to become nurse-midwives (*sage-femmes*) and visiting nurses (*infirmières visiteuses*). Unfortunately, the production of graduates from the school was very slow, in part because the educational system feeding into the medical school was so weak to begin with. In 1925, the total number of doctors awarded degrees was thirteen. The number of women training to become *sage-femmes* that year was only forty-eight.[5] Obviously, the health system overall had, in the wake of the war, very little to offer the African population. In 1914, there had been fifty-six civilian doctors serving in the Indigenous Medical Assistance (IMA); in 1926, there were only thirty, of whom only sixteen were actually at their posts. They were far outnumbered by the forty military doctors serving in the IMA (ANOM FM 1AFFPOL 3058 Merly 1926).

The accumulating information on the state of the health system prompted Governor General Jules Carde to develop strategies to rework and improve the existing system. In February 1926, Carde directed his lieutenant governors to develop and orient the IMA so that it focused not only on healing but also on preventive and social medicine. The failure of the native "races" to increase in numbers, he argued, was a problem of mortality, not of natality. The solution would be better care for newborns and a continued emphasis on infectious diseases and especially "social diseases" among adults. The focus of the services, therefore, in the domain of infant mortality would be on the education of mothers and the "progressive penetration of notions of childrearing [*puericulture*] into family life" (Carde 1927, 5). Carde's instructions were remarkably detailed: *sage-femmes* should not become too distant from the people they are to serve, *matrones* or traditional birth attendants should be taught "notions of hygiene and cleanliness," the visiting nurses should be drawn from among the peoples they were to serve and should, beyond seeking out pregnant women and infants,

Table 4.1 FWA Indigenous Medical Assistance 1926

	French Sudan	Guinea	Dahomey	Mauritania	Niger	Côte d'Ivoire	Senegal	Dakar	Upper Volta (Burkina Faso)	Total
Health service establishments devoted to indigenous medical assistance	1	1	1	1	1	2	20	2	1	30
Hospitals	2	1					1			5
Military doctors	4	7	145	1	6	5		9		177
Civilian doctors		6	6	1		7		1		15
Auxiliary doctors	7	6	3	2	6	7		1		32
Indigenous nurses				20						20
Aids					34	144				178
Ambulance drivers			3			5				8
Urban hygiene monitors	6	7								13
Dispensaries	30		5	2	3			2	1	43
Maternities	7						4	1	5	17
Sage-femmes (French)								2		2
Auxiliary sage-femmes (African)	12	6	10			15		1		44
Medical establishments	50	9	9		5	16	9		5	94

Source: ANOM FM AGEFOM 384 AMI 1926

be on the lookout for epidemic and social diseases (10–13). The precision of Carde's requirements for this medical staff appears in retrospect—and certainly from the vantage point of a distant colony such as Niger—far out of keeping with the actual numbers of medical personnel available.

Finally, Carde reiterated the Colonial Ministry's request for statistical data: "the increase in the population being the goal of all our efforts, it is important that demographic changes be followed as precisely as possible, and if there is a decline, the causes be sought and redressed immediately" (20). Accordingly, each year the Health Service (Service de Santé) was to draw up statistical tables with the following information broken down by gender: the current population of infants under three, children from three to fifteen, young people and adults, the elderly over fifty, all deaths according to the same categories, and all births (noting stillbirths as a separate category). It was then to be collected for each district by ethnic group and accompanied by explanations of any year-to-year variations in population. An annual ritual developed in the form of the production of tables recording the total number of medical "consultations" provided and how that figure had increased over the preceding year.

Carde's lofty goals notwithstanding, the situation for the administrator far from Dakar had not changed. His priority continued to be collecting taxes, finding labor, and meeting the needs of the military; he had to accomplish all this with insufficient revenue and an absurdly small staff. The reports documenting field visits are full of details showing how slippery the collection of such population information continued to be. In Maradi, the nomadic Fulani population was nearly impossible to count: "They live in a willful state of utter anarchy," despaired the commandant. "They keep to the margins, and if this situation continues we will lose contact with them altogether" (ANN 1 E 10 30 Author unknown 1926). In Tillabery, another administrator complained, "it is impossible to gather this information in a satisfactory manner; it is repugnant to the natives to make reference to any children who died in their compounds. And since the census was not taken using names it is impossible to follow one individual from birth to death" (ANN 1 E 10 35 Pambrun 1927). Populations continued to move in search of a preferable chief or, better yet, total autonomy (ANN 1 E 10 73 Pambrun 1928). It was not clear how to count populations in the small semi-temporary settlements to which farmers moved during the farming season (ANN 1 E 10 68 Perrault 1928). Much energy was expended in trying to come to terms with suitable categories for a highly mobile and ethnically fluid population—categories went in and out of being without any evident rationale.

The focus on the ground, then, continued to be on counting taxable units and securing male labor rather than on promoting maternal health. In order to build any infrastructure at all, the administration required labor; furthermore, to attract capital investment, it needed to be able to promise investors that labor would be available. Paris pushed Dakar to encourage the production of raw materials, in particular cotton. Dakar then encouraged the same of each colony. Within some forest zone colonies, notably Côte d'Ivoire, there was already an export economy based on tree crops such as cocoa and coffee. In those settings, the urgent question was how to obtain sufficient labor to service private capital investment. Within the larger structure of FWA, Niger was seen as a labor reserve—it was unlikely to become a wealthy colony, and therefore its most important contribution to the whole would be in the form of labor.

Forced Labor versus Obligatory Labor

Population issues arose therefore most acutely in the context of debates about the recruitment of male labor or, to be more precise, the question of "obligatory" labor. In a characteristic exchange of the era, Governor General Carde sought Lieutenant Governor Brévié's response to a report commissioned for the French Textile Service that suggested alarmingly that Niger was losing its labor force to British Nigeria as a result of the overuse of forced labor for public works projects.[6] The relevant workers would have been Hausa-speaking farmers from the regions closest to Nigeria. In his lengthy rebuttal in June 1926, Brévié retorted that, indeed, there was a great deal of short-term movement of laborers from Niger to Nigeria during the dry season to earn wages, as well as seasonal movements of merchants to sell millet and cattle (FM AGEFOM 395 8bis Brévié 1926). This trade was, he pointed out, quite profitable—the prices were higher in Nigeria, and the exchange rate worked in favor of the migrants. Herders moved south during the dry season to find pasture and returned to Niger when the rains returned. None of this in any way affected labor during the farm season—indeed, it was beneficial to the economy as a whole. While it was true that at times the indigenous chiefs in Nigeria attempted to lure farmers to settle on the other side of the border, farmers generally came back because, in the end, the powerful chiefs in Nigeria had more capacity to extract wealth from poor farmers than did the more constrained chiefs in Niger.

Finally, Brévié declared, while it was true that in the past there had been military demands for food and labor that had caused some unrest, ever since he had sent out his circular of July 26, 1922, the situation had been carefully regulated. The annual labor "contribution" was not very heavy, he explained, as no one was obliged to provide more than ten days per year. Like Carde, Brévié resisted seeing this obligatory "contribution" as forced labor—it was rather to be thought of as a kind of tax (Conklin 1997, 212–45; F. Cooper 1996, 25–56).

Brévié seized on the opportunity to complain about what he did see as a problem—namely, annual military recruitment in the Hausa-speaking region, which the textile report had not mentioned. In general, it was easier for colonial governments to make the case for obligatory military service (common in Europe) than for forced labor, which didn't appear to be different from the slavery the colonial powers had in theory abolished. Each year, he reported, before the recruiting board arrived, most of the young men of age to be incorporated into the army left for Nigeria. Once the required number of recruits had been reached and the peril had passed, they returned. But if he were to apply the rules strictly and pursue these unexcused absentees mercilessly to force them to perform military service, there would indeed be a mass departure across the border, not only of those of military age but also of their entire families. Brévié pointedly made the case that military recruitment could not be conducted blindly; it had to be alert to the willingness of local populations to take part in the army. In the case of Hausa farmers, it was in everyone's interest to respect their preferences.

Administrators of the Sahelian colonies were squeezed from two different directions. On the one hand, they were encouraged to promote the production of raw products, notably cotton. On the other hand, the unwelcome attention of the International Labor Organization on colonial territories (and in particular the newly mandated territories turned over to France after the war) made it difficult to justify certain kinds of forced labor. Jules Carde warned his lieutenant governors, "increasingly the great colonial issues are not contained within the national domain; whether we like it or not, international organizations have a tendency to seize upon such issues, a reality there is no point in denying" (FM AGEFOM 382 Carde 1928). The varieties of coerced labor were multiple. The *"prestation"* ("service provision") could be paid either in labor or in cash. This obligation fell to those of lower social status, as the more influential could simply buy their way out or send a proxy. Prisoners could also be called on to perform heavy labor as part of their punishments. The military recruitment that prompted such abrupt population movements among young Hausa men was cast as a civic duty despite the fact that subjects were not citizens; former slaves were far more likely to have to perform military service than others.

Administrators habitually requisitioned pack animals and provisions; by an extended logic, they could also requisition labor for such collective projects as experimental cotton fields or road building. Such labor was called on in large numbers to build the new residence for the lieutenant governor in Niamey in 1931. The administration could also requisition crops at absurd prices to secure the provisions necessary for colonial employees and the peacetime army, as also happened in 1931. In the event of any reluctance on the part of the native, the *indigénat* could be invoked. In light of the increasing scrutiny of colonial labor practices, administrators of FWA were careful to establish, at least on paper, guidelines for the proper work conditions of natives "engaged" to work for the administration (ANOM FM AGEFOM 382 JO 1927 [clipping]; AGEFOM 382 Carde 1928). Carde had already begun in 1929 to prepare for the day when some of the forced labor France had relied on in the past could no longer be defended. His intention was to rely even more heavily than before on the labor of the military conscripts who were assigned to the reserve unit known as the *deuxième portion* (ANOM FM AGEFOM 382 Carde 1929; Bogosian 2002).

There was, therefore, quite a tension between the rhetoric of racial improvement and the ever more extractive practices of the colonial administration, particularly as the Great Depression deepened. The very first sign of the calamitous famine of 1931–32 in Niger appeared in the medical report for Niamey for the month of May 1931. Tellingly, the first to notice a serious problem were the nurse-midwives. The medical officer reported cases of severe starvation leading to death among both adults and children, adding, "the sage-femmes and the visiting nurses report that women do not want to have any more children because they can't feed the ones they have. Miscarriage and pre-term births are also more frequent" (ANOM FM 1AFFPOL 592 Sol "Rapport" n.d.). The famine presaged by that medical report killed thousands of people and dislocated thousands more.

In report after report written during the famine, local-level administrators had noted the deaths of very young children, the elderly, and women abandoned by husbands who had migrated. Administrators who solemnly reported populations eating leaves, roots, and the hearts of the doum palm tree nevertheless continued to collect taxes. The well-regarded Djermakoye of Dosso was rebuffed when he sounded the alarm and asked for relief and seed grain. Despite the intelligence coming in, the newly arrived lieutenant governor Louis-Placide Blacher blamed the troubles on the laziness of the Zarma and Songhai farmers who should have established grain reserves—this would be a lesson for them. By the time Blacher did attempt to provide some relief grain it was far too late. Blacher's successor, Théophile Tellier, estimated that twenty-six thousand had died in the Niamey, Dosso, and Tillabery regions and that another twenty-nine thousand had left to try to find food (ANOM FM 1AFFPOL 592 Commission d'enquête n.d.)

Colonial Inspector Bernard Sol, who was to write up a report for the inquest commission, placed the blame squarely on the shoulders of Lieutenant Governor Blacher and local-level administrators who mindlessly estimated crop yields and tax receipts based on formulas that bore no relationship to the farming realities of the region: "The tax is too high, far too high. There's no point in emphasizing now that just because it is collected without resistance that doesn't mean that [the tax level] has any relation to the native's abilities. If the tax comes in, that doesn't tell you much of anything. On the other hand, the day when it doesn't come in, and you keep pushing to collect it, then disaster is not far off. And that's what happened here" (ANOM FM 1AFFPOL 592 Sol "Rapport" n.d.). Sol argued that exorbitant taxes prohibited farmers from building up a reserve of grain and livestock against years of poor harvests; the farmers were left without any safety net.

The inquest commission was, partly as a result of Brévié's intervention, less harsh in its judgment of Blacher than was Sol. The commission noted that the commander of a colony twice the size of France with a million and a half inhabitants and staffed by a tiny personnel could hardly be expected to know everything that was going on. Furthermore, the governorship of the colony of Niger had been handed off six times in the period between 1929 and 1931. The commission called for more experienced administrators, fewer shifts in their postings, the elimination of requisitions, the adjustment of taxes and labor recruitment in light of local conditions, the development of an alert system to discover famine conditions early on, and the establishment of reserve granaries and savings societies. In the future, famine should be treated as seriously as endemic and epidemic disease (ANOM FM 1AFFPOL 592 Commission d'enquête n.d.).

The crisis in Niger set the tone for the priorities across France's African territories for the remainder of the interwar years. Food security had become a central preoccupation for the first time; despite the famines of 1900–03 and 1913–14, food production had not previously been a major preoccupation in light of the push to produce raw materials for French industry. Albert Sarraut, the minister of colonies, announced to the heads of all the African territories in 1933 that although the major public works would continue, agricultural education must be the key to the future. Sarraut presented most of the recommendations of the *commission d'enquête* as aims to be taken up by all the colonies: the gradual elimination of requisitions, a careful balance between food crops and export crops, famine warning systems, and a commitment making protection against famine a priority on par with countering epidemic and endemic disease (ANOM FM 1AFFPOL 591 Sarraut 1933).

Paper Pushing

Nevertheless, by the late 1930s, administrators were juggling ever-increasing obligations: their usual tasks of raising revenue; counting people, crops, livestock, and now reserve granaries; preventing child mortality and the spread of sexually transmitted diseases; encouraging cash crop production; and promoting innovations in food production and animal husbandry. Doing a good job with this far more complex set of tasks called, once again, for detailed accounting. Tellier's replacement, Maurice Bourgine, was confident that the population would soon be happier knowing that they would now pay only what they *actually* owed in light of an exhaustive inventory of all the resources of their villages: population, livestock, crops, wells, and natural resources (ANOM FM 1AFFPOL 591 Bourgine 1934). The new assessments could document that even a growing population might have fewer taxable members and therefore would pay less in taxes than at the time of the famine (ANN 1 E 16 35 Author unknown 1934).

This new exhaustive counting of various kinds did not meet with universal enthusiasm, however. In the Zinder region, once the villagers saw that the French were actually counting the animals rather than taking the chief's word for the figures, they all ran off so that they wouldn't have to explain why the real numbers were so much higher (ANN 1 E 16 55 Vincens 1934). In Agadez, the main concern of the nomads, as reported by Lieutenant Quint in 1934, had little to do with food reserves as the French

Table 4.2 Niger Livestock Census 1937

District	Horses	Cattle	Sheep and Goats	Donkeys	Camels
Agadez	321	10,900	157,454	16,243	17,916
Bilma	85	86	2,196	942	1,457
Dori	3,243	38,434	77,838	5,638	37
Dosso	3,611	39,290	63,993	6,722	494
Fada	3,050	29,300	38,400	2,700	
Goure	7,405	84,557	225,416	19,135	1,745
Konni	5,112	58,130	155,750	14,485	6,197
Maradi	7,562	74,946	345,768	19,358	681
N'Guigmi	1,270	34,680	49,000	3,630	2,478
Niamey	4,849	76,129	103,500	6,132	964
Tahoua	3,625	135,290	671,212	24,173	19,451
Tanout	1,887	29,676	125,150	10,091	2,544
Tillabery	6,914	92,244	287,785	9,261	339
Zinder	13,775	66,278	345,000	22,650	1,067
Totals	62,709	759,940	2,648,462	161,160	55,370

Source: ANOM FM 1AFFPOL 591 Court 1937

understood them. The Tuareg felt that their traditional pastureland in the south was being encroached on and degraded by Fulani herders, whose animals consumed all the wild grains on which the Tuareg traditionally relied in times of drought (ANN 1 E 16 71 Quint 1934).

All this data was of mixed value. Certainly there was a greater investment in staff and energy to conduct these *recensements*, and much more paper was produced as a result. However, of the 1937 table above, the lieutenant governor of Niger was to offer the following caveat: "The counts given [above] were established through the census and obviously do not provide accurate figures. As a rule the underreporting is on the order of a third among the sedentary populations and by more than two thirds among the nomads. Accordingly the real figure for cattle is on the order of 1,500,000 to 2,000,000 head, while the number of sheep and goats is on the order of 4 to 5 million" (ANOM FM 1AFFPOL 591 Court 1937). In other words, despite the new and purportedly reassuringly accurate count, administrators had little confidence in the numbers and continued to work through a kind of presumptive common knowledge. Much of the information related not to human population per se but to taxable units, as in the past, and therefore was not forwarded to the Health Services. The figures were generally sent in raw—there was no analysis of trends. This is not surprising, because the categories administrators counted constantly shifted, and the population itself was constantly moving. It was extremely difficult to compare spatial units, population units, or even individual colony totals from year to year.

The requirement that the human population figures be set down by ethnic group spawned an endless reconfiguring of groups—new ones added in, others taken out—as the administrators "discovered" something new about the subtle lines of alliance and distinction among their subjects, or as shifts in status became marked by changes in naming. In 1926, there were twenty-three ethnic categories in the tables; by 1937, there were thirty. Five categories were eliminated and then mysteriously reinstated. Religion complicated the picture immensely, as did the racial and ethnic intermixing that, whether new or not, further confused the matter of counting (CAEF B-0057576/2 Afrique Occidentale Française [AOF], dénombrements de 1926–1937).

By 1938, the Colonial Ministry felt it needed a firmer grasp of the demographic situation. Governor General Léon Geismar sent a memo requesting that each of the colonies of FWA produce a study of the "causes of the failure of the population to grow" (ANS 1 H 122 versement 163, Geismar 1938). While population was rising elsewhere on the continent, he announced, for some reason it was not rising in FWA. Why? The table below casts doubt on the perception that the population was declining everywhere—if anything, the figures seem to have been going up in Niger rather than down.[7]

The governor general's request prompted a flurry of skeptical reports by medical officers working at a variety of scales within the colonies. Doctor Lieutenant Colonel Lefrou in Upper Volta (contemporary Burkina Faso) noted dryly that statistical analysis "is the art of computing precisely information that is imprecise" (ANS 1 H 122 versement 163, Lefrou 1938). In his experience as a doctor, he remarked, whenever he set out to perform screening for sleeping sickness in the villages, the population size never matched the census figures. The chiefs always claimed the men were off in Gold Coast. However, when the populations gathered for the examination, he could see that "most of the young women carried an infant on their backs," suggesting that the birth rate was strong. If the population was declining, he averred, it must be due to out-migration, not a decline in births. Given the great numbers of Mossi soldiers, offering incentives to soldiers to have more children could make sense. Contracts would need to be revised to encourage them to have even more children rather than to take more wives.

Table 4.3 Niger Population by People Group 1926–37

People Groups	1926	1928	1930	1936	1937
Aderawa			150	79,424	66,000
Aderan Gabes					9,000
French Equatorial Africa					660
Arab	2,158	2,689	4,708		4,953
Aza					509
Aznas		76,267			20,000
Bazolies		8,200			
Beriberi	88,763	76,802	69,827	45,935	46,105
Boudoumas		1,347		712	1,092
Cadots and Azas	25,128	500/	36,730		84,325
Courteys	11,802	24,300	24,964		
Dagas	13,592	12,142			
Dagara					16,815
Dahomeens			44		
Dendi	6,500	7,840	7,840		12,500
Dietkos		955	971		
Europeens	260				
Goubeye		3,000			
Gourmantche				124,965	125,164
Hausa	492,943	508,374	591,923	526,932	549,542
Kanembu	2,607	3,180	1,892		2,739
Kanuri			1,953		
Kourfey					28,068
Kourteyes/Sudie					23,380
Libyan					153
Mangas	19,084	31,987	31,692	34,894	33,688
Maouris	91,974	63,817	87,668	77,570	74,322
Métis	65	169	115		
Mobeurs	10,693	9,801	10,611	31,105	11,654
Mossi					55,722
Nigerian					1,056
Ouagos and Dagaras	8,000	7,389	20,198		7,939
Fulbe and Rimaybe	115,575	161,214	161,859	254,289	257,619
Songhays	4,603	100,477	55,700		5,018
Songourtis		956	1,166		
Soudies	9,849	24,544	1,802		
Foreign subjects		2,050			
Tiengas	6,044	2,485	2,500		
Touareg and Bella	115,347	125,424	138,924	149,929	187,107

Table 4.3 (*continued*)

People Groups	1926	1928	1930	1936	1937
Tubu	3,542	6,420	6,459	2,834	7,354
Various	177,532	19,916	22,777	276,044	3,884
Various Chad					2,199
Zarma	172,636	158,844	174,916	160,869	184,751
Total	1,378,697	1,433,200	1,457,389	1,745,427	1,815,379

Sources: CAEF B0057576/2 Afrique occidentale française (AOF), dénombrements de 1926–37

A bit more credulous, Paul Dechambenoit, the auxiliary medical officer reporting from Kindia (Guinée), pointed to a mix of cultural and medical problems as the source of the lack of growth of the population there. First of all, he suggested, the abstention from sex during nursing could be seen as the source of several obstacles to population growth:

> Any new mother who has a baby during this period of abstinence damages the honor and social standing of her family. She is treated as a prostitute by the other women of the village and loses all her social relations. They treat her as an animal and she is rejected by her family. To that moral issue one should add excision, performed on future mothers between 11 and 13 years old in order, they say, to reduce their genital sensation. I have even seen on rare occasion pregnant women in this situation [improperly pregnant] use every means they can find to prevent the birth. And if none of those abortive methods work, the woman will run off into the forest at the first sign of labor to give birth and to get rid of the baby. When she returns the villagers will be surprised that her abdomen has gotten small again, and she will say that she had a stomach illness, but that it was miraculously healed by the marabout. (ANS 1 H 122 versement 163, Dechambenoit 1938)

One solution, he proposed, would be to have an annual celebration in which the commandant, the chief, and the doctor would honor women who become pregnant during the period of abstinence. He also proposed a festival for large families and a reduction in tax for those with five children or more.

The report by Doctor Lieutenant Colonel Campunaud for Côte D'Ivoire pointed out that the local populations were more likely to report a death that reduced the tax rolls than to declare the death of a baby that had died before it was even named: "It's as if it had never existed" (ANS 1 H 122 versement 163, Campunaud 1939). Campunaud did not see any evidence of a decline in population but did suggest a number of ways in which growth might be encouraged through the improvement of education, hygiene, and record keeping; he also suggested a greater medical emphasis on social diseases, particularly syphilis and gonorrhea. He noted tartly that all these recommendations had also been made previously in reports to Roume as early as 1905.

The ever-increasing demand for reports on population prompted Lieutenant Governor Joseph Court from Niger to observe irritably that the real issue was the insufficient medical personnel. Rather than generate yet another report, he passed along verbatim the words of a subordinate stationed in Tahoua protesting the expectation that he expand syphilis testing into rural areas: "The [urban] maternity and post-natal services are massively overworked and the dispensary is already almost entirely devoted to servicing the soldiers and those who are ill. Is it a good idea to neglect the known for the unknown, which includes weekly efforts to extract unwilling villagers from their huts, like foxes from their dens?" The harried doctor closed his report with the sharp rebuke: "here, as in all branches of administrative activity we must either simplify and reduce the bureaucratic formalities required . . . or increase the number of functionaries" (ANN 1 H 2 23 Court 1937).

These reports were almost all written by military doctors, for France continued to rule the Sahelian zone largely through a military apparatus. The demands of the military were very much at the forefront of the concerns of the medical services. It was essential to meet the *tirailleurs'* needs first—the actual French presence in Niger continued to be quite small by comparison. Furthermore, as Lefrou proposed, the soldiers and their families were exemplary populations, both for others to emulate and for the French to employ in their experiment with a kind of positive social hygiene.

Niger, it appears, did not manage to produce anything at all in the way of a direct response to the request for a demographic study. In the months preceding the outbreak of World War II, Niger's beleaguered lieutenant governor Jean Rapenne was chastised by Governor General Pierre Boisson in Dakar for failing to send along the requested studies of birth and death in proper table form to contribute to an overview of demography in FWA. Rapenne in turn expressed his dissatisfaction to his own subordinates, some of whom, he observed, did not appear to have made much of an effort to respond to this important matter. He urged his commandants to pressure the doctors in their ambit to produce the requested reports (ANN 1 H 2 10 Rapenne 1939). It emerged that the matter was complicated by the fact that administrative districts (*cercles*) didn't necessarily correspond with medical circumscriptions. Administrators often had little authority over the medical personnel.

Rapenne suggested a variety of ways in which commandants should work to improve birth rates, such as enforcing "a minimum age, below which the consummation of marriage would be forbidden" and setting a maximum level for the key marriage transaction offered by the family of the groom to the family of the bride. The idea was that the younger and presumably more fertile men would thereby be in a position to marry and contribute to the growth of the population. These suggestions were marked off with a pair of red question marks by at least one reader, probably the chief medical officer. Certainly the mechanism for enforcing these prescriptions was not at all clear.

Rapenne also had some thoughts about the duties to be expected of African medical personnel. The feeding of children at weaning deserved attention from visiting nurses; these junior nurses were also to keep an eye out for cases of syphilis and gonorrhea, which might be contributing to low birth rates and infant mortality. Both visiting nurses and *sage-femmes* ought to insist on postpartum rest for mothers; in addition, they should provide oversight of traditional birth attendants.[8] He also requested that commandants suggest practical solutions to the problem of overseeing the health of prostitutes. Rapenne was evidently unduly optimistic about what his male European personnel could accomplish through these female African intermediaries. His request went entirely unanswered. With the outbreak of the war, any policy directed at enhancing the well-being of the African subject population fell by the wayside in favor of an energetic effort to provision France during the war. As large numbers of FWA doctors were recalled to serve in Europe, the already understaffed health services shifted into crisis mode.

After the fall of France in June 1940, Governor General Boisson instructed his lieutenant governors throughout FWA to concentrate the dispensaries in a limited number of locations near markets and transport and to focus exclusively on contagious diseases. Anything that was not contagious was to be handled with dilute medicines in the hope that patients might benefit from the power of suggestion (ANN 1 H 3 9 Boisson 1940). By December, Rapenne had been replaced by Maurice Falvy, who as a brigadier general was seen as more suited to defending Vichy France from the encroachments of the "enemy" territories of British Nigeria, Italian Libya, and Gaullist Chad. Falvy closed the borders, prohibited migratory labor, and embarked on a program of increased production, taxation, and requisition with a view to redirecting all Niger's production toward France. His regime's unvarnished appropriation of labor and commodities (peanuts, livestock, millet, and oils) reduced Rapenne's lofty colonial enterprise to a business of forcible extraction that contributed to yet another series of famines across Niger (Fuglestad 1983, 139–41).

The unrelenting pressure of the war brought into visibility the ambiguous status of the Bella, who as the former slaves of the Tuareg were expected by both the French and the freeborn Tuareg to continue to bear the burden of any labor demanded by their masters or any requisitions demanded by France. They were to be listed in the census within the household of the master, who in principle paid their tax for them. Many Bella preferred to become heads of household on their own account and to pay their own tax; tax payment had in a sense become the mark of free status. Large groups of Bella wandered off into neighboring circumscriptions in order to be listed as household heads at census time. Their masters then sought the support of the French administration to force their laborers to return. In the context of a census in 1943, a hapless administrator named Texier attempted to reduce the tensions that had erupted in Tillabery between errant Bella and their masters by drawing up an agreement through which the services of Bella "domestics" would be delimited and the tribute to be offered to their "patrons" clarified. The convention implied in effect that the Bella were free agents capable of entering into a contract. His efforts were met with fury by the colonial inspector, who informed the lieutenant governor that the "primitive and backwards population" of Bella could under no circumstances exhibit such independence and that the census would have to be redone (ANN 5 E 2 5 Author unknown, inspecteur du cercle Tillabéry 1943).[9]

The dilemma of how to handle the former slaves of the Tuareg threw into high relief the essentially political character of the census and the undeniable relationship between taxation and population counting. Within the census tables, the Bella were bundled into the category "Tuareg and Bella," but such figures were very misleading. The Bella were far more prolific than their former masters. It was becoming clear that, in demographic terms, the Tuareg were soon going to become insignificant next to their former slaves and that the status quo could not stand forever (ANN 5 E 2 5 Reeb 1947). The only real reason to establish the "race" of any given subject was to make clear the line of indigenous authority through which colonial exactions could be made. If the Bella were not under the authority of the

Tuareg chiefs, to whom would they deliver their taxes? What kind of *justice indigène* would they answer to? And, crucially, how could their labor be exploited?

Soldiers and the Threat of "Venereal Disease"

Although the relationship between population and venereal infection was unclear, medical officers were clearly concerned that sexually transmitted infections (STIs) might contribute to patterns of low population growth. A variety of quasi-demographic studies conducted by the medical personnel in Niger suggested to the administration that in some regions population size remained stagnant. A variety of reasons were adduced to account for this pattern: the polygamy of impotent wealthy men with multiple nubile young women, damage caused by premature commencement of sexual activity of young brides, high sterility rates in some regions, and miscarriage caused by syphilis (IMTSSA 62 Saliceti 1941, 95–96). Another factor proposed was the premature aging of women who were overworked far into pregnancy (IMTSSA 62 Saliceti 1943, 112). Women were also assumed to engage in induced abortion, which in addition contributed to sterility (IMTSSA 62 Saliceti 1943, 113). In the absence of good epidemiological data, this broad set of potential contributing factors was difficult to assess.

Certainly, much of the energy of the medical services across FWA during World War II was devoted to handling syphilis cases in posts with large numbers of soldiers. In 1943, General Medical Inspector Ricou, who oversaw both public health and the military medical services, drew up what appears to be the first study of STIs across FWA. Ricou's conclusions, based on the previous five years of hospital records, were grim: "venereal diseases are extremely widespread in FWA. Syphilis weighs heavily in the demographic future of the local populations" (ANN 1 H 29 26 Ricou 1943, 1). The question of STIs was clearly a central preoccupation because it affected soldiers. Field-testing techniques of the time could not reliably detect gonorrhea, which contributed to the emphasis on syphilis in most reports, including Ricou's. We also know now that venereal syphilis, endemic syphilis, and yaws are very difficult to distinguish and that diagnoses of syphilis without blood tests may have been inaccurate. Ricou worked with the data that was available at the time, not all of which would have been reliable.

In urban centers, the problem appeared at least approachable. The medical and policing infrastructure in Dakar in 1943 was such that the twenty-three to thirty European prostitutes, grouped into five "permitted houses" were visited twice a week by a doctor and each given a blood test every two months to test for STIs. The inspector noted that "the number of these pensioners is notoriously inadequate for the number of clients (particularly the French soldiers and their allies)"—a recognition that where there were soldiers, there would necessarily be prostitutes. Of course the numbers of indigenous women engaging in sex with soldiers in the city was much higher and difficult to oversee: "the women that the police have been able to identify disappear, change their names, move to another house, and escape all medical screening and treatment. . . . Indigenous women," he continued, "present the most dangerous disease reservoir for treponema, gonococcus and Ducrey's bacillus" (Ricou 1943, 23). Attention to STIs among the African population was a matter of self-interest on the part of the military hierarchy.

Outside Dakar, the situation was difficult to assess and impossible to control. Only Dakar had the benefit of the laboratory of the Pasteur Institute to run regular blood tests on prostitutes and to confirm the diagnoses made in the hospitals and clinics. In the absence of blood tests, Ricou relied on hospital records to gain a sense of the proportion of individuals who came in for treatment following a diagnosis of venereal disease. On closer inspection, Ricou found that a great deal of the syphilis appeared to have been congenital—of the 73,952 children under two who were brought in for consultations in Senegal (excluding Dakar), 3,193 were diagnosed as having syphilis (4.3%). Of the 84,147 children from two to five brought in for treatment, 5,005 were treated for syphilis (0.58%); of those, 83 cases were fatal (Maladies Vénériennes, 4). In French Sudan, the figures were similar. Syphilis far outstripped gonorrhea or chancroids there as well: 4.2 percent of children under two who came in for consultation were treated for syphilis. In the schools, if the figures are to be believed, there were 774 cases of syphilis, which would represent 10 percent of the student body. Many of those cases may actually have been yaws. Ricou noted that within French Sudan, it was the nomadic Fulbe, Tuareg, and Maure populations that were most affected.

Niger, for once, appeared to have a modest advantage over the other colonies (with the exception of the city of Dakar) in that the persistence of military rule had enabled administrators in the northerly towns to maintain medical surveillance over prostitutes. In 1942, among the 610 prostitutes examined, 275 (45%) were hospitalized for a venereal disease (Maladies

Vénériennes, 13). Children under two brought in for consultation were treated for syphilis 4.4 percent of the time, a figure very close to those in French Sudan and Senegal; however, children from two to five were also treated for syphilis 4.4 percent of the time, suggesting that hereditary syphilis was having a particularly big impact in Niger (12). Beyond these figures based on consultations and diagnosis, Ricou also reported the results of a study done in Zinder among Hausa women. Among the 165 women over forty-five years of age, there were 22 who had *never* been pregnant—a startling 13.33 percent. Among the 143 women who had had pregnancies, there were a total of 526 pregnancies, of which 34 miscarried and 11 were stillborn. That meant that 8.55 percent of the pregnancies did not produce a living child. In a similar study done in Tanout, 69 of the 1,256 pregnancies completed resulted in miscarriage or stillbirth, a failure rate of 5.49 percent (13).

Ricou did not draw the plausible inference that the soldiers also had a very significant role in spreading disease among indigenous women. Certainly, after the war, medical administrators struggled with the public health consequences of demobilization, for it was no longer possible to dictate the behavior of the soldiers with the postwar elimination of the *indigénat*. In officially sanctioned sites of prostitution known as Military Field Bordellos, the military could require soldiers to be checked for sexually transmitted disease before entry. Administrators wondered whether demobilized soldiers could be forced to accept treatment should they be known to be infected, whether they could be prosecuted for knowingly transmitting such diseases, and whether their families should be encouraged to declare fatalities due to serious contagious illness (ANN 1 H 3 25 Commandant de cercle Fada 1946; ANN 1H 3 25 Toby 1946).

Ricou recommended that the health service reinforce and expand its work in the face of venereal diseases by drawing from the successful model used to combat sleeping sickness by Eugène Jamot. The Mission Jamot had deployed mobile crews equipped to screen populations and to treat those infected with a view to eliminating the disease reservoir in France's mandate territory of Cameroon. Jamot's approach had been authoritarian, experimental, and—given the treatment options available at the time—risky for the patients treated. Setting up a similarly invasive and ambitious screening for STIs in the FWA would have been extremely difficult in both financial and political terms (Bado 2011, 201; Lachenal 2013).

In fact, something more like the reverse occurred. With the end of the war, it was more difficult to justify the institutionalization of prostitution in Military Field Bordellos. Within France, a growing antipathy for the licensed houses of prostitution that had been frequented by German soldiers during the war led to the passage of a 1946 law rendering prostitution illegal and criminalizing pimping. Once the law eliminated them, a fairly significant sector of the economy—particularly in cities and towns frequented by large numbers of soldiers—was disrupted (ANN 1 F 2 20 Barthes 1946). The practical epidemiological implication of the law was that there was no longer any way to require prostitutes (or their clients) to undergo regular check-ups and treatment for sexually transmitted disease.

In Niger, single women (generally divorced or widowed) typically rented rooms in the home of an older woman known in Niger as a *magajiya*. This female homeowner did not serve as a pimp in any way, although she did ensure the safety of her renters and provided a convivial environment by selling things like cola nut and locally brewed beer. In Tahoua, women designated a particular male trader to represent them in conflicts with the administration. But he did not replace the *magagiyas*, and his compensation consisted of serving as unofficial purveyor of cloth and perfume to the prostitutes (ANN 1 F 2 20 Chiramberro 1952). Such women were not particularly difficult to find, as the houses of *magajiya* were well known in their neighborhoods. Thus, although there were not official military brothels across Niger, the health services had been able to use the law to keep track of the spread of STIs. This health inspection had had a policing dimension; in Niger, the security forces had worked together with the health services to make periodic checks among known prostitutes. From the vantage point of the health services, the new law eliminated health controls without actually eliminating prostitution. In fact, it appeared that prostitution was on the rise and that women were far more mobile in the knowledge that the health inspection was no longer required. The upshot was a 45 percent increase in diagnosed syphilis cases across the medical services between 1942 and 1948 (ANN 1 F 2 20 Espitalier 1950).

In Niamey, the medical services worked with the police to pressure prostitutes to undergo testing and treatment, focusing particularly on the village of Gamkale near the military camp and then by seeking the cooperation of the known *magajiyas* within Niamey (ANN 1 F 2 20 Mathurin 1951). For a time, this collaborative approach appears to have worked fairly well and was replicated elsewhere in the pre-Saharan zone where the hardest-hit groups were to be found: Manga, Tubu, Arabs, and Fulani. The newer treatment with penicillin was far more effective and appears to have attracted nomadic populations to the health centers. The doctors were alarmed by what they were finding: 10 percent of the prostitutes in Niamey and Ayerou had contagious syphilitic lesions (ANN 1 F 2 20 Lorre 1951). In a climate in which French intrusions into African private lives was particularly resented, the efforts to regularly test prostitutes were falling apart (ANN 1 F 2 20 Bocce 1952; ANN 1 F 2 20 Cassagnaud 1952).

Military doctors were inclined to threaten to close down any *magajiyas* who did not cooperate with inspections, but the governor of Niger was wary of the possible anger such a move might provoke in an increasingly militant political environment. Indeed, it did not take long for African soldiers and functionaries to step in protectively on behalf of their favored *magajiyas* and prostitutes (ANN 1 F 2 20 de Boisboissel 1952). There was a clear limit to how intrusive the administration could be, particularly as these "free women" were often recruited to events sponsored by the emerging parties in the leadup to the 1956 territorial elections.

Notes

1. A perusal of the *Annuaire statistique des territoires d'outre-mer* of 1948 setting out data from the 1930s is sobering. The sheer level of activity in the single colony of Madagascar far outpaces that of the entire FWA. Institut National de la Statistique et des Études Économiques (1948).

2. The métis son of a French colonial administrator and his Fulani mistress, Condat was raised as an "orphan" in the Hausa-speaking east of the country. After a brief career in the colonial military, he went on to become a politician and was elected deputy to the French National Assembly from 1948 to 1959. His alliances shifted with the political winds, enabling him to become president of the Territorial Assembly, then an ambassador to Germany, and later the United States. Fuglestad (1983, 154–55, 161–62, 180–81); Saidou (2012); Idrissa and Decalo (2012, 134).

3. Mauritania, which also levied taxes by "tribe," had absolutely no good reason to conduct a census of its highly mobile population; figures for Mauritania in the file consist of one telegram sent on May 1, 1907, reporting that their best guess was 190,000 Maures and another 103,000 "blacks." ANOM 22 G 20 Statistiques Télégramme 163 May 1, 1907.

4. Gado cites both French colonial documents and geographer Michael Watts on British northern Nigeria (1993, 72–76). The famine is known in western Niger by the Zarma expression *Ize-Neere*, which could refer to the pawning of a slave or criminal or to the exchange of a child for food in time of famine. The practice generally entailed the exchange of a child by his or her maternal uncle. Sometimes a girl would be offered in marriage in exchange for food.

5. I shall refer to biomedically trained nurse-midwives as *sage-femmes* with the Americanized plural throughout. Where traditional birth attendants are referred to as *matrones* because they have a formalized association with medical structures, I will use

the italicized French term *matrone*. ANOM FM 1AFFPOL 3058 Table effectifs des diverses sections de l'École de Médecine 1921–26.

6. The report in question would have been by Robert H. Forbes, an American cotton specialist who served as an adviser for France's cotton policy, particularly in the context of the Office du Niger in French Sudan. Roberts (1996, 35, 147).

7. The request was prompted by an essay by two experienced colonial doctors, Frank Cazanove and Alexandre Lasnet, on the demography of the French colonies produced for the Office International d'Hygiène, a precursor of the World Health Organization. Despite the imperfect data, the two respected authors appear to have been confident that the population of FWA was not growing. They suggested that it would be useful to study a number of issues of a cultural nature as well as the effects of military service and labor migration. Health-related causes of a decline in birth rates might include syphilis, gonorrhea, malaria, poor food, overwork of women, umbilical cord infections, pulmonary infections, lack of clothes, gastroenteritis, and parasites. ANS 1 H 122 versement 163, Cazanove and Lasnet 1930.

8. In the absence of adequate numbers of *sage-femmes*, Niger made a push to make more use of the *matrones* by offering inducements for better handling of birth conditions and postnatal care. Without oversight, it is hard to see how this solution could have had much effect. ANN 1 H 2 10 Maternité: Actes officiels Arrêté no. I.I41/SS.

9. Interestingly, all the ANN 5 E 2 5 documents appear to have been assembled by Jean Toby in 1951 in order to craft a response to a UN questionnaire on servitude and slavery. The marginal notes suggest that he found Texier's solution quite promising.

5

PERILS OF PREGNANCY
AND CHILDBIRTH

FRANCE'S CONCERN TO MANAGE THE REPRODUCTION OF THE Africans under its domination took two forms. On the one hand, the attention to population prompted the impulse, seen in the preceding chapter, to count people and to record the practices of ethnolinguistic groups. On the other hand, it entailed improving the African "races" in quantity and quality (Schneider 1990). In this chapter, I set out the halting growth of the medical services relative to reproductive health in French West Africa (FWA) up to 1950 to draw attention to the striking absence of health infrastructure in Niger and much of the Sahel. Prior to 1920, the major thrust of health interventions was directed at measures to protect European populations in cities. In the interwar years, a significant infrastructure (named for Pasteur) was developed to address infectious disease (Azevedo 2017, 243–82). However, in terms of primary health care and reproductive health, the impact was very slim.

Certainly, in the interwar years, the concern to foster population growth prompted greater attention to women and children. However, scholars sometimes mistake France's pronatal rhetoric and colonial accounting for a fully realized policy. The rapid growth of numbers of prenatal consultations from 6,104 in 1929 to 470,000 in 1937, for example, gives the illusion that visible progress was occurring on the ground (Conklin 2002, 150). But French West Africa was not a single colony; it was a vast federation in which a government medical corps growing at a glacial pace could not keep up with the urgent and growing needs of the population, particularly in the landlocked region of the Sahel where (unlike the coasts and North Africa) precious few missionaries were present to fill the void.

Practices related to pregnancy, childbirth, nursing, and weaning were shifting during this period as a result of the expansion of Islam and the unresolved tensions between Islamic therapeutics and local ritual practice addressing spirits. In this chapter, I hope to convey what childbirth was like in the early decades of the twentieth century and how it was gradually changing. Childbirth was a rite of passage into adulthood for women. It has to be understood against the backdrop of the socialization of boys and girls in general and in the context of the deepening relevance of shame. As the century progressed, the decline in conjugal abstinence that accompanied the expansion of Islam complicated immensely the timing of conception, nursing, and weaning. Some of the resources previously available to women and men to control their fertility were gradually being undermined with urbanization and colonial rule. Those resources included skills learned in adolescence to inculcate sexual restraint and noncoital sex, temporary relocation of mothers while nursing, and, of course, infanticide. While a premium on the capacity to withstand pain continued to be part of the disciplining restraint of shame, how pain was experienced was shifting in tandem with changes in practices marking the transition to adulthood of young men and women.

In the midst of all this change, the traditional birth attendant was a constant. In the absence of sufficient African and European medical personnel, the traditional birth attendant continued to be the first and often the only figure to whom pregnant women could turn. Unlike traditional midwives in some other parts of the colonial world, these women had very little empirical knowledge to assist in delivery; they were generally simply postmenopausal women who had received no systematic apprenticeship other than their own experiences.[1] Because shame required that women labor silently and alone, the midwife generally only entered the scene after the baby cried. Unlike Ammanite birth attendants in colonial Vietnam, for example, they had no repertoire of practices regularly deployed during labor (Nguyen 2016). In this chapter, I attempt to establish the significance of these women, often referred to as *matrones*. Silence, secrecy, and restraint, all linked to the concept of shame, were of the utmost importance to women in the context of the ever-changing perils of pregnancy and childbirth. The *matrones* understood this to a degree that European-trained *sage-femmes* and doctors could not. The occult skills of the *matrones* were far more important to women than any practical empirical knowledge they might have brought to delivery.

A Child's-Eye View of Childbirth

For three days Aissa, Madame Kandalla, has been in pain. She cries, she screams, and she repeats over and over "I am lost, forever!" The poor little thing is accompanied by her neighbors who attempted to console her. Childbirth. . . . [*sic*] In the morning, sitting in the village gathering place under a shade tree I hear cries and long deep moans. The fateful moment had arrived when Aissa was to give birth. I watched the home of the suffering woman anxiously. Soon an old woman, Toko, the *matrone* [traditional birth assistant] of the village, entered into the shelter. All the other women immediately left the room. That's strange, I thought. I wondered how and under what conditions this procedure [*opération*] would occur. (C 71 Jean-Louis Méon n.d.)

One of the most striking of the student memoirs from the École Normale William Ponty was written by a Nigerien by the name of Jean-Louis Méon at the close of the 1930s. This autoethnography of the Zarma was rich in description of the many different status positions and specialized forms of labor encompassed by one ethnolinguistic tag. This variety of activity (farmers, warriors, fishermen, hunters) and nomenclature frustrated his teacher's desire for a unitary narrative; the marginalia reveal a great deal about the limits of the French colonial imagination. Rather than see all this diversity as a predictable part of an environment in which activities related to the river, to hunting, to farming, and so on coincided with complex histories of immigration and long-standing fissures in social structure, the professor complained that Méon contradicted himself.

In structure, such student memoirs typically began with broad generalities and progressed to personal narratives about individuals, often without a clear transition to account for the shift or an explanation of the nature of the narrative (fiction, memoir, folktale?). Following this pattern, Méon offered a lengthy and vivid description of a birth he had witnessed:

Aissa was on her knees, arms stretched out, and her fingers squeezing tightly the fine sand of the floor of the house. This was no longer a woman but a monster; and this was not a birth but some kind of operation—something damaging, complex, nameless, and bizarre—there were no rules, no method. This procedure is just based on the often fanciful experiences of old women, governed only by cabalistic symbols and koranic verses. Toko approaches the suffering woman mumbling some prayers. She pushes hard against her lower stomach to reduce the pain but most of all to push the baby out . . . Then suddenly, as if struck by vertigo [Aissa] collapses onto a pile of cloth red with her blood. Toko herself seems afraid. She leaves, calls another old woman who is more expert and returns.

An old woman of perhaps seventy, bent trembling over her cane, her eyes half closed, enters. . . . With the assistance of Toko, she has the patient lie down with her belly against the log. As Toko continued to massage Aissa's upper and lower back, Hawa repeated a prayer over and over with an air of contrition "*Yaladifou! Yaladifou!*," which means "Oh, Merciful God!" Then after every imaginable effort the baby came out.

The two old women cried out in one voice "*Alhamdulillah!* Thank God!" Toko, with a light in her eyes came out and called to the uneasy and impatient relatives, "*A don a bon*: she has had her head," meaning that she is free. (C 71 Jean-Louis Méon n.d.)

Méon's teacher, skeptical from the very outset that a woman could be in labor so long, noted in the margin, "Three days? You are exaggerating." Nor was he convinced that the moment of birth merited the characterization as *fatale* or "fateful."[2]

Shifting to the ethnographic present, Méon explained that the *matrone* would wash the baby and then have the baby drink cow's milk, which was "generally more nourishing for the baby." For three days the baby would "absorb" milk in this manner and only on the third day would it be put to its mother's breast. The father would be informed of the birth, and he would seek out powerful Muslim marabouts or traditional priests for amulets to protect the baby from witches, Satan, and malevolent magicians.

Méon and the other male students of the École William Ponty seem to have taken far more interest in issues related to childbirth and infant care than did their teachers.[3] Typical assignments often focused on the socialization of children in the context of colonial concerns about male education and indigenous authority. Those assignments never posed direct questions about childbirth or infant care so far as I can tell. For example, the memoir of Maurice N'Diaye Mody Diabe included verbatim the full assignment for the essay topic, "the child in its family milieu." It required demographic observations of a particular place, a discussion of beliefs about the child prior to its birth, observations about how a child is named, and an account of who has authority over the child (C 3 N'Diaye Mody Diabe Maurice 1948–49). As we have seen in the preceding chapter, teachers prompted the students to think in terms of "population" and demography, which makes sense in light of the bureaucratic imperative to count and codify populations.

Nevertheless, the memoirs are surprisingly rich in material on beliefs and practices related to pregnancy, childbirth, and infant care. Oft-repeated assignments related to the upbringing (*éducation*) of the child in the family gave rise to observations by the students related to the behavior of the mother well before the child had even been born. By their understanding, the human child was already in social and moral formation well prior to birth; that social and moral formation would continue during the birth process and into infancy. These sources give us a rare glimpse into this intimate realm. Colonial-era ethnographers, regularly working explicitly to provide information perceived to be useful to colonial administration, did not generally take much interest in the affairs of women (Walentowitz 2003, 21).

Enduring Pain, Cultivating Fertility

The Cahiers Ponty reveal some of the many ways in which adolescents were taught self-restraint, tolerance of pain, and submission to authority—all necessary for the successful birth and rearing of a recognizable social person (cf. Davison 1989). Diakite Mamadou, a Muslim Malinke from Guinea, was bitterly sarcastic about the abusiveness of his own ritual initiation. He reported in 1945 that both boys and girls underwent genital cutting. Boys would be circumcised at about fifteen. Although the practice was understood to be required by Islam, it was performed by the blacksmith, a powerful occult specialist. During a period of three months, the blacksmith would teach the young men never to cry, to be "obsequiously polite" to elders, to rise early, to pray regularly to Allah, and to suffer pain and hardship with resignation.

Diakite reported that "the elders required excision of women, supposedly to make them less sensitive to love [*sensibles à l'amour*] and therefore less likely to commit adultery" (C 14 Diakite Mamadou 1945). A girl would undergo excision between the ages of six and fourteen; only after this could she be married. It is not clear that men saw much difference between male circumcision and female excision; for example, another Guinea student commented that the two ceremonies were conducted at the same time and that "the operation [for young 'women' of about twelve] doesn't differ very much from circumcision. The treatment is the same" (C 33 Samoura Sinkoun n.d.). Both young men and young women were taught during these ceremonies that above all they must make good on their responsibility to have children. Women were to be docile "like a sheep" while men were to "multiply the blood" of their family line by producing many children. If they failed to do so, they were warned that "the ancestors are abandoned and the family extinguished" (C 14 Diakite Mamadou 1945).

Circumcision and excision were explicitly intended to be experienced as martial and painful; surmounting the pain stoically marked a youth as particularly admirable (C 30 Diouck Sanor 1949; C 30 Diallo Seydou 1949; C 30 Oumar Diouf 1949). The centrality of pain and endurance to the ritual prompted Jean-Louis Méon to express contempt for the faddish practice of infant circumcision of male babies, which seemed to him to be of no utility; a boy should be circumcised at eight, to prepare him to pray properly and to have a pure body. Only once he was ready to pray five times a day at about age ten would a boy be given adult male clothing and become recognizably Muslim (C 71 Jean-Louis Méon n.d.).

These were the perceptions of young men in a highly Islamized region, not those of women, and one suspects that women might have had other interpretations of such ceremonies. Among Bamana, the capacity to endure pain was linked to a profound valorization of silence and controlled speech. Silence and verbal discretion, Brett-Smith notes, ensured the safety of villages vulnerable to slave raiding and could therefore be highly valued among non-Muslims. Cutting rituals emphasized the endurance of pain for both men and women. Men were being hardened, in principle, to be warriors, while women were being hardened for the difficulty of childbirth. This gendered pairing of men with war and women with childbirth is nicely captured in the common Sahelian adage "childbirth is war" (Olivier de Sardan, Moumouni, and Souley 2001; Brett-Smith 2014, 223). While in some settings genital cutting was practiced, in many others it was not, even within the same ethnolinguistic group.[4] Other ritual markers could mark restraint in the face of pain, including painful scarification or tattoos on highly sensitive parts of the body, such as the lips.

As the colonial enterprise set in, participation in the colonial military in effect became a related stage of passage into male adulthood in some settings. Numerous Ponty memoirs mention that marriage for young men was now displaced until after the completion of military service (C 3 N'Diaye Mody Diabe Maurice 1949; C 14 Caba Sory 1949; C 30 Amadou Badiane 1949). A young Zarma man in Niger might prove his manliness by undertaking a difficult period of migratory labor to the cities along the coast. Restraint in the face of pain would mark the difference between the mature and the immature, the old and the young, those who could command the labor of others and those whose labor could be commanded, and, in this case, those who could pray and dress as a Muslim adult and those who could not.

Sustaining the Life of the Infant: Sexual Restraint, Nursing, and Polygyny

Despite what might appear at first to be restrictive sexual mores, Sahelian girls and boys in the early decades of the century were permitted—indeed expected—in many societies to have romances prior to marriage, with the strict understanding that such intimacy must never lead to pregnancy. Fulani girls in some settings were permitted to engage in sexual play with boys prior to puberty. The shame for a girl was not in engaging in sexual play but in losing her virginity to anyone other than her husband (Wilson-Haffenden 1967 [1927], 260–62). Such arrangements cultivated the appropriate boundaries of sexual restraint while providing youth with an initiation into sexuality. The virginity of the bride at her wedding attested to her proper upbringing, her powers of self-restraint, and her respect for the desires of her parents (who often did *not* intend to marry her to her boyfriend). Not surprisingly, Diakite Mamadou observed in the context of Malinke that the question of the virginity of unmarried girls could become "the cause of a great deal of trouble in some families" (C 14 Diakite Mamadou 1945). When a Fulani girl became pregnant by her fiancé, it might be regarded as a happy sign of her fertility and pass without opprobrium. However, if she fell pregnant by someone else, the scandal would reduce her value as a potential bride. An abortion might be attempted, or her boyfriend might be compelled to both repay any gifts that had already been offered by the fiancé and to provide bride wealth to marry the girl and gain paternal rights to the child (Wilson-Haffenden 1967 [1927], 263).

These memoirs and early ethnographic studies provide important evidence that sexual experimentation could, and often did, coincide with a premium on female virginity at marriage and with genital cutting. Furthermore, neither cutting nor virginity were directly related to Islam. Among some urban Muslims, such as the Wolof of Saint Louis, girls were understood to be more flirtatious than boys and were therefore subject to more scrutiny and restrictions to their mobility (C 30 Magatte Fall 1949). In other settings in which Muslims lived alongside non-Muslims, adolescent sexual latitude could be unexpectedly permissive so long as it did not include intercourse. In a strict Islamic setting such as Futa Jallon, where the illegitimate child was understood to be excluded from both inheritance and paradise, a girl whose lover refused to recognize the child and to marry her might be pushed by the elders to commit infanticide (Dupire 1970, 153, citing Vieillard 1939, 60).

When Baba of Karo explained to Mary Smith the Hausa practice of adolescent cuddling known as *tsarance*, she situated it within the context of sleeping arrangements and space in family compounds. When children began to "have sense" (at about six years of age), they were no longer permitted to sleep in their mother's hut when she and her husband engaged in sexual relations. Small children were sent off to the hut of an older grandmother, such as Baba herself. Such children therefore clustered together and invited their friends, male and female, in what were undoubtedly festive sleepovers under the supervision of an elderly woman. If the elderly woman tired of having the children's giggles keep her from sleeping late into the night she, too, might shoo them away. These older children, between eight and twelve or so, then would invite others in the neighborhood and sleep together in "the hut in front of some compound," where they would light a lamp, tell stories, and laugh. "They laugh and joke," she reported. "They don't lie together a great deal" (M. F. Smith 1954, 178).

Baba asserted that girls were more likely to fall pregnant in the villages than in the larger towns. "If she should become pregnant before she is married her lover, if he is a good man, will say he wishes to marry her. There is a feast and everyone rejoices" (178). However, given the premium on virginity at marriage, and the possibility that the lover would not or could not accept responsibility for his actions, the girl could try to abort the pregnancy by drinking a solution of henna or indigo. Failing that, she might decide to kill the baby once it was born or to run away to a town and rely on sexual favors to survive until she found a marriage partner (178–79).

The frankness with which Baba recounts the continuation of *tsarance* within the territory that had been absorbed into the caliphate of Usman 'dan Fodio reveals the tacit approval of it in rural areas because it conveyed sexual practices and habits useful for preventing pregnancy. As recently as the 1970s, lamented one middle-aged Zarma man, "we could dance and sleep together without having sex at all, we were more disciplined, that's all gone now" (Monsieur A., Niamey, May 29, 2014). Saskia Walentowitz observes that permissiveness toward the night visits to Tuareg girls in the Azawagh prior to marriage is best understood as a means to teach both sexual pleasure and restraint—an "apprenticeship" into responsible sexuality for both men and women (Walentowitz 2003, 359).

Among Hausa speakers in the first half of the twentieth century, young men and women were grouped together in rough age sets referred to as *samariya* groups in which participants had playful titles. Members were fined for various infractions, enabling the groups to gather enough money to hire drummers to dance. The *samariya* groups competed with one another and were called on to participate in work parties at major moments of the farm season, in particular at harvest. Young men would show off their prowess cutting the millet while the girls encouraged them with songs and dancing. Beer might be provided as compensation for the work of the day (M. F. Smith 1954, 60–61, 260 note 6). Baba's account shows the ambivalence urban Muslims could feel about these practices. She had to sneak out to watch such dances as a girl, and as an adult she prevented girls in her charge from taking part in *samariya* activities, especially at night (M. F. Smith 1954, 60–61, 179).

In Hausa settings, genital cutting was limited to the circumcision of boys well past infancy, although some Hausa households in Nigeria long exposed to Fulani practices did introduce a kind of nicking of the clitoris of a girl baby. In such settings, the relationship between pregnancy and excision was not nearly as relevant as it might be in regions in which the cutting was featured as a major rite of passage prior to marriage and childbearing. On the other hand, one senses that the status of a boy's circumcision relative to his first sexual act might well be noted less with opprobrium than with humor. The 1934 Bargery Hausa-English dictionary reveals the richness of the Hausa words and expressions that captured the sexual experimentation of young men: *tsaranci* ("fornication between children," derived from *tsarance*); *do'bane* ("sexual intercourse by uncircumcised lad"); *kurkuda* ("precocious sexual indulgence after circumcision"); *shashe bakin aska* ("indulge in sexual intercourse as soon as healed after circumcision. To fail to do so will, it is urged, be severely punished in the next world"); *'dugulle* ("a form of precocious sexual indulgence"). The terms notably distinguished between sexual behavior by uncircumcised, unhealed but circumcised, healed and recently circumcised, and simply "normal" sex by a young man who has never married.

The premarital sexual experimentation of girls, on the other hand, did not receive the same degree of nuance—either a girl fell pregnant or she didn't. The vocabulary in Bargery related to women focuses far less on sexuality than on pregnancy, or, to be even more precise, on the exact timing of conception. If premarital sexual play was condoned, it implicitly had to be noncoital, but the burden of that obligation fell to girls. The pregnancy of an unmarried girl of course deserved its own name, *giribtu*, suggestive of the public loss of her virginity as evidenced in her pregnancy. But the vocabulary for married women's pregnancies was also quite specific. For example, a woman who fell pregnant while nursing would be said to have *rurrutsa*; the word is an intensive conveying excessive speed or an overflowing vessel. A child born of such a pregnancy might be referred to as *kwanika*, implying shamelessness or unseemliness. If such a pregnancy took a woman by surprise because she did not believe she could fall pregnant yet, it was referred to as a *dunhu*, a hard calabash. A pregnancy that occurred while a woman was still nursing and had not yet experienced the return of her menses was known as *bunk'u*, a word suggestive of the bursting forth of a shallowly planted seed or the cracking of the ground by a root crop.

Why such attention to the *timing* of conception among married women? A woman who became pregnant while still nursing had violated a strong prohibition against conjugal sex while nursing; that violation was just as evident to others as a pregnant girl's loss of virginity. Across the Sahel, the norm up until the middle of the twentieth century was that a woman would nurse a child for two years before becoming pregnant again. Maurice Delafosse claimed in 1912 that across the region from the upper Senegal river to the Niger, sexual relations were forbidden while a woman was menstruating, during pregnancy, and during nursing for two to three years, "such that a man who had only one wife would often be either constrained to endure an intolerable chastity or obliged to throw himself upon the wife of his neighbor—the custom of polygyny was designed to reduce as much as possible this disruption of family and society" (Delafosse 1972 Vol. III, 59–60). A later 1930s ethnographic overview of marriage practices of the Sudanic zone suggested that both Muslims and "fetishists" abstained from marital sex during nursing, a practice that appeared to be linked to polygyny among both communities (Delafosse, Poutrin, and Le Roy 1930, 367). From these studies it is clear that the practices of polygyny and sexual abstinence during nursing predated the spread of Islam in the region and were taken for granted in the early colonial period (Delafosse, Poutrin, and Le Roy 1930, 367, 377, 386). Not every man, however, would be in a position to take on multiple wives, nor would he necessarily feel inclined to refrain from sex with a favored wife for so long in any case. Among the largely monogamous Tuareg, men could resolve this problem in the context of female domestic slavery through their access to concubines (Delafosse 1972, Vol. III, 63; Walentowitz 2003, 247 note 75). But men without female slaves or the wealth to take multiple wives would require tremendous sexual restraint.

Among Hausa speakers, this restraint was enforced by the constant scrutiny of others conveyed through the mockery of undisciplined mothers and untimely babies. Conjugal abstinence for two years would be quite difficult to maintain; the restraint learned in *tsarance* provided couples with tools that made it easier to have sexual intimacy without necessarily falling pregnant. Bamana women as well adhered to norms of sexual restraint in part to avoid the mockery of other women (Brett-Smith 2014, 245). Men also experienced opprobrium for failing to adhere to norms. Walentowitz found that Tuaregs in Azawagh today disapprove of men who get their wives pregnant before the proper two years of nursing enjoined in the Koran, despite the ending of conjugal separation after only forty days. Such a man has proven himself incapable of proper sexual restraint; he should practice *intra crura* (non-penetrative "thigh" sex), coitus interruptus (withdrawal), or abstinence. Precipitous pregnancy leading to early weaning is, in their view, shameful and ignoble, the sort of thing that only sedentary peoples and slaves would permit (Walentowitz 2003, 244–47).

The failure to show sexual restraint or at least some mastery of fertility *within marriage* could be the cause of not simply mockery but very public scolding, as Baba tells us occurred when one of her "granddaughters," Dantambai, began having sex with her husband, Musa, only five months after her baby had been born; this was particularly shocking as he had another wife and therefore no excuse. The scandal became a crisis when Baba's granddaughter fell pregnant. The pregnancy posed such a danger to the nursing baby that the elders encouraged the couple to abort the fetus. The couple refused, imperiling the health of the nursing child, who either had to be weaned quickly so that he would not drink the milk that now "belonged" to the growing fetus, or he had to continue to nurse milk that was no longer suited to him until the normal time of weaning arrived. The story ended happily, for Baba performed a ritual for the older child using the stomach of a freshly slaughtered bull each week for several weeks to successfully protect him during an accelerated weaning (M. F. Smith 1954, 148–49).

This norm of conjugal abstinence ensured that a woman would avoid becoming pregnant while caring for an infant. From a medical standpoint, it is easy to see how pregnancy while nursing would be extremely taxing for the woman and possibly dangerous for both the infant (who might suffer from a reduction in milk supply) and the fetus (whose nutritional needs necessarily competed with the demands of nursing). Whether or not the practice of refraining from marital sex was a conscious choice to protect women and infants, the taboo certainly would have had that effect (van de Walle and van de Walle 1988). In the early colonial period, birth spacing in the region was quite commonly three years as a result of long nursing and this taboo (Cross and Barker 1992, 100, 137).

Corinne Fortier's research on "vital substances," including milk, sperm, and blood, would suggest that the belief that pregnancy "spoils" the milk derives from an ideological anxiety to establish firmly the primacy of the male contribution to a particular pregnancy (in facilitating conception, gestation, and the production of milk) through his sperm (Fortier 2001). If the milk was understood to continue to form the nursing child, and the child was indelibly the product of one lineage, it followed that the father must have a role in promoting the vital substance transmitted through the milk (Fortier 2001, 120). The necessity to wean a nursing infant immediately once a woman falls pregnant results, in a sense, from the incoherence of these imaginings if the sperm must be understood to be redirected toward the new fetus. The fetus must inevitably become jealous of the nursing child; jealousy is everywhere in the Sahel understood to be the source of misfortune. The fetus will, through its envy, somehow poison the milk, and the nursing baby will die (Fortier 2001, 111). Better to give in to the desires of the fetus and wean the nursing child.

Baba of Karo explained to Mary Smith her rather different understanding of the practice among Hausa-speaking peoples:

> If she only sleeps with her husband and does not become pregnant, it will not hurt her child, it will not spoil her milk. But if another child enters in, her milk will make the first one [the nursling] ill. . . . It is not sleeping with the husband that spoils her milk, it is the pregnancy that does that. But if her husband desires her, then in the day she carries her child, at night she carries her husband—*this is what pleases Allah*. He does not like argumentative women. But it is not right that she should sleep with her husband. (M. F. Smith 1954, 148, emphasis mine)

According to Baba's account, it had become more difficult for women in northern Nigeria—the heartland of the Islamic jihad of Usman 'dan Fodio—to enforce this two-year abstinence, even within a polygamous household, in the 1950s. Evidently, it had become acceptable for a man to argue that Islam conferred on him the right to begin sleeping with his wife again after only forty days. Jacqueline Rabain observed a similar shift occurring among Muslims in Senegal in the late colonial period (Rabain 1994, 43 note 5). Maliki judicial practice gave men the right to up to four wives without any reference to childbirth or nursing. A man's "need" for multiple wives became detached from the question of the welfare of mothers and babies and was increasingly treated as both a right and a sign of status. The length of time in which a woman could expect to "rest" after giving birth was reduced to forty days, despite Islamic arguments in favor of *al-azl* (withdrawal) to prevent pregnancy while nursing (Omran 1992; Bousquet 1950).

Perhaps because of the difficulty of childbirth and the extra strain produced by in-law avoidance as a part of proper comportment, in parts of Nigeria a young woman in the 1920s might return to her own kin to give birth and remain there until the three years of nursing had been completed. To have conjugal relations during this period was understood to spoil the baby's milk (Wilson-Haffenden 1967 [1927], 136, 278). The arrangement explains in part why patrilateral cross-cousin marriage was common in some regions, whereas a strong matrilineal component to social organization might prevail elsewhere (Dupire 1970). The rigor with which the separation of the parents was overseen may also account for why Fanne Fodé announced proudly that the Fulani women of Casamance were particularly prolific. His 1949 memoir suggests that these women managed very effectively to space their births three years apart, which would have protected both infants and mothers (C 3 Fanne Fodé 1949).

So long as the proscription on conjugal sex while nursing was treated seriously, as in Baba's account, the general pattern of three-year birth spacing between babies could be maintained through the fear of public humiliation of those who violated it. Among Hausa, women whose lactational amenorrhea was known to all because they had not returned to postmenstrual washing might be referred to as *bara'kuma* or *wangila*. Until they washed, their husbands could not, in principal, return to the marital bed. The richness of this vocabulary, alongside Baba's account of Dantambai and her pregnancy, suggests that it was not always possible for women to maintain conjugal abstinence for the full period of nursing, whether their periods had returned or not. The quite public weaning of such a child would be the occasion of commentary, for the weaning of a baby required the support of a mother's kin to take the baby while it "forgot" the breast. Of the nursing child being weaned, one might say, *an sa masa laifi*, meaning "he has been weaned through no fault of his own," implying that there was fault to be attributed elsewhere.

Critical to the survival of a child was the success of the mother in nursing the infant. Gayego Leopold accounted for the widespread practice of polygamy as being linked to nursing: "Why is Polygamy the norm? There are many reasons but the main one is procreation. The native generally does not have the means to feed children other than mothers' milk, and so he is obliged to wait three years before taking up sexual relations with the mother of a child. And so he prefers to have several wives" (C 14 Gayego Leopold n.d.). His teacher, evidently finding it hard to follow the logical flow of the paragraph, wrote a question mark in the margin. But the link between polygamy and nursing was probably self-evident to most students; consequently, Leopold didn't explain the taboo on a couple having sex while the woman is nursing. Practically speaking, abstinence ensured the continued flow of milk, since pregnancy can "dry up" the milk.

In her study, Denise Savineau reported that European males tended to see conjugal abstinence among Africans as resulting from a kind of insubordination on the part of the wife that forced men to seek out other women. Observing (somewhat implausibly) that conjugal abstinence could last as long as five years, these Europeans felt that "women [refused] their husbands and, what is worse, [took] off to live with their mother, abandoning the monogamous husband" (Savineau 2007 [1938], 20). But the African men Savineau spoke with about polygyny emphasized rather their desire to have many children. To them, having multiple wives guaranteed that some would bear children even if one proved to be infertile. Chiefs in particular felt obligated to have large numbers of wives as a mark of wealth and prestige and to do the work of cooking for a large entourage (Savineau 2007 [1928], 21). Clearly, the rapid expansion of Islam had complex implications for fertility. On the one hand, it endorsed the "solution" of polygamy for extended nursing. On the other hand, it justified the reduction in the period of marital abstinence, thereby threatening the survival of nursing babies.

Childbirth Proper and the Mystical Role of the *Matrone*

However, not all practices were altered by the expansion of Islam. The mystery and uncertainty of childbirth contributed to the resilience of practices that had no apparent origin in Islam. Maurice N'Diaye Mody Diabe complained in 1949 that the customs among his people in the largely Muslim Bambara village of N'Gologougou were "still too imbued with mysticism":

> Mysticism is the primordial source of [the Bambara's] great naiveté. Of limited imagination, he turns everything he doesn't understand into a divine being. The child is for him a supernatural being, a consoling messenger sent

from the heavens to particular privileged households, of which others are obviously going to be jealous; and it is that [jealousy], they say, that is the origin of enmity between families. The length of life of the child, they add, is a function of how it was received and how he is treated during infancy. That's why, during the nine months of the child's formation the Bambara alternately makes offerings to fetishes and prays to God [*la divinité*], in order to protect its life. (C 3 N'Diaye Mody Diabe Maurice 1949)

N'Diaye's memoir captures the ambivalence of Muslim populations that continued to draw on multiple kinds of expertise to protect wealth and well-being.

Childbirth appears to have been a domain particularly resistant to any rigid and exclusive monotheism. The child was sometimes believed to be the reincarnation of a virtuous ancestor or family member (C 14 Gayego Leopold n.d.). Georges Condat remarked that in the Hausa-speaking region, the death of an elderly person was understood to herald the birth of a future child: "The death of an elderly person will be received with as much joy as the birth of a child." The task of announcing the death throughout town would be left to small children who would run through town singing:

Grandmother is dead
We are hungry no longer
We will have the funeral millet drink to drink
May God increase me
May God increase us[5]

According to N'Diaye, the Bambara *matrone* generally succeeded in bringing the baby safely from the world of the dead and the spirits and into this world. Reversing his earlier portrayal of local practices as backward, N'Diaye remarked, "Few babies die at birth because of the supernatural techniques of the *matrones* who not only intuitively know the child, but no matter how the baby presents itself at birth they know how to skillfully exploit the situation to protect its life. Additionally they perform the traditional ceremonies of 'Sonni' through which the new creature is entrusted to the protective genies of the neighborhood" (C 3 N'Diaye Mody Diabe Maurice 1949). The mother might also make a sacrifice at the family altar, asking the protective genies to look out for the health of her child and promising to make a sacrifice of a red goat, a red dog, and a red cock if the child was born alive. She would do all this to ensure that the baby would be born normally, beautiful, alive, and "looking like the rest of the family." The concern that the genies permit the child to look like the rest of the family signaled a fear that the father or his family might reject the child. The implication was that any ugly, deformed, or simply unusual child had resulted from either adultery or from a malevolent spirit. If, happily, the child was recognized by the father, there would be a public naming ceremony in which both the family's bard (*griot*) and the family's Islamic authority (*marabout*) would have a role.

Pregnant women were to adhere to a host of prescriptive rules to prevent harm to the fetus. The unfortunate corollary was that a woman who had a miscarriage, stillbirth, deformed infant, or simply a difficult labor was assumed to have done something that angered the spirits or ancestors (or to have failed to do something that pleased the spirit world). A woman who died in childbirth was particularly likely to have occasioned the anger of the spirit world, and her body had to be handled with care. In the Hausa-speaking region, Condat tells us, "such women are buried at least three kilometers from town. This is because the local people believe that such things only happen to evil people, sorcerers, who kill their own children. And if they are not distanced [from the living] their souls will return to massacre the family" (ANN 1 G 4 6 Condat Georges Mahamane 1938–39).

Alioune Sarr noted that the Diola of his village of Nyassia in Senegal had a deep belief in the power of the caste of sorcerers, who protected the pregnant woman and her fetus in a host of different ways. Rather than remain naked, the mother would from the fifth month of pregnancy begin to wear a large blue or black cotton cloth blessed by the sorcerer. The cloth would serve as "a kind of barrier between the future baby and the undesirable gaze of others." Such dress would mark her as well as a woman who had proven to be fertile. For the first time, she would wear shoes to protect the baby from urine that might undermine the efficacy of her protective charms. She would stay within the compound and avoid contact with hideous people and ugly animals that might affect the appearance of the baby once born. She would be kind to animals and the elderly because custom holds that "women who are unkind and disrespectful will be punished with a painful and unproductive labor" (C 3 Sarr Alioune 1949).

Like N'Diaye, Sarr believed that few women or babies died during childbirth; he averred that because pregnant women go about their difficult tasks, their organs are trained for the upcoming labor. After the birth, the female "sorcerer" would wash the newborn with a cloth soaked in a liquid that would protect it from evil spirits, and later she would attach amulets that would protect the child forever. This birth attendant would also give the mother a white drink that would make her milk abundant and cause the baby to crave her milk alone. When it was time to name the child, the female sorcerer would choose the name on the basis of the time of birth, and the father would announce the name to the gathered community. That name would be the official name "without which," Sarr noted dryly "it would be possible to escape the obligations of military service and taxes" (C 3 Sarr Alioune 1949).

Sarr's use of the French word *sorcière* (female sorcerer) highlights the occult significance of birth attendants, although his choice of terminology is unusual. In Casamance, that translation reflected the coincidence of the therapeutic work of a particular clan with occult powers with the role of birth attendant. More typically, the students adopted the more prosaic French term *matrone*, which by the 1940s had become the generic term for any elderly woman who assisted in childbirth. However, as Sarr's choice of terminology suggests, the task of such women was not primarily delivering the baby. Their role was to protect the baby and the mother prior to and after delivery through prayers, charms, ablutions, and potions. Recall that the elderly women in Méon's childbirth account appear to have been called in only because of the extremely long time the mother had been in labor.

Baba of Karo, who served as a traditional midwife to many women in her family, provided this description of how her "daughter" 'Yardada gave birth:

> It was one day about noon that the people of Sarkin Yelwa's compound sent for me, they said her head was aching; I went over and found her lying on her bed. The kinswomen came, then late at night they got up and said "May Allah preserve us", and went home. 'Yardada lay down on her bed, then in the middle of the night I saw that she had got off the bed and was kneeling down; I said 'Are you all right?' She replied 'Yes, quite all right'. A little later I heard 'Ya-a-a-a-a!' I opened the door of the hut and called 'Kande, Rabi, Kwari—see here's the child, a boy!'" (M. F. Smith 1954, 249)

Baba's role was largely to take the grandchild and wash him and then to subject the new mother to a painful washing therapy for forty days using extremely hot water to clean her vagina. A woman who did not endure this painful washing silently would be treated with contempt and called a bastard (249–50). Baba had much more to report about this ritual washing than about the childbirth itself. The account underscores how a woman's capacity to endure silently during childbirth and the period of washing established her as freeborn and legitimate. The ultimate shame for a woman was to render her physicality—her bestiality—visible or audible to others. The practices of such women and of their traditional birth attendants were not necessarily Islamic in character, although they could become integral to how a community understood the proper comportment of Muslim women.

Laboring Alone

Through a variety of amusing tales, *sage-femme* Aoua Kéita conveyed the diversity of sexual and birthing practices to be found in late colonial French Sudan. Within that diversity, however, she emphasized the shared bodily and moral habits of women across a broad range of ethnic groups: "Songhai, Bambara, Wolof, Malinke, Kassonke, Serer, Samoko, Pehlhs, Diolas, Sarakoles and Bobos that I have had the occasion to assist in my long career as a midwife have all had the same behavior in the face of the pain of labor.... All these women had an admirable capacity to bear the pain caused by contractions" (Kéita 1975, 261). Her admiration was tempered by a concern about the vigilance this required on the part of the *matrone* or the *sage-femme*, because such women were likely to attempt to give birth at home without letting anyone else know—"their kin would proclaim proudly that the traditional birth attendant only woke up when she heard the cries of the baby" (Kéita 1975, 261; see also ANOM 17 G 381 Savineau Rapport 15, 1938, 37).[6] To fail to bear such pain with self-restraint and dignity could be a source of deep shame to the woman, her mother, and even her close friends (Kéita 1975, 262). Women did not take part in wars, hunting, fishing, or other dangerous activities: "their battlefield being childbirth, it was their duty to bear the pain of labor with courage and dignity.... For them, it was a test to be borne with honor" (Kéita 1975, 262; see also Belloncle 1980, 60).

This largely sedentary norm was not necessarily shared by nomads and pastoralists. Childbirth in Tuareg communities does not appear to have required the same degree of stoicism on the part of the birth mother as we see among agriculturalists. When births do not go well among Tuareg in Aza-wagh today, it may be the husband who is blamed for failing to protect his wife from the dangers of the space outside the tent, for overworking her, or for providing the wrong foods (Walentowitz 2003, 203). This takes the burden of enduring pain or failed reproduction off of the woman and opens the way to a far more communal experience of childbirth. When a pregnancy approaches its term, a woman, particularly if she is young, will return to her own mother's tent to give birth. Avoidance relations with her in-laws would make giving birth near them extremely difficult, for she would not be able to ask for help or cry out. In her mother's home, she could cry out without shame and she would receive the best of care from her maternal kin (Ag Erless 2010, 235). In addition to her own mother, she might have maternal aunts and a woman of slave ancestry from her family to assist her, someone before whom she would not need to show restraint (Walentowitz 2003, 172).

Among Tuareg in the past, a slave woman would have been likely to become the wet nurse for the child of a noble woman. This practice gave rise to complex milk kinship ties between the children of the slave woman and the noble children she has nursed. The use of wet nurses resolved the potential problem of nursing while pregnant (Walentowitz 2003, 252). Here nobility and respectability were marked far less by silence in childbirth than by the performance of restraint in marital sexuality and by showing reserve in the presence of in-laws. Noble women were enclosed in protective womb-like spaces (Ag Erless 2010, 180). While a woman might be surrounded by kin while giving birth (unlike women in sedentary societies), the grandmother was simply to catch the child with her hands by reaching under the pregnant woman's clothing when given the signal; there was no expectation that she would either examine or touch the mother or the child during labor (Ag Erless 2010, 180).

When she was young, *sage-femme* Aoua Kéita was present on two occasions when her own mother gave birth. Her mother, she reports, "always gave birth entirely alone without any assistance" (266). On the first occasion, Kéita only awoke when she heard the baby cry. The second time, in 1925, when she was about thirteen, she returned from school and her mother attempted to send her off to the kitchen. Seeing that her daughter was not willing to leave her alone, her mother had her face the wall. Like Méon, Kéita could not resist looking as her mother labored on all fours:

> When she started to push I turned towards her but I couldn't see anything, for her cloth was draped over her and covered her lower body. I could only see her naked torso. The size of her abdomen stretched to the limit, the skin of her belly of the palest brown—an indescribable color—these made a huge impression on me. I thought that this skin, so stretched, and shining so strangely, would open up to make way for the baby. At that age, I really believed that that was how things happened. I sensed from the grimace on her face, the swelling of her neck muscles and the hardening of her arm and thorax muscles, that she was making a tremendous effort. I could neither help her nor find someone to help; powerless, I began to cry hot tears, smothering my sobs. Paying no attention to my tears she continued to push. At around 10 at night she shifted

upwards gently. And just then I heard a piercing cry. My brother had arrived!
(Kéita 1975, 266–67)

If this fortitude in the face of labor was honorable and admirable, it had the effect of diminishing the practical knowledge and experience of women who were called on to assist. A woman who had never actually assisted women during the first stage of labor would have few resources on which to draw in handling more complex cases. She might not be called on to help until, like the woman viewed by Méon, the labor had continued for days. By that time, the fetus might be firmly lodged in an adverse position or the mother so exhausted that she could no longer push. Under such circumstances, birth attendants had little to offer other than prayer and brute force, which, as Méon suspected, could itself be dangerous.

In the mid-1950s, Kéita attempted to learn more about how traditional birth attendants were trained and the nature of their actual practices. Her local assistant Sokona explained:

> When the birth attendants of my land find themselves facing a breech presentation, or a shoulder, or a face presentation, they expect the worst. They go crazy, they pray to God and all the saints to protect women against these fetuses that are set on killing their mothers. These children, believed to bring misfortune, are neglected—no one worries about their survival. Marabouts and charlatans give holy water, amulets and charms to protect the life of the mother. You hear everyone say "Better to lose the water than the jar" or "better to save the container than the contents." In other words, it's better to save the mother, who has at least a chance to have other children. Unfortunately that often means the death of both of them. If the child lives, it dies within two weeks of its mother's death. It's a rare family that is attentive to the orphan. (Kéita 1975, 278, my translation)

Sokona asked Kéita to teach her the secrets she used to handle such presentations to save the mother and baby. Kéita explained that these skills had been earned at great length through schooling but that Sokona and other traditional birth attendants could have an important role in teaching hygienic practices, using sterile instruments to cut the cord, disinfecting the newborn's eyes, bandaging the cord, cleaning the mother, and keeping watch over the mother and baby to call on a trained midwife in a hospital setting in the case of complications (Kéita 1975, 279).

Successfully Wooing the Infant

Islamic therapeutic traditions contributed to but did not entirely displace the array of protective words and substances women might draw on prior to, during, and after childbirth. Fanne Fodé emphasized the importance of the advice and protective charms provided by a marabout to Fulani women during pregnancy. But the mother of a newborn also had to be very careful to prevent the baby from being exposed to any woman "carrying the horn of a special small deer known as the Mancara" who could inadvertently undo all the work of the marabout (C 3 Fanne Fodé 1949). The account is suggestive of a kind of conflict of interest between traditional occult powers held by women and mystical powers held by male Islamic specialists. Intriguingly, it appears that the ambiguous magic horn could be more powerful than the charms of the marabout. N'Diaye also remarked that once a baby's milk teeth had come in, it was no longer necessary to protect the child from genies, who evidently were no longer interested in it (C 3 N'Diaye Mody Diabe Maurice 1949). Having protected the infant up to the age of two or so, nothing in the occult arsenal of women or marabouts could combat the dangers facing the child.

N'Diaye estimated that roughly two out of six babies would die at weaning. Fodé, like N'Diaye, was quite forthcoming about the reality of infant mortality. Often, he noted, the children of one family die one after the other. In such a case, the mother would not give her sons traditional names, but instead she would call them things like "Forage," "This One Is For God," and "Ashes"—"expressions that [conveyed] her skepticism" that the child would remain (C3 Fanne Fodé 1949). The problem was that the spirits were very successful in persuading a particular ancestor/child to return to the afterlife. Gayego Leopold explained that "if a woman keeps losing babies, people assume . . . that it is the same child that keeps coming back, so to make it stay they give it a meaningful name: Yewayan, which means 'here he is back again, it's still him, we recognize him'" (C 14 Gayego Leopold n.d.). Issa Kalapo reported that when the children of a Bozo woman in French Sudan died regularly, they might name the infant "Who Has No Shame" or "Under the Tamarind Tree," and a boy might be disguised with a nose ring such as those worn by girls (C 24 Kalapo Issa n.d.).

The emphasis on protecting the boy child could reflect the greater value placed on them as heirs. Savineau recounted the assessment of a Fulani teacher in the Futa Jalon that a girl was "a kind of stranger, who would soon enough leave to live with future husband" (Rapport 15, 7). On the other hand, if infant mortality among boy babies was perceived to be higher than among girl babies, disguising a child as a girl would make sense. In any case, dismissive names were a common ploy throughout the region to prevent the spirits from taking a liking to the infant and enticing it back into the spirit world. According to Issa Kalapo, such ploys were successful. Who would want to seduce a child that had names that suggested that it might be a bastard child, with no capacity to feel shame, destined to be abandoned under a tree? Who would steal a child that is so worthless that it is feed for animals, ashes, or given up already as dead? Who would steal a girl baby?

Enticing the ancestor/child to enter and remain in the human world required attention to the desires of the fetus, which in turn entailed meeting the requests of the pregnant woman, however unusual. This was not because pregnancy in itself was understood to cause women to have strange cravings. It was because the fetus could only have its desires met through the medium of the mother. This attention to the desires of the fetus ran contrary to other common taboos dictating what a pregnant woman could and could not eat. Throughout the region, she was not to eat sweet things, such as honey, nor was she to eat eggs. She was not under any circumstances to eat the meat of a pregnant cow or her child would be deformed or stillborn (ANN 1 G 4 7 Garba Labo 1938–39; ANN 1 G 4 8 Kano Ibra 1938–39).

Women were trained to restrain their desires because it was shameful for a woman to be greedy or ungenerous; it was particularly unseemly for a woman to claim too much meat. Often women ate less than men and children, particularly during times of food shortage (ANN 1 G 4 8 Kano Ibra 1938–39). Thus, this attention to the desires of the fetus via the mother is particularly striking. A grisly folktale related by Gayego Leopold in the post-war period provides a depiction of the tensions generated by this logic:

> Once there was a king who had a beautiful white horse that he dearly loved. His queen was pregnant and one day said coldly to her husband, "I want to eat the liver of your white horse." The king refused and her health got worse and worse. The best counselors of the king became concerned and learned of the queen's request. The king relented and gave the order to slaughter the horse and give the liver to the queen. But his skepticism caused him to commit an odious act. "We shall see if it is my son who demands the liver of my white horse." He called the executioner, who was surprised to learn that he was to cut off the head of the queen. He nevertheless sadly did his duty. As the blood of the victim spewed in great spurts through the severed neck, [the executioner] solemnly opened her womb. And there the king and his assistants found a fragile baby sucking the incompletely ground up debris of the liver. (C 14 Gayego Leopold n.d.)

The moral to the story was not that it is wrong to kill one's wife. It was that her desires belong to the baby, and in particular to the male child, and therefore they must be honored.

The primacy of the needs of the legitimate infant, therefore, could come before the preferences of others and in particular those of the father of the child. The illegitimate child, on the other hand, could be subject to the wrath of a woman's husband, particularly if the child was male in a patrilineal context and therefore threatened the purity of the paternal line. An illegitimate girl child might at least bring in a bride-price once married. Gayego Leopold commented rather startlingly that "when the husband is furious he kills the baby at birth. I hasten to say that this is condemned by indigenous morals, and it revolts quite a few people. But it is still the case that the husband has unlimited power over the child and can do with it as he sees best" (C 14 Gayego Leopold n.d.). Although women were more often charged with infanticide than men, his observation suggests that it is very likely that when the mother was a married woman, her husband had either killed the baby or compelled her to do so.

This pressure was not limited to instances of a known illegitimate birth. Savineau described the case of an imprisoned woman in Gaoual in the Futa Jallon in 1937: "In the prison a poor woman little more than a child. She had given birth to a deformed baby. Her husband criticized her so much that she slit the baby's throat. Or anyway, she says she did. There was quite a lot of emotion in Gaoual over this case. There was evidently some inconsistency between the woman's account of the matter and the facts determined at the time of the exhumation. Was she really the guilty one?" (Rapport 15, 30). A great deal rested, therefore, on the attitude of the husband toward the mother of the child. The legitimate child might indeed be the man's ancestor or grandparent; he had a great interest in producing such children and could presumably be very deeply disappointed at any sign that the child did not conform to his expectations that it "look like him."

The Upending of Hierarchies: Disruption and Opportunity

All the complex shifts of the interwar years gave rise to greater uncertainty about how to live up to the obligations of transgenerational entrustment. Across the territory of FWA, administrative posts gradually emerged, sometimes attached to older centers of trade (such as Zinder along the old trans-Saharan trade routes), sometimes planted anew on sites that appeared particularly promising (such as Niamey on the Niger River). Troops took up residence in barracks for longer or shorter periods. Agadez and Zinder grew in the context of this prolonged military presence. Where there were soldiers, there were women who catered to their sexual and domestic needs. Ambiguous marriages and prostitution became common in such centers, as did mixed-race children whose fathers frequently abandoned them when they were posted elsewhere.

Savineau noted in the late 1930s that in some places neither slavery nor pawning had been entirely eliminated, despite the claims of chiefs and district commanders. Court cases revealed the continuing attempts of masters to reclaim children of their "former" slaves (Rapport 15, 21). Where Zarma men, whose social and political structures had been built on slave labor and trade in slaves, lost control of their former captives, they had to take over farming activities themselves. Their freeborn wives were constrained to take up domestic tasks they had never done in the past and to abandon the remunerative activities, such as spinning thread, that had previously been the mark of a noblewoman. With the rise of peanut farming to earn cash, such women also took up some farm tasks, notably shelling peanuts. For the first time, Savineau remarked, one could see the former slave-owning class in rags (Rapport 5, 14).

Little wonder, then, that whenever masters could find ways to restrict the autonomy of the formerly captive population, they did so. Everywhere she went, Savineau recorded traces of the resilience of servile status. Without access to land of their own, the Bella farming land nominally owned by Tuaregs had to provide tribute in grain, milk, or cash; sometimes they were sent to perform labor for hire by their masters (Rapport 4, 5–6, 11–12). Some Bella women were "unmarried" and their children technically "fatherless," although one suspects their children automatically belonged to the master. Rank was reinforced through new mechanisms; for example, the Djermak-oye of Dosso insisted that the administration must not train the children of noble families in crafts such as smithing, carpentry, or weaving. These should be reserved for the children of former slaves (Rapport 4, 15). A blacksmith, when asked whether the demands on his labor (*corvée*) were manageable, responded frankly, "*Corvée* all the time." This nominally freed man worked three days for himself and three for his master (Rapport 15, 6). Savineau encountered a perplexingly large number of suicides, one of whom was a young man who killed himself after being repeatedly designated for forced labor by the head of his household (Rapport 5, 25). Even quite trivial titles and positions tended to be assigned to the children of those in power (Rapport 5, 31).

In the sedentary villages of RimaiBe, former slaves of Fulani, it was the masters who were to arrange the marriages of the RimaiBe and who in principle "owned" the children and any property of the villagers (Rapport 5, 30). The continuation of marriage exclusively within status groups ensured that "free" Fulani and "captive" Rimaibe would forever be distinguished from one another, as would Tuareg and Bella. The willfulness of youth who wanted to choose their own partners risked undermining not only paternal authority but also a host of other socioeconomic relations as well. Such marriages and divorces were opposed at all cost by older men and women in the colonial courts. The elimination of slavery and the insubordination of the young were, in the minds of the elite, linked to one another (Rapport 15, 7–8).

In the administrative centers that Savineau visited, the myriad processes underway provoked a great deal of anxiety and in particular anxiety about the sexual behavior of women. Zarma parents believed that girls who go to school "don't listen to their parents anymore, they go out without permission, they marry who they want or become streetwalkers [*filles de rue*]. As soon as they are 13 or 14 boys will run after them, and there will be bastards and dishonor" (Rapport 5, 15). Familiar hierarchies by gender were in danger of being upended. Savineau related at length the account offered by Balde Saikou, a teacher in Dalaba (Guinée), of the changes to Fulbe society, which I paraphrase below:

> With the arrival of the whites and the suppression of slavery noble women had to give up their idleness. Their husbands, destroyed by the loss of their slaves, could no longer provide clothing, and the women became dyers, traders, and farmers, and they did needlework to earn money. With it they bought themselves the light-colored muslin cloth and bright white enamel dishes that so charmed them.

> When the depression hit, the men, who cultivated cash crops for export, were destroyed. Women who sold only locally lost very little. They fed their deeply humiliated husbands, who had to make concessions as a result. Fulani women dressed themselves in the new "Senegalese" or "civilized" styles and mimicked the verbal exuberance and shamelessness of the Soussou and the commercial savvy and the loose behavior of the Malinke. But they did so without taking up the housekeeping skills of the first or the wifely compassion of the second. Husbands lost patience; some women reformed, but others resisted and won out. Many were repudiated or ran off. They headed to major towns. They sought proximity to the camps of *tirailleurs* [colonial African soldiers], where the abandoned husband dared not go. (Rapport 15, 6–8, my paraphrase).

As a teacher, Balde Saikou was confident that with time and in particular with female education couples would begin to enter into more balanced arrangements in which power would be shared. But education was not embraced evenly. In some settings, chiefs had initially sent only the children of the poor and powerless in a ploy to protect their own sons from unknown dangers. Often schoolchildren were "orphaned" *métis* over whom the administration had parental authority. Eventually, some were the children of chiefs and functionaries, who had no interest in the agricultural training provided in the curriculum. Their parents hoped their sons would become bureaucrats or office workers (Rapport 5, 25). Some boys enjoyed the agricultural training, but many would never be in a position to apply the methods back in their villages for want of oxen and ploughs (Rapport 5, 7–8). Girls did not receive instruction in the kinds of skills expected of a proper wife. Still, one chief sent a daughter to school with a view to having her become his secretary and keeping a close watch on the translators (Rapport 15, 14–15, 17, 21, 22, 26–27).

Parents and chiefs consistently objected to the mixing of boys and girls in a single school. There were so few girls presented for schooling across FWA, however, that frequently they were simply integrated into already existing classes for boys. Parents, and in particular mothers, were wracked with worries that their daughters would become insubordinate and loose (Rapport 15, 27–28). This led to a vicious cycle, for parents were reluctant to send their girls to such schools, and as a result there were rarely enough girls to justify a girls' school, or even a girls' class, for them alone. Well-placed Africans, such as the Chef de Canton of Tillabery in Niger, felt that schooling for sons was useful to train future chiefs, but it was of no use for girls (Rapport 5, 4). A schoolteacher declared to her that he had no interest in marrying an educated woman because he wanted to be the master of his household (Rapport 5, 6). Schooling was valued for providing entrée for men into medicine or the administrative bureaucracy, but the idea of educating women was deeply unsettling. Female education took a back seat to other concerns. This was to have profound implications because it once again undermined the potential to train African women to staff medical services to serve women and children.

Notes

1. This is in contrast to the findings of Nancy Rose Hunt for the Belgian Congo (1999). Jonathan Cole argues that professional midwives and *matrones* were in tension from the very

outset in Senegal, despite the necessity of depending on the older women for lack of sufficient personnel (2012).

2. The teacher wrote similarly dismissive notes elsewhere on the memoir, characterizing as "infantile" the instructions a grandmother might give to her small charges "to love their parents, to prefer death to shame, and to respect the elderly."

3. The assignment in this instance was not related to children or family life; it appears to have been to describe the history of a people group. "You have only talked about your family," objected the teacher, "there is not enough history."

4. At the time of colonial conquest, speakers of Fulfulde were to be found across the entire Sahel region, some sedentary, some nomadic, some highly Muslim, others indifferent to Islam. In some settings, girls underwent genital cutting, in others they did not (Wilson-Haffenden 1967 [1927], 259). In late colonial Casamance (Senegal), when a young Fulani man was circumcised at about twelve, his bravery would be rewarded with the gift of a bull (C 3 Fanne Fodé 1949). In another setting, circumcision might have no direct temporal relationship to collective initiation into adulthood, which nevertheless involved painful punishment and deprivation (Wilson-Haffenden 1967 [1927], 259). Fulani men in entirely nomadic populations might engage in painful and dangerous stick fighting in preparation for warfare, games that sometimes left scars (C 14 Sow Ibrahima n.d.).

5. ANN 1 G 4 6 Condat 1938–39. Condat suggests that the last two lines of the song imply first a single person and then more than one. In the Hausa version, the final line reads "*Allah karo*," which is suggestive of going to collect something and bring it back, very much in keeping with the circulation of souls.

6. Hereafter when citing from the archival documents of the 1937–38 Savineau reports in ANOM, I will cite only the report number and page.

6

PRODUCING HEALTHY BABIES AND HEALTHY LABORERS

COLONIAL HEALTH OFFICERS KNEW BY MIDCENTURY THAT INFANT mortality was quite high and were not convinced that infertility and sterility alone could account for the low population growth in all regions (IMTSSA 62 Saliceti 1941, 97). In Niger, during the war the head of the medical services, Lieutenant Colonel Saliceti, resorted to the notion of *débilité congenitale* (congenital infirmity) to account for this high rate of infant mortality.[1] The theory was that, as a result of generally poor hygiene, close birth spacing, and the overwork of women, children were born with a kind of physical retardation that contributed to their vulnerability to illness. The notion dovetailed nicely with the neo-Lamarckian inclinations of French social hygiene (IMTSSA 62 Saliceti 1941, 97; IMTSSA 62 Saliceti 1943, 114). "Reprehensible customs" were, he argued, also important contributing factors; these included washing babies too often in the cold, failing to dress them properly, and permitting them to become filthy once they were crawling (IMTSSA 62 Saliceti 1941, 97). In addition, some practices of traditional birth attendants were seen as particularly dangerous, such as cutting the umbilical cord with dirty instruments and using premasticated juices as astringents, leading to tetanus and septicemia (IMTSSA 62 Saliceti 1943, 115). Interestingly, infant feeding practices were subject to particular scrutiny:

> Cercle de Fada-n-Gourma: The gourmantché infant is ... nursed at the breast. Additionally twice daily there is a forcible feeding of an infusion of tamarind and "sesseguéri" to "strengthen the child". If the mother should not happen to produce milk, a relative—but only a relative—will place the child at her breast. If this isn't possible then the child is only fed the herbal infusions. The child is nursed for at least one year, often longer. At that time suddenly [*brutalement*] the child is given millet paste with a lightly spiced sauce. This shift, without

any transition, from milk to adult food obviously can cause occasionally severe gastro intestinal problems. (1941, 97)

Cercle de Zinder: The child is exclusively breastfed for a year or until the mother becomes pregnant again. From one year the feeding is accompanied by an uncooked millet paste to which a bit of sour milk is added. The mother continues to offer milk for up to 21 months for boys, 20 for girls. The child is placed at the breast at all hours of the day or night, without any limit. Nevertheless digestive problems are rare, as mother's milk is the best protection against gastro enteritis. The sour milk added to the millet flour produces lactic acid which also serves as an effective intestinal antiseptic. (1943, 106)

Cercle de Tanout: Early and brusque weaning or solid foods fed too early and in too great quantity (millet paste from the sixth month) are the cause of many cases of gastro enteritis, which, when aggravated by the cold, becomes a major cause of mortality. (1943, 115)

For Saliceti, a number of factors accounted for the low population growth rates across the *cercles* of Niger, including syphilis, gonorrhea, and malaria. But more important were a variety of customs that produced the "feeble child" (*enfant débile*), who could not withstand illness and the climate (1943, 117). The goal, therefore, was to address these unfortunate customs and in particular those related to nursing, infant feeding, and weaning. It is possible that this emphasis had particular salience in a period when the Vichy government was celebrating motherhood and family, although such a link is not clear from the documents (cf. Slobodkin 2018, 67; Simmons 2015, 129).

Women's failure to schedule infants' nursing perplexed medical officials, even though, in some instances (as in Zinder) this didn't appear to cause problems. Saliceti objected to feeding children adult foods at six months in Tanout but was equally perturbed by the Gourmantché practice of nursing for a full year. In Zinder, the addition of fermented milk to infant foods was noted approvingly, whereas elsewhere it was seen as a pernicious local custom (IMTSSA 62 Morvan 1946). In other words, local practices appear to have been objectionable in regions with seemingly low population growth rates and commendable where there was growth.

While Saliceti and other medical administrators were interested in questions related to infant care and women's reproductive health, they simply did not have enough staff to undertake ambitious efforts on those fronts. French doctors and teachers with a colonial ambition were far more interested in going to the Maghreb or Indochina. To attract them in large numbers, French West Africa (FWA) would have had to offer highly competitive compensation far out of keeping with the limited territorial budgets (Barthélémy 2010, 26). The solution to "saving the African race" would have to come from less expensive and more approachable African professionals; "making Africans" would require making African health workers first. One is struck by just how much the postwar medical system for the civilian population would come to rest on the shoulders of the very small numbers of African graduates from the medical school in Dakar.

The Medical School and the School for *Sage-Femmes*

The medical school was established in Senegal in 1918 after the recruitment drives of World War I revealed just how ravaged the African population was. In principal, the school was of a piece with the pronatal public hygiene movement of the interwar years in France; however, the approach in French West Africa focused less on individuals than on the African "race" (Conklin 2002, 149). Accordingly, the school trained young African men to become "auxiliary doctors" to work alongside European doctors focusing initially on the health of male labor. Women were trained to become "auxiliary *sage-femmes*" to staff dispensaries and maternities dotted across FWA. The overall approach did not envision a dense network of primary care clinics but rather systematic vaccination through mobile health units and better maternal and infant health services in a handful of maternities. In general, the push to vaccinate against smallpox, among other things, was more effectively structured, staffed, and successful than the effort to develop maternity care.[2]

Many of the early students in the medical school and the school for *sage-femmes* were of mixed-race background, having been left by their European fathers in the care of their African mothers. Such children were more numerous in places such as Zinder and Agadez where there had been a long military presence. The French education these girls received provided them with access to the emerging educational structures to train as nurses or teachers, particularly in the interwar years. By 1934, for example, sixty-six *métisse* girls from across FWA had become *sage-femmes*, visiting nurses, or general nurses.[3]

In some parts of the Sahel, such as Upper Volta, girls raised by Catholic missions after being abandoned when their mothers had died in childbirth also received schooling in French.[4] The regions that had benefited from the presence of largely Catholic mission schools produced many of the early candidates for the school.[5] Such religious schools had been in operation for far longer in coastal regions, such as Dahomey and Senegal, than in the Sahel. Unlike Great Britain, Belgium, and Portugal, France did not encourage the development of mission schooling in its West African territories and indeed did much to impede its development in the period prior to 1945 (B. Cooper 2006; Zorn 1993; Salvaing 1994; Benoist 1987). France's attitude toward mission schooling in West Africa was at best counterproductive. Where the numbers of secular schools were small, the figures to build on were not promising: in Niger in 1931, there were only twenty-one schools in total, all secular. Of the 1,447 students enrolled that year, only 71 were girls.[6]

Pascale Barthélémy's magisterial historical study of the elite female graduates of the medical school and the teacher training school in Senegal reveals that barely 2 percent of those exceptional women came from Niger. Over a period of close to four decades, the two schools produced a total of eighteen Nigerien graduates in all (Barthélémy 2010, 292). Like Upper Volta, Niger was distant from Dakar, landlocked, and undesirable as a posting, resulting in a vicious cycle of lasting significance. There were very few French present in Niger in the first place, much less civilian teachers. The establishment of missions had not been encouraged prior to the close of World War II. Niger's state schools produced very few graduates, of whom only a pitiful number were girls. As an index of the significance of the presence of religious schooling, in 1921–22 there were 328 girls enrolled in state schools in Dahomey and 830 enrolled in private schools. At the same moment in Niger, there were a total of 53 girls in school, all of whom attended the handful of public schools (Barthélémy 2010, 36, Tableau 1). The colony was therefore never in a position to send its underserved students for higher training to Dakar. By comparison with other territories, very few Nigerien children were equipped to even take the entry exam, much less pass it.

In turn, because so few of the medical school graduates were originally from Niger, very few had any interest in serving there. Niger colony had an extremely difficult time recruiting teachers and medical personnel even once the school generated graduates. A leitmotif of the medical reports for Niger is the frustration expressed by the medical personnel that the colony was doing such a poor job of training Nigerien girls to go on to become health personnel rather than housewives (B. Cooper 1997, 116–19). While the territories of Dahomey, Senegal, French Sudan, and Côte d'Ivoire succeeded, little by little, in leveraging their growing educated population to generate a modest educational and medical infrastructure staffed by Africans, Niger fell further and further behind.[7]

The overwhelming majority of educated and skilled women posted in Niger were ethnically and linguistically "strangers." In 1934, Niger had not yet sent a single student to study to become a trained *sage-femme*. The eleven women posted there came from other territories within FWA. Because Dahomey had produced far more graduates than any other colony, Dahomeans were stationed where they were most needed, often in Niger. At a time when young women across FWA were beginning to imagine going to school and becoming professionals as well, girls in Niger were confronted with women with whom they were far less likely to identify—very different from them in language, religion, and culture.[8] Rather than making it more familiar, this simply underscored the foreignness of French education. Niger was regarded as a difficult and undesirable posting for both French medical personnel and the women trained in Dakar. Such graduates preferred their home regions or better-off colonies for their placements. As their careers progressed, most women managed to gradually make their way back to their home territories (Barthélémy 2010, 176–80). Niger, so desperate for educated staff, was particularly ill-favored when it came to the distribution of those precious resources.

By 1946, the medical school in Dakar had trained four hundred African auxiliary doctors, more than four hundred auxiliary *sage-femmes*, and a modest number (sixty-two in all) of visiting nurses (trainees whose academic performance was not adequate to continue to become *sage-femmes*).[9] Gradually, small numbers of these graduates scattered very unevenly across FWA began making their presence felt. It was a *sage-femme* and her visiting nurses who first noted the signs of famine in western Niger in 1931 (FM 1AFFPOL 592 Crise alimentaire 1931–32). These small numbers of women graduating from the École de Sage-Femmes in Dakar quietly attempted to meet the needs of pregnant women under what can only have been very difficult conditions. Most were little more than twenty-one years old when they graduated and had not had children themselves (Barthélémy 2010, 175). Some of the very earliest graduates, unmarried and childless, faced considerable resistance due to their youth. In a letter to the house mother of the École de Sage-Femmes, one graduate wrote of her reception, "An adult woman who has never had a baby shouldn't see a birth, much less a young woman" (Mme. Nogue 1923, 454–55). Many recounted the painstaking work required for them to gain the trust of women, often through the mediation of chiefs and administrators (Mme Nogue 1923, 457–59). Another recounted a typical struggle with the traditional birth attendants or *matrones* in French Sudan:

> I had a woman who labored for at least ten hours, it was her first baby. . . . [T]he *matrone* whispered to me that this woman had had her baby with someone other than her husband, and so long as she refused to name that man she would not be able to give birth. . . . I felt so sorry for the poor woman that I begged the old women to leave me with her for a moment so that I could talk to her. Alone with me she gave me a grateful look, I examined her and had her walk a little in her room, and within an hour she had given birth to a beautiful little boy. Afterwards the old ladies ran in to ask me the name of the real father—I told them that it was because of them that she had had so much trouble and that this [long labor] was normal with young women having their first babies. (Mme Nogue 1923, 455)

Often the graduates did not speak the local languages and found the local customs perplexing and even disturbing. Even when they, at length, managed to gain the trust of the communities, it was an ambiguous truce, gained through a certain amount of pressure from the administrators and chiefs and enforced tacitly through their proximity to the police and military.[10]

These graduates had not been trained to handle venereal diseases, nor were they pediatricians (Barthélémy 2010, 113). Often the facilities in which they worked were poorly constructed, understaffed, and undersupervised. The construction of actual maternity buildings and dispensaries only began in the 1930s. As a result, much of their early work was conducted in the homes of women whose relatives called on them for assistance. The visiting nurses did not always serve as liaisons with local communities, as had been intended. Instead, they served as assistants to the auxiliary *sage-femmes*. Once facilities were actually built, there were not enough doctors to oversee all the maternities and dispensaries. African medical staff were regularly called on to take on tasks that would otherwise be assigned to someone with more training. Some auxiliary *sage-femmes* were not above attending more closely to "paying clients" in their homes than they did to the general population in the clinics (ANS 1 H 102 versement 163, Cayla 1940). Consequently, after 1938, the *sage-femmes* were discouraged from assisting in home births.

The Halting Growth of Colonial Medical Services

In late 1937, Denise Savineau encountered a well-oiled health service in Tillabery, in western Niger. It was staffed, happily, by Dr. and Madame

Wilson—a Togolese auxiliary doctor and his wife, a *sage-femme*. Having been raised in a coastal setting where numerous protestant missions operated, they had had mission schooling, spoke French well, and had advanced to the heights of the education system available to Africans within FWA at the time. The two had served in this locale for seven years, long enough to have learned to speak Zarma and to establish a rapport with the local population. Savineau accompanied them on one of their periodic medical visits to a village named Sakouare, where a large straw hut had been constructed for the purpose of these consultations. Pregnant women and their children lined up, holding their medical record cards: "The doctor examined them. His wife updated the individual record for each one. All moved along in an orderly, efficient, attentive and good humored fashion. . . .This [prenatal] consultation took up the morning. The actual medical visit would occur in the afternoon" (Rapport 5, 3).

This model service was not at all typical. Savineau remarked that Madame Wilson seemed to her to be more professional than many of the doctors she had encountered on her mission. The couple had replaced a European doctor, Doctor Sousonzof, whose legacy to Tillabery was "the memory of his lack of commitment and a *métis* boy he [had] abandoned" (Rapport 5, 3). The admirable work of the Wilsons was facilitated by the fact that the couple remained together in one place for an extended period of time rather than being posted to separate sites, as was typical. Kéita noted that even though doctors and nurses were often married to one another, "the cynicism of the colonialists went so far as to split longstanding households" (Kéita 1975, 45). Personnel consequently moved from post to post in search of the best of a variety of unsatisfactory family situations. The ability of the Wilsons to combine their resources and materials probably improved the services they could provide. Unlike many of the doctors Savineau observed, they managed to make visits to neighboring villages. Many doctors and *sage-femmes* complained that they lacked a service vehicle suited to the terrain and that when they did have a vehicle they had no petrol (Rapport 5, 18).

Although the health services in the capital of Niger were more developed than in other regions, Savineau's remarks on them ranged from neutral to critical: two *sage-femmes* seemed "lackluster and uncommitted," the timid visiting nurses were "utterly unsuited to what is expected of them," and the *matrones* had to be given economic inducements to follow protocol (Rapport 5, 8–9). Women in the local population had a similarly dim assessment of the services. Savineau had been told that the *sage-femmes* "[were] not always welcoming." Women preferred the charitable service that had been overseen by Madame Gosselin, the wife of a prominent administrator. This activity quickly died out, for "European women come and go, and not all are energetic" (Rapport 5, 9).

If the services in the capital were less than ideal, in a smaller town such as Dogondoutchi they could be extremely difficult. There being no *sage-femme* stationed there, the male doctor had little success in persuading pregnant women who did not see themselves as ill that they should come in for consultations. Furthermore, women often went to the homes of their mothers to give birth, where the male doctor could not reach them. Even when the roads were traversable, the station vehicle was aging and there was no gas. The medicines were in inadequate supply, and the promised budget never materialized (Rapport 5, 18–19).

The *sage-femmes* posted to Gaya complained to Savineau that they had no beds to sleep in. No one had made any arrangements for their lodging because it had been assumed that the women would be married to male functionaries with access to government housing. The two were sharing a traditional hut, which Savineau deemed "damaging to their prestige" (Rapport 5, 22). When Aoua Kéita first arrived in Gao in 1931 to take up her first posting, there was no actual maternity building and no obstetric supplies. The doctor could offer her only two clamps, a pair of scissors, a bit of tincture, some alcohol, cotton, compresses, and some bandages (Kéita 1975, 31). Graduates from the medical school only received a medical kit if they graduated at the very top of the class; others had to simply fend for themselves or depend on the generosity or foresight of others. It took three years of persistent requests on Kéita's part for the administration to supply the funds to build an actual maternity building in Gao (Kéita 1975, 45).

By contrast, when Kéita was exiled to Bignona in the favored colony of Senegal, she found the cost of living lower, her wages higher, and her ability to earn income on the side by offering treatment to *métisses* and European women profitable (Kéita 1975, 212). When she was reassigned back to French Sudan to the town of Nara in 1953, "the little room that served as the maternity hardly merited the name. The single room that was to serve for both births and consultations was so narrow that the *sage-femme*, patient, and nurse's aide, could barely move around one another. There was no waiting room. When two women arrived in difficult labor during the hours for prenatal and postnatal care, all the assembled mothers had to wait in the courtyard until the risky delivery was completed." She added with some bitterness, "After the beautiful maternities that I had managed elsewhere, especially in Ziguinchor, my previous posting, I was truly unhappy to be forced to work under such conditions."[11] The graduates of the medical school took pride in their skills and were eager to use them. However, in marginal colonies like French Sudan and Niger the working conditions were almost intolerable.

Savineau's reports reveal the unevenness and unpredictability of the health services of FWA in the interwar period. Sometimes there was a doctor or a *sage-femme*, sometimes there was not. With luck, a traditional birth attendant with some medical instruction (*matrone instruite*) might stand in for them (Rapport 5, 28). Sometimes there were medicines, vehicle, and gas, often not. Nowhere was there provision of food for the patients. The maternity and clinic might be in very good shape, while the wards themselves were squalid (Rapport 4, 20). The staff understood the local language only rarely, for they moved from station to station (Rapport 3, 14–15). There was in all this little evidence of a linear forward march toward an effective health system and nothing to suggest that pronatalism in the metropole translated effectively into attention to the reproductive needs of African subjects far from the coast.

In this ever-changing context, the relationship between formally trained midwives (*sage-femmes*), traditional birth attendants who had received a bit of training (*matrones*), and those birth attendants who simply went about their business as they always had (*accoucheuses*) was never consistent or clear. Given the enormity of the territory to be served and the tiny numbers of women trained at the École des Sage-Femmes, the system could not even come close to working effectively without collaborating with the elderly women traditionally called on locally to assist in birth. Yet, even in settings where these birth attendants worked very well with the medical staff, they generally received no remuneration at all: "they do truly lovely work," observed a *sage-femme*. "Without them we could do absolutely nothing here" (Rapport 15, 28).

Ideally, traditional birth attendants would handle all uncomplicated cases themselves, sending along more complex cases to the *sage-femmes*. But the message purveyed by the health services was necessarily muddy; their unspoken goal was to eventually replace the *matrones*, whose practices were seen to be dirty or dangerous. If they could not be replaced immediately, they needed to be disciplined to approximate birthing practices more familiar within the European biomedical tradition. However, the interface between the different systems was imperfect. *Matrones* might wait a very long time before making the decision to intervene in a delivery or to alert the *sage-femme*: "The sage-femme handles roughly half of the births in Ouagadougou. Sometimes she is called upon too late, after the *matrone* has attempted dangerous maneuvers. One woman who had been in labor for five days, the baby completely destroyed [*pourri*], died a half hour after the sage-femme arrived, and the two deaths were blamed on the maternity by the women of the village" (Rapport 8, 25). In Dire, a doctor remarked to Denise Savineau that the traditional birth attendants of Songhay and Bozo women "have the women give birth sitting down. This often results in tearing because excision reduces the elasticity of the tissue" (Rapport 4, 9). It is possible that the doctor's objection to squatting simply reflected Western bias toward labor on the back, which is easiest to manage for the medical practitioner. Certainly, the *sage-femmes* had all been trained to deliver in lithotomy position. Barthélémy's interviews with *sage-femmes* trained during this period suggest, however, that in settings where many women had been excised, the *sage-femmes* did everything they could to protect the scarred tissue so that it would not tear, which would have been significantly easier to accomplish if the woman adhered to Western norms. Unlike the traditional *matrones*, *sage-femmes* actively intervened in delivery earlier, sometimes simply by following their medical training but very often by improvising in light of local circumstances (cf. Livingston 2012).

Childbirth in Colonial Niger

Where a maternity benefiting from the presence of a *sage-femme* existed in Niger, the services were reported in 1942 by Médecin Lieutenant Colonel Saliceti to be doing very good work. *Sage-femme* Koulibaly in Maradi and *sage-femme* Souma in Tahoua attracted particular praise. On the other hand, the young and less rigorously trained visiting nurses seem to have posed a bit more of a problem: "One visiting nurse, whose conduct leaves much to be desired," he noted, "seems to have turned to prostitution (nothing is for certain—she will be transferred to Agadez and fired if the allegations turn out to be true)" (ANN 1 H 3 12 Saliceti 1942). The disappointing experiment with training such young and academically weak visiting nurses in the interwar years had already been abandoned by 1939 (Barthélémy 2010, 291).

Thanks to the growing corps of medical personnel, immediately prior to World War II Niger was poised to make strides in health and hygiene. Medical staff increasingly consisted of a mix of European military doctors, African auxiliary doctors, auxiliary *sage-femmes*, male African nurses, female African visiting nurses, and the occasional European female nurse or *sage-femme*. These modest but growing efforts to reach out directly to women with children in the interwar period were supplemented by the wives of various administrators, who volunteered with the women's groups affiliated with the Red Cross. In her 1914 call to French women to join local Red Cross committees, Andrée d'Alix had emphasized that the Red Cross was "an authorized auxiliary to the army" to be organized with military discipline (d'Alix 1914, 54). Child and infant care only gradually emerged as a secondary concern with a view to directing existing resources (many developed in the context of the antituberculosis campaign) toward preventive care (258). These hygienic concerns, d'Alix suggested, were "truly feminine" in nature (266–69).

After World War I, such lay volunteer activities provided colonial women with a sense of purpose. Hygiene activities were directed not to the soldiers already covered by the medical services but to African mothers and children. In the early 1930s, Governor General Jules Brevié's wife oversaw baby clinics with an emphasis on weighing infants so that if they appeared to be doing poorly, their mothers could be encouraged to take them to a dispensary.[12] Similar clinics were held in the larger administrative centers across FWA. With the precipitous decline in military medical personnel during World War II, such volunteer efforts in Niger would have been all the more precious and the value of indigenous medical staff all the more urgently felt. Such ad hoc interventions depended on the postings, whims, and interests of the untrained wives of white male administrators. Baby weighing was encouraged through the giving of small gifts of clothing, millet, soap, and milk to the mothers who attended (IMTSSA 62 Saliceti 1941, 76).

During World War II, the charitable activities of Red Cross volunteers in Niamey were noted regularly in annual medical reports, as if to absolve the Service de Santé of its inability to adequately attend to maternal and infant health across the vast territory of Niger. In his 1943 report, Lieutenant Colonel Saliceti declared implausibly, "The activities of this charity meet very nearly all the needs relative to the protection of small children" (IMTSSA 62 Saliceti 1943). In any case, by the 1950s the Red Cross, preoccupied with reconstruction in Europe, was no longer functioning in Niger, leaving a hole in the already threadbare outreach to women and children (IMTSSA 62 Lorre 1951, 21).

The government health services were strained to the limit during World War II, with the unfortunate consequence that the fragile rapport with local populations was put in jeopardy. In 1940, the European nurse posted to Zinder appears to have had such a rigid and insensitive approach that she alienated women, very much as Mor Ndao suggests occurred in Senegal (Ndao 2008). Lieutenant Colonel Guillaume, the medical director, commented in his annual report that although the nurse appeared quite qualified on paper, "her rather dictatorial character unfortunately prevents her from entirely gaining the confidence of the natives" (IMTSSA 62 Guillaume 1940, 36). The question of the approachability of the medical staff, in part as a result of their association with the military and with the policing of prostitutes, was to prove an important and enduring problem.

One gains the sense that, at least in Niger, an authoritarian medical culture, growing out of the longer history of French colonial medicine's roots in military medicine, generally prevailed over the charitable or humanitarian approaches that might have attracted women more quickly, even in the interwar period (Savineau, Rapport 4, 10).[13] During and after the war, some positive inducements such as gifts of baby clothing were offered, and in Maradi women were briefly urged to come stay at the maternity a full week before they were expected to give birth, with the costs to be supported in principal by the Société de Prévoyance (IMTSSA 62 Morvan 1946, 55). Yet, when one reflects more deeply on the social effect on a pregnant woman of abandoning her children and husband for that long, it is less clear that such "generosity" would have been welcome. Such efforts generally entailed a degree of coercion. In Zinder, indigenous women's "natural repugnance" to seeking prenatal medical care was at times overcome through "more effective arguments," such as the possibility of administrative sanctions: "At one point a system of punishments was applied here: women who gave birth at home without immediately informing the maternity from the beginning of labor were transported to the maternity in the subsequent days and remained there for some eight days for care. This practice provoked incidents and was eliminated. But mere persuasion and obligating the traditional birth attendants to inform the *sage-femme* as soon as they are called for a birth are not sufficient to overcome resistance due to custom, religion and atavism" (IMTSSA 62 Morvan 1947, 62). Some administrators in Niger were inclined to see "resistant" women as criminals and to deploy hospital stays as a kind of punishment. Despite more positive efforts to attract women to give birth in clinics, such as raising the bonus offered to local birth attendants for bringing women to the maternity, attendance at maternities in Niger in the late 1940s actually went down rather than up (IMTSSA 62 Kervingant 1948, 31). The work of building an effective maternal and infant health system had clearly still barely begun.

The Absent Middle Figure: The Quandary of the *Matrone*

The colonial administration consistently had a problem staffing and enforcing its medical and hygienic initiatives, turning to its troops and veteran soldiers to assist in the task with the unfortunate consequence that the medical services were necessarily linked in people's minds to the coercion of the colonial state. This was not limited to the interventions in the realm of venereal disease discussed in chapter 4, for Savineau reported in 1937 that in Dori it would have been better not to recruit the *gardes sanitaires* who were to enforce public hygiene from among former soldiers whose approach had more in common with policing than with medicine. She went on to add that the uniforms used by health inspectors should not look so much like those of the district-level police (*gardes de cercle*), for they scared people away (Rapport 4, 27). The postwar medical services struggled to link the emerging obstetric services located in fixed sites to rural populations that more often than not hoped only to evade them.

In principle, the visiting nurses were to bring pregnant women into contact with the maternity services; however, they were often quite young, did not necessarily speak any local language, and in any case were not sufficiently numerous. Consequently, periodic efforts were made by the medical services of FWA to liaise instead with the *matrones* despite the fact that *sage-femmes* trained at the medical school were often in direct competition with these traditional birth attendants. In theory, such elderly *matrones* could be taught to improve hygiene, refer difficult cases to medical centers, prevent tetanus through the use of clean blades to cut the cord, and prevent eye infections in the newborn. But it quickly became clear that not all were suitable candidates: "the most apt are not always the oldest," observed Leon Cayla in his directives to the medical services of FWA in 1940. Cayla felt that *matrones'* services should be discouraged wherever there were actual maternities in place, for "their activities, often destructive, run counter to the advice of the medical and administrative authorities, who patiently and consistently encourage African notables to bring clients instead to the maternities" (ANS 1 H 102 versement 163, Cayla 1940).

By 1948, General Medical Inspector Peltier frankly proclaimed the experiment with the *matrones* to be a failure. Peltier felt they should no longer be encouraged to assist births at all but should rather simply refer pregnant women to the closest medical center (ANS 1 H 102 versement 162, Peltier 1948). However, women among sedentary populations in the Sahel did not expect or desire the presence of other women at the actual moment of labor; the task of the traditional birth attendant was to deliver the placenta and bury it. Ideally, she only entered when she first heard the baby cry. Furthermore, the general reserve about revealing a woman to be pregnant would have made it inappropriate for an elderly woman, susceptible to witchcraft accusations, to draw attention to another woman's condition even if only to prompt her to go to a maternity for prenatal care.

The gradually emerging maternal and infant health system in much of the Sahel and certainly in Niger developed in a context in which neither the visiting nurses nor the *matrones* could effectively serve as mediating figures with the local populations. Under the circumstances, it is not surprising that well into the postwar period the services in urban centers remained mysterious and unappealing to most rural women. In his 1950 report on the progress in maternal and infant health in Niger, Doctor Lieutenant Colonel Kervigant declared discouragingly, "Niger is a new country, whose population is little evolved [*est encore peu évolué*]. The medical services experience the greatest difficulty in conveying any notions of maternal and infant hygiene to the masses without running up against their customs. It will be a long-term undertaking which only the devotion of the corps of *sage-femmes* and nurses will succeed in bringing to fruition" (ANS 1 H 102 versement 162, Kervingant 1950). Niger was not alone. The unevenness of the distribution of the health infrastructure across French West Africa was by this point glaringly obvious. Pierre Queinnec, the head of the medical services in newly reconstituted Upper Volta, gave a scathing report on the condition of maternal and infant health services there in 1950. From 1933 and throughout the war, Upper Volta had been treated as a labor reserve to be carved up in the service of "peopling" other territories, in particular Côte d'Ivoire. Condemning the exploitation of the region, Queinnec noted acerbically that all the financing and staff had been directed to the coast, leaving an impoverished health service to the reconstituted northerly territory in 1948 (ANS 1 H 102 versement 162, Queinnec 1950). Like Niger, Upper Volta had benefited very little from the development of medical services compared to the coastal colonies.

Tellingly, what little care was available to vulnerable infants in Upper Volta appears to have been offered in the context of the military camps and charities, most notably through the work of the Catholic missions: "for this [work] a particularly devoted staff is called for, which is difficult to find outside of missions" (ANS 1 H 102 versement 162, Queinnec 1950). Queinnec's insistence on the unreliability of charitable work done by French women (increasingly drawn to careers of their own) and his emphasis on the utility of missions evidently struck the director of health services in Dakar, who marked the passage with a red exclamation point. Yet Queinnec's observation echoed sentiments expressed again and again by medical staff in their administrative reports: if the medical services for the African population were to have any real meaning, either there would need to be a much larger, better equipped, and more reliable personnel or there would need to be many more religious missions.

Only quite late in the colonial enterprise did France fully understand the implications of the exclusion of missions from the development of education in the interior. A folder on Niger between the years of 1948 and 1959 in the archives of the French Ministry of Economics and Finance included a study entitled "Enseignement situation en 1948" (CAEF B-0057586/ 2). Tellingly, this proved to be an intelligence document on education policy in British Nigeria from 1912 to 1948. "From these figures," noted the author, "one discerns the very significant role of religious missions compared with the government, the lag in the north relative to the south, and the differences between Christian missions and Islam with regard to education." In contrast to French policy in Niger, a significant proportion of the British colonial schools were private schools subsidized by the colonial government, which was providing an ever-increasing budget for education. Particularly striking to the author of the report was the emphasis on training institutions for teachers in anticipation of a rapid expansion of schooling. Even in the neglected north of Nigeria, directly across the border from Niger, there were already 14 missions engaged in educational activities and 164 subsidized schools, 86 of which were functioning in local languages.

The contrast with circumstances in Niger, where only one mission, the Sudan Interior Mission, was working outside the capital, and where the mission's requests to set up vernacular language schools had regularly been rebuffed, must have been quite startling and not a little alarming. After World War II, France began to encourage missions to undertake work in its colonial territories as the yawning gap between the civilizing ideal and the impoverished reality of the medical and educational system for Africans became ever clearer.

Evangelical Ambivalence

In her study of the late colonial medicalization of childbirth in the Belgian Congo, historian Nancy Rose Hunt characterizes missions as "agents of a hygienic form of 'indirect rule'" (Hunt 1999, 6). Belgium systematically turned over the work of generating an infrastructure of health and educational institutions to Catholic and Protestant missionaries, and, in the waning days of colonial rule, pointed to that same infrastructure as evidence of the beneficence of the colonial order. Similarly, British colonies benefited tremendously from the educational and medical institutions produced by missions. Both Belgium and Britain were far more pragmatic than France in their approach to the business of what Sara Berry (1992) has aptly referred to as "hegemony on a shoestring." Both were historically far less anticlerical in disposition than France—indeed, the church held an important place in national and political culture in both imperial contexts. As a result, the reliance on mission structures to begin some of the work of building educational and health infrastructure seemed fairly natural, which is not to say that colonial administrators and missions were never in conflict. If missions were not specifically encouraged in northern Nigeria, they nevertheless made their presence felt there in a host of ways, not the least of which was promoting Hausa literacy through the Roman alphabet.

The Catholic orders working in West Africa were focused on coastal stations started in Côte d'Ivoire, Dahomey, and Senegal well before colonial rule. In the interior, most Catholic efforts in FWA were focused on French Sudan, where France's most ambitious irrigation project, the Office du Niger, had been established. The Catholic Church had been slow to establish major efforts in Niger, although it had taken on the staffing of an orphanage in Fada N'Gourma, the portion of Upper Volta that briefly fell to Niger. By and large, the Catholic presence outside of major cities was only felt in Niger in the aftermath of World War II. Thus it was, paradoxically, the largely Anglo-American protestant Sudan Interior Mission (SIM) that was to take the lead in this French colony.

During the interwar period, SIM had struggled and failed to gain permission to establish schools and medical institutions in Niger. The French administration did not regard the missionaries as equivalent in qualification to secular French teachers and French trained medical personnel, much less in commitment to French civilization and *laïcism*.[14] For one thing, the missionaries taught not in French but in the local vernacular (in this case, Hausa in Roman print). Their priority was presenting populations with the Gospel in their own languages, not to produce French-speaking functionaries. Prior to 1950, most of the missionaries who volunteered were not trained in medicine. It was only after World War II that the French "opened up" Niger to vigorous mission activities in social services, attracting many single women trained as nurses into the mission field. By the lead-up to decolonization, SIM had a major hospital at Galmi; a leprosarium at Danja; countless dispensaries dotted across the southern edge of the Sahara; schools at Tsibiri, Soura, and Dogon Doutchi; and a network of bible training centers.

Given this rather unique opportunity, why didn't SIM fill the void by developing a vigorous maternal and infant health infrastructure? The letters of an SIM nurse, Elizabeth Chisholm, who was stationed in Niger from 1953 until her retirement in the mid-1980s, offer a glimpse over a forty-year period of the kinds of issues evangelical missionary medical workers—and in particular women missionaries—encountered in their work in this Sahelian setting.[15] Like many women missionaries of her generation, Chisholm never married and never had children; she would say that although she never gave birth she certainly regarded many of the children raised or schooled by the mission as "her children."

In her earliest letters, Chisholm dwelt on the sexual sinfulness of "the locals." The conviction that her patients were sexually profligate was informed by the very high numbers of syphilis cases she treated. In an interview with me much later in her life, she was to remark wryly that she eventually discovered that the Hausa word she and other missionaries had taken to refer to syphilis was so broad that the diagnosis of syphilis was frequently misplaced (Interview with Elizabeth Chisholm [Sebring] November 16, 1990). In the absence of labs, it was very easy to mistake yaws for syphilis. Many customs appalled her, as they had appalled military doctors such as Saliceti:

> Half-starved babies suffering because of the pernicious superstition that mothers' milk is poisonous for two weeks after delivery. We give the

mothers, if possible to get hold of them in time, any harmless medicine and assure them that the milk will do no harm. Otherwise the little wee thing is fed on unsterilized cow's milk and mortality is high due to indigestion and diarrhea. . . . Another malignant custom of Mohammedan origin, which fosters infidelity and polygamy is the habit of the pregnant woman returning to her mother's compound for delivery and remaining there until the child is almost a year old. Meanwhile the husband is on the loose to get a second wife or make what other arrangements he can afford. (ERC 1/A 3 April 19, 1953, Tsibiri)

These two issues—infant feeding and marital sexuality—were to mark both missionary and government perceptions of the "cultural" problems of Hausa-speaking women in particular (B. Cooper 2007, 2009).

Interpreting maternal and infant health problems as having their origin in "custom" may have made them seem less amenable to specifically medical intervention; such problems were simply further signs of the urgency of Christian conversion. Her thoughts on the *bori* spirit possession activities so typical of women suffering from infertility in the region is revealing in this regard: "Despite his 16 wives the chief has very few children, one of the reasons being this head wifes [*sic*] jealousy for the chieftainship for her son & to prevent competition she casts a spell on any of the pregnant wives so they leap into the air with a scream & fall violently to the ground & abort. . . . They say it so effects the mind as to dull it & that the majority of African women are so affected by it as to be incapable of learning much" (ERC 1/A 3 August 14, 1953, Tsibiri). Given the centrality of *bori* to women's reproductive concerns, the mission's consistent demonization of spirit practices could not have made its services enticing to women struggling with underfertility, even those who were nominal Muslims. Thus, the SIM's medical missionaries had a variety of ideological predispositions that probably hindered their medical work with women.

Chisholm's evangelical convictions prompted her to turn first to prayer to counter perceived evils and only secondarily to her medical training. Converting Africans to evangelical Christianity was far more important than improving their health. In response to a query from a young mission recruit who asked whether Chisholm recommended seeking midwifery training as part of her course of study to become a missionary, Chisholm gave the following rather surprising response: "I believe your time and money would be far more profitably invested in Bible School. I wouldn't exchange my one brief year there for all my nursery experience. We battle not against flesh and blood but principalities and powers and our armour must be intact. Our medical knowledge is only a means to an end whereas our knowledge of the Lord and His Word is our only offensive weapon" (ERC 1/A 3 December 13, 1953, Tsibiri). She may have even discouraged women from coming to her for assistance with childbirth: "I really don't have too many deliveries nor do I try to encourage them as I have no place to keep the patients here as a maternity ward and it would be impossible to treat many in the villages as the time involved in being with them and making rounds would prohibit all other work" (ERC 1/A 7 July 11, 1955, Tsibiri).

Seven years into her career, however, she did seek out midwifery training after witnessing several fatal gynecological incidents including the death of a beloved pastor's wife due to a ruptured tubal pregnancy (ERC 1/A 7 September 27, 1955, Tsibiri). Shortly after independence in 1960, she took time off from her work in Niger to gain midwifery training in Switzerland and to enter a new phase of her life. Her training completed, by Christmas of 1964 she jubilantly wrote home about delivering "the chief's" baby, sharing new observations about the local handling of infants, and full of excited plans for the new maternity she would establish. After the depressing setbacks of conventional dispensary work in Tsibiri, the maternity she took over in Guescheme had given her a new lease on life: "I did have a real good time with those [first three] deliveries—I love it & it was so sweet to see the three new mothers sitting on their little wooden stools bathing their babies" (ERC 1/B 21 December 25, 1964, Guescheme).

This kind of work, while deeply rewarding in its affirmation of life, exposed her to deaths of a kind that could not readily be attributed to carnality or sin. Deaths of innocent babies and helpless young mothers could give rise to feelings of doubt and inadequacy. In a searching letter to her parents in 1966, after the harrowing delivery of a dead baby, she wrote: "[God] really brought out the question to a crisis making me admit I will praise Him whatever the outcome" (ERC 1/B 23 July 5, 1966, Guescheme). Maternity care had brought her to a moment of spiritual reckoning of the meaning of her work. Despite the evident satisfaction maternity work sometimes gave to Chisholm, it was emotionally draining and led to few conversions. While Chisholm was but one nurse among many, her experiences give evidence of the challenge that maternity care presented to the evangelical vocation to save Africans from eternal damnation by bringing them to Christianity. Much more energy, money, and staff were devoted to the work of the leprosarium at Danja and to the full-service hospital at Galmi, where prospects for conversions were much better. A systematic approach to mission work through maternal and infant care was never a priority for SIM in Niger and could not as a result fill the considerable gap between government rhetoric and the realities of childbirth on the ground.

Postwar Nutritional Science and the Problem of Infant Malnutrition

Of course, improving the health of African subjects and encouraging population growth were not exclusively a matter of improving maternity care. The recurrent famines in the region and the work on nutrition in Europe led by the League of Nations had already raised food security to a major priority in the interwar years, with little practical impact (Slobodkin 2018). After World War II, French colonial scientists turned to the problem of nutrition with greater attention, for the realities of war-related food rationing and lengthy blockades creating severe food shortages had generated a great deal of data on the effects of malnutrition. Postwar circumstances made it possible to track the health of subpopulations that had survived on different kinds of rations and supplements (Carpenter 2003d). With the implementation of the Marshall Plan in Europe, the United States and eventually the United Nations became increasingly interested in monitoring nutritional health globally, with a particular concern that colonial territories not be neglected (B. Cooper 2016).

France's postwar effort to address the nutritional status of colonial subjects was initiated in the wake of the first organizational meetings for the Food and Agriculture Organization (FAO) in 1943. The title of the new research effort formed in 1945 reflects a mix of postwar optimism and French colonial ambivalence: the Investigative Body for the Physical Anthropological Study of Indigenous Populations of FWA Food and Nutrition. The colonial system in FWA had been predicated on a sense that African subjects were members of different "races"—more or less ethnically and linguistically configured societies that differed in fundamental ways from French society—hence in need of civilization. The priority up to this point had been to understand these populations as ethnically or "racially" defined subjects with particular hierarchies, customary practices, and legal norms through which they could be governed. Nutrition and food had, by this way of thinking, to be mapped in ways that conformed to the kinds of categories that had been used to collect tax and census information: ethnolinguistic groups seen as separate "races."

The head of the mission, Dr. Leon Palès, was assistant director of the Musée de l'Homme natural history museum and had conducted previous anthropometric research (anatomy, physiology, and comparative pathology) in French Equatorial Africa and among African soldiers stationed in Marseille in 1938 (IMTSSA 162 Palès 1945, 2).[16] Much of the initial work of the Mission Anthropologique bears the marks of his penchant for measurement, X-rays, and careful drawings. It also echoed a tenacious model of "raciology" that called for the measurement of noses, jaws, and necks and the administration of intelligence tests (Bonnecase 2011). The choice of Palès to lead the mission reflected the continuing significance of military medicine in FWA well after the initial conquest had been completed. France's relationship to local societies had been shaped by the need to recruit soldiers and the concern to characterize the various African "races" in order to control them militarily (Lunn 1999; Echenberg 1991). Palès's previous work had made use of convenience samples of soldiers, traditionally a useful population for social science and medical researchers (IMTSSA 398 Palès 1949, 5).[17] But the medical interest in soldiers in FWA, as in other parts of the colonial world, also had to do with their capacity to perform a particular kind of labor. The goal was to have healthy and effective soldiers and, by extension, to find ways to improve the productive capacity of African male labor more broadly (IMTSSA 162 Mayer 1954, 8).

Palès knew that the sample he had from among soldiers would not be representative of the population as a whole. In effect, he used the relatively robust and well-fed male soldiers as an ideal "norm" against which to measure the actual physical and nutritional shortfalls among civilian members of their respective ethnic groups. Palès inventively used the military population to try to gain insight into the condition of civilians of the same ethnicity: "the soldier becomes thereby physically an index of what could be but is not . . . it is he who gives us the measure of how much change perceptible improvements in food and essential nutrition can bring about in African populations" (IMTSSA 398 Palès 1949, 20). To do so, he measured large numbers of adult male military and civilian subjects to establish how robust they were. Palès's measurements also served as a means of gaining a more rigorous taxonomy of the degree of racial intermixing of Negros, Ethiopians, and Arabs in order to skirt the "false" self-designations of populations in this extremely hybrid region (IMTSSA 398 Palès 1948, 8–9). Ironically, among the important discoveries of this comparative work was that hypoglycemia, which Palès had hypothesized to be the "normal" condition of the African, did not exist among soldiers on a good diet—as Palès was to note, "in this respect, human physiology is one" (cited in Bonnecase 2011, 129). Overall, his research established that in fact race was of little utility in understanding disease.

In 1952, the mission's name was changed to the Research Organization on African Food and Nutrition (L'Organisme de Recherches sur l'Alimentation et la Nutrition Africaines, better known by the acronym ORANA), more in keeping with the mandate to respond to the urgings of the FAO. Not long after the publication of its major findings in 1954, the research agenda of the mission was for all intents and purposes disbanded. A new phase of implementation was, in principle, to succeed it (Collignon and Becker 1989). In producing recommendations for improved diets, the ORANA researchers were operating from a newfound awareness of just how impoverished the local diet actually was across much of French West Africa. The final report found diets deficient in calories and poorly balanced all across the territories. It accounted for them in a variety of ways (purchasing power, seasonal shortfalls, a mixture of the two), but the overall picture was one of a population straining to meet even the most basic caloric needs, much less a varied and balanced diet.

A variety of not entirely congruent explanations were adduced to account for this shortfall. One focused on the "native nutritional errors" or the poor eating practices that purportedly contributed to malnutrition. The native was, above all, seen to be improvident—"the overwhelming majority of blacks are lacking on foresight. They don't know how to save either foodstuffs or money" (IMTSSA 398 Bergouniou 1951, 15). Native diets were poor in animal products such as the milk and meat so "indispensable for the nursing mother and the child at weaning—it is at that moment that ravages of gastro-enteritis are felt and that kwashiorkor appears among small children whose livers begin to fail" (IMTSSA 398 Bergouniou 1951, 15). Some French nutrition specialists were inclined to see the "failure" of natives to eat more meat as irrational attachment to cattle: the challenge would be to "convey to people that herds must be exploited and should not remain unproductive capital" (IMTSSA 398 Bergouniou 1951, 15; cf. Wiley 2001).

Resonating with the rising fear of "detribalization" in British Africa, Palès's studies also suggested that with Westernization and modernization, Africans were losing their "ancestral knowledge" of rurally based and ethnically inflected food practices most visible not in staple foods but in condiments and snacks such as wild fruits (IMTSSA 398 Palès 1948). Implicit in the admiration for highly nutritious indigenous foods was a criticism of Africans' foolish abandonment of this rich diet in the chimerical pursuit of the status that would come with a more Westernized lifestyle. The role of ORANA was not to discover something new but to persuade the native to return to the riches of Africa's natural wealth: "West Africa, the land of malnourishment, is also the land of the richest sources of vitamins: vitamin A (and D) in shark liver oil, vitamin B 1 from the pomme du Cayor, vitamin C from the Detarium tree and from the Bauhinia" (IMTSSA 398 Palès 1948, 27). This approach had the advantage of costing very little while placing the burden on Africans to "choose" to change (IMTSSA 162 Palès 1954, 225–26).

By the early 1950s, the earlier colonial concern to increase the size of the African population had begun to give way to unease about the implications of a population that, following the decline of major epidemic disease, was growing rapidly. With the expansion of education, farming was becoming less appealing. Fewer producers were increasingly expected to feed larger numbers of urban consumers. Turning to mechanized agriculture and fertilizer, the intensive approach in European farming, was unknown and in some ways impracticable in the Sahel. Far more likely would be an ever more extensive agriculture at the expense of fallow periods, potentially aggravated by the promotion of animal traction (IMTSSA 162 Palès 1954, 28). In his final report, Palès expressed his fear that this shifting agriculture was a luxury in the land of the poor, sustainable only so long as the population remained sparse and land plentiful.

Gendering Nutritional Science: Female Knowledge and Male Labor

The mission's emphasis on maximizing potential male labor through interventions tailored to different regions and ethnic groups rendered the needs of women and children largely invisible. Despite an initial effort to take careful measurements of children's growth, the research mission quickly lost interest in the subject given the extremely poor development of birth and death registrations across FWA and the inaccuracy of the ages offered by potential subjects (IMTSSA 398 Palès 1948, 11). Similarly, after a single early study of bloodwork among a convenience sample of soldiers, civilian men, and women in Dakar, attention to women as potentially distinct subpopulations was completely dropped. It was dropped precisely because the women most accessible for scientific study were women attending a postnatal clinic: 90 percent of the women were found to have a vitamin A deficiency as compared to only 8.3 percent of the soldiers and 46 percent of the civilian men. Women's pregnancy and childbirth rendered their blood samples difficult to interpret: Were the women's diets poorer than the men's? Or were they simply losing their nutrients temporarily to the fetus? No one pursued the question of why pregnant women were not consuming the local sources of iron or whether they managed to bounce back while still nursing (IMTSSA 398 Palès 1948, 17–18).

Another study of women's breast milk was abandoned because not all the women in the study were eager to give up their milk, and the research subjects had a habit of disappearing before researchers could determine whether shark's oil improved their milk: "it is useful to emphasize that women generally go out only on the eighth day after giving birth, and that because of various superstitions, we ran up against difficulties in the course of taking milk samples. In particular there is a belief that an infant will die if his mother gives his milk to another child" (IMTSSA 398 Auffret and Tanguy 1947, 230). Rather than explore the meanings of milk and why it was so important to women to protect it, the researchers turned to other issues.

Nevertheless, Palès forthrightly confessed that the ideal informant for his study of native diets would be a French-speaking wife of a polygamous chief (IMTSSA 162 Palès 1954, 106). Puzzlingly, researchers ignored women's role as the producers of food and as contributors to a complex food production system that went well beyond the staple millet, rice, and manioc fields. While researchers had to have been aware of women's food processing and marketing activities (after all, they sampled women's wares in the market), the studies of diet didn't attempt to make sense of how women acquired the elements of meals, what they did with the profits of food sales, or how those kinds of foods (unlike the family meals cooked by wives of soldiers) circulated. The "social relations of consumption and exchange" fell very much outside the purview of that schema (Moore and Vaughan 1994, 47).

Ethnos Theory: Faulty Feeding and the Neglect of Political Economy

French colonial science read the space of FWA in ways that documented bodies as fundamentally ethnic, with little attention to gender, social status, or history. The ideal body was a male body. Although preventive rather than purely curative medicine was recognized as important, the focus of most interventions in nutrition touched only African workers and soldiers (largely male) and their families (Domergue-Cloarec 1997, 1233). Neverthe-less, by the late 1940s, scientists were increasingly attentive to the health effects of protein shortfalls, although they did not entirely understand how amino acids actually worked. In the late 1940s and 1950s, kwashiorkor had been identified as a specific problem thought at that time to be largely the result of inadequate protein consumption. By the 1960s, this emphasis on protein had led to the declaration of a "world protein problem."[18] Discus-sions of the prevention of kwashiorkor ignored the implications of the intro-duction of cash cropping for nutrition; the explosion of peanut production for export, for example, was not explored as a significant dimension of nu-tritional well-being. In particular, no attention was given to how such shifts might have affected women's nutrition or that of children. Women came into visibility only in the context of the handful of medical centers devoted to the health of pregnant women and small children. While valuable, they could never adequately address the problem of nutrition in FWA.

From the records of the Service de Santé for Niger, one is left with the impression that the innovations in improving infant and maternal care that were to come to Senegal in the wake of ORANA's work, however limited and problematic, entirely bypassed Niger (Ndao 2008). By 1955, Niger did have a service for the protection of children's health, but it was reported to be "embryonic and barely functioning except in major centers" (IMTSSA 62 Author unknown 1956). In the lead-up to independence from the mid-1950s, annual medical reports for Niger were dismal affairs, dominated by uniform tables enumerating vaccinations delivered, consultations held, surgeries performed. More rarely they included perfunctory explanations of mortality that simply repeated previous reports: "the principal causes of mortality among infants and children between 1 and 4 are the same as in the past, that is, gastro-enteritis, malaria, respiratory infections, and small-pox" (IMTSSA 62 Author unknown 1956). Medical officers in colonial Ni-ger were acutely aware of the problem of infant mortality and were attuned to the question of how nursing, weaning, and food might be implicated in infant and child health, but they had neither the technical nor the budget-ary means to begin to address it. It was only after independence, with the creation of a dense network of centers for the promotion of maternal and infant health under the Hamani Diori and Seyni Kountché regimes, that a consistent effort to invest in the health of women and children was made.

Notes

1. In some ways, the term *débilite congénitale* was a catchall statistical category for infant deaths in general (Bertillon 1900, 107–8).

2. William Schneider's 2013 overview of the "long history" of smallpox eradication illustrates some of the important dimensions of France's more successful campaigns: centralized production of vaccine in specialized continental facilities, collection of surveillance data, targeted interventions in regions of likely outbreak, and efforts to contain the spread through quarantine. The Achilles heel of the programs was the mobility of populations across colonial boundaries, particularly through Chad and Nigeria.

3. ANS 1 H 102 versement 163, Protection maternelle et infantile "Mesures législatives et administratives en AOF" 1934.

4. ANS 1 H 102 versement 162, Protection maternelle et infantile: organisation I "Haute-Volta" 1950.

5. Aoua Kéita began school at the Orphelinat des Métisses in Bamako in 1923; her father recognized early on the significance of education for women, in part because as a member of the chiefly elite he had been encouraged to send his sons and daughters (1975, 24–26).

6. 1 H 102 versement 163, Protection maternelle et infantile "Mesures législatives et administratives en AOF" 1934.

7. Frustratingly, just as Niger began to produce larger numbers of graduates in the late 1940s and 1950s, the entry requirements into the medical school were raised (Barthélémy 2010, 76).

8. Barthélémy's interviews with graduates of the school show a clear link between girls being exposed to professional women they could admire and their determination to go on to attain a higher education (2010, 63–69).

9. ANS 1 H 102 versement 162, Protection maternelle et infantile "Documentation" July 13, 1948.

10. One woman reported that once the Bobo she served in Upper Volta saw that she had had success in assisting in births, the children gave her a military salute when she passed (Nogue 1923, 461).

11. Kéita (1975, 258). Kéita's political activism clearly affected her medical postings—this assignment was probably intended to be particularly unpleasant for her.

12. ANOM FM 1AFFPOL 541 Affaires Politiques de Coppet 1936, 15.

13. Dr. Gultzgoff in French Sudan reported to Savineau that doctors in Dire had used guards to enforce vaccination in 1928, but by 1937 ideally the chiefs themselves reported epidemics. The picture was shifting, and not all regions were moving toward a less militarized approach at the same rate.

14. French secularism, known as *laïcism*, has often been less amenable to religion than American secularism. The former protects the population from religion, the latter protects religion from government.

15. I knew Liz Chisholm personally and interviewed her several times in Sebring, Florida, where she served generously as my host and liaison to other retired missionaries who had served in Niger. She died at the age of seventy-four in 1999, having lived out the end of her very active life with her sister Ruth Chisholm in the SIM retirement community. The documents I draw on here are letters she wrote home, largely to her mother and to Ruth, during her long missionary career, which were donated to the SIM archive. For a fuller

exposition of this argument on mission medicine and childbirth in Niger, see B. Cooper (2018a).

16. Palès authored a celebrated thesis on paleopathology, using the study of ancient bones to study disease in prehistoric times (Palès 1929). Palès went on to do celebrated work on the rock art of the Grotte de la Marche in France together with his partner Marie Tassin de Saint-Péreuse.

17. Nutritional science has historically depended on research subjects whose diets could be bureaucratically controlled—notably sailors, prisoners, soldiers, and orphans. See Carpenter (2003a, 2003b, 2003c).

18. Carpenter observes that this emphasis on protein was to give rise to a great deal of impractical and highly theoretical nutritional research on fish protein concentrates and other "high-tech" solutions to the "world protein problem" (2003d, 3337).

7

FEMINISTS, ISLAMISTS,
AND DEMOGRAPHERS

JUST AS HEALTH PRIORITIES IN NIGER PRIOR TO independence tended to favor male labor (and in particular soldiers) over women, so also in the realm of politics after World War II the interests of organized male laborers structured the French colonial approach to the demands of West African subject populations. The central labor demand—family allowances such as those earned by workers in France—conceived of the household as headed by a man supported by male wages. Mirroring the demands of French trade unions, salaried activists in French West Africa (FWA) demanded compensation that could support the male breadwinner in maintaining an urban "evolved" lifestyle. In an agricultural economy such as Niger, the proportion of such households was very small compared to longer-established coastal colonies. Yet, the logic of family allowances held in Niger as elsewhere.

Eventually, in 1956, family allocations became a required component of any formal-sector employment. Workers earned more for producing more children. But as Fred Cooper notes, "the corollary of the support given to workers' wives was their submission to surveillance—to the certification by doctors, nurses, and teachers that they were raising their children correctly" (F. Cooper 2003, 135). In other words, women were visible politically and bureaucratically primarily as wives and as bearers of children. Proper citizenship implied being "good" mothers as measured by outsiders. At the time of decolonization, Nigerien women were firmly constrained within a paradigm of citizenship in which women's rights to vote and to have a public presence were linked to their functions as mothers and as the protectors of "tradition." The earliest debates about female suffrage in the French West African territories proposed the vote exclusively for women who had served the public good by producing four or more children; this was convenient since such women were already legible bureaucratically as the beneficiaries of special government benefits for large families (Djibo 2001, 96–99). Women's very franchise was bound up not only with their capacity to bear children but with high fertility. Eventually, party politics rendered single women useful as emblems of modernity, but it was woman-as-mother who remained the focus of serious discussion of women's issues in the decades that followed independence.

Under the circumstances, women had no immediate incentive to focus on fertility control, and their political demands emphasized maternal concerns from the very outset of Nigerien independence. Salaried women did articulate the priorities of female civil servants (primarily teachers and *sage-femmes*). However, access to contraception was far from being a central concern; limiting fertility appeared to fly in the face of the ambient fear of infertility and the high mortality of small children. The notion that "too many" children resulted in food shortage and famine (the presumption of many in the West, see Brown and Eckhom 1974) was not self-evident in the Sahel, where consumers were more closely attuned to issues of access and pricing. Far more significant than food shortages were the periodic and highly seasonal epidemics of childhood diseases, particularly measles and meningitis (Fargues and Nassour 1988). Addressing the causes of child mortality through vigorous vaccination programs would have made more sense to most mothers than controlling fertility.

Therefore, just as the discourse of overpopulation gained traction in the West, concerns of women in Niger and much of the Sahel were articulated not in terms of individual rights but rather in terms of the family as a male-headed unit and motherhood as a dimension of citizenship. The externally driven insistence on population control that accelerated in the years after decolonization struck a discordant note in Niger, compounding the existing reticence toward maternal health efforts under colonial rule. Any discussion of women's reproductive rights in Niger today inevitably runs up against a legacy of overburdened services, mismatched priorities, and distrust. As a result, emotions surrounding women's reproductive practices and the use of any kind of "Western" medicine in the context of reproductive concerns in Niger can run very high. It is very difficult for the modest numbers of female activists to initiate debate about family structure, paternity, or reproductive health without being seen as members of a fifth column bringing danger and contagion into Niger.

This chapter will trace the growing postindependence debates in Niger about population size, available resources, and contraception. Colonial-era demographers and policy makers—the "counters"—had begun to raise concerns about population growth immediately prior to decolonization. After independence, those discussions about how best to further the interests of Niger as a nation, how to preserve and protect women's fertility, and whether to take demographic considerations into account in addressing the needs of Nigeriens grew in intensity. By the 1990s, these debates regularly pitted female activists and Islamic reformists against one another in an interminable dialogue of the deaf.

Decolonization and the "Population Problem"

By the 1950s, the need for plausible statistics for planning had become acute. In the postwar environment, France was expected to report to the UN on education and health in its colonies. This oversight produced flurries of paper for reports on FWA as a whole and on the overseas territories in general. Accurate information was not simply a matter of international prodding or budgetary planning, although both were important. Data was needed to anticipate and respond to social and political problems. Understanding population was, as in the past, necessarily bound up with questions of labor. It was becoming increasingly clear that there was no system in place to match the production of African graduates to appropriate posts. The minister of overseas France informed his personnel: "Employment for graduates is henceforth a question that must be approached with as much precision as possible in order to resolve the problem properly. The social and political dangers of a negative perception of the employment prospects for the future native elite prompt me to place the greatest importance upon the conditions and probability of employment in the overseas territories" (CAEF B-0057578/1 Ministère de la France d'outre-mer, September 20, 1955).

Making any kind of population prediction was complicated by the perennially undeveloped civil registry system across FWA. Predicting population growth from the scant existing records would be hazardous given the tendency of individuals to report certain kinds of deaths (the death of a father in the context of an inheritance) and not others (the death of a baby girl after one month) and to report some births (boys who might need to register for school) but not others (girls who would stay home to assist their mothers). Similarly, only civil servants and soldiers tended to report marriages and divorces; even then the status of a marriage that had not yet produced a child might not be promising enough to merit registration (CAEF B 0057576/2 "Remarques" May 19, 1951).

With the 1956 Overseas Reform Act (known as the Loi-Cadre) individual territories gained greater autonomy to manage infrastructure (schools, medical services, and public works). Electoral politics were gradually introduced through elections at multiple levels; parties were scrutinized by France and either nurtured or thwarted. In many ways, the signal event of the period was not the formal independence of Niger in 1960 but rather the highly contentious 1958 referendum on the French constitution of the Fifth Republic under de Gaulle.

Guinea, under the leadership of Sekou Touré, and Niger, under Djibo Bakary, were the only territories in danger of voting "no" to the proposed constitution. In Niger, resentment toward the privileges of the chiefly class under colonial rule had crystalized into support for the populist Bakary, particularly in the breadbasket of the Hausa-speaking regions that had benefited relatively little from French rule centered in Niamey. He and Sekou Touré hoped instead for immediate independence leading to the reconfiguration of the political structures of the region in ways that might retain a stronger federal structure while providing greater political voice for the "little people" who were neither highly educated nor part of the free-born aristocratic elite. France, with a vindictive bad grace, let Guinea go but was unwilling to lose control of Niger, despite its marginality (Schmidt 2007; van Walraven 2013; Lefebvre 2015).

As World War II had made clear, Niger sat at a geostrategically critical juncture between France's interests in North Africa, West Africa, and Central Africa. France was loath to lose access to Niger's untapped oil and uranium. French meddling in the referendum and subsequent election resulted in the ousting of the populist Djibo Bakary (leader of the socialist party Sawaba, the majority in the Assembly) and his replacement by the Francophile Hamani Diori (the head of the Nigérien Progressive Party, PPN-RDA), largely through the mobilization of the traditional chiefs. The Sawaba Party was forced underground and eventually crushed. The independent regime that emerged was marred by its repressive authoritarianism, as the illusion of party politics gave way to the Françafrique reality under Diori's PPN (Lefebvre 2015, 382–97).

In the wake of the referendum, all the colonies of FWA (except Guinea) continued to be part of the French overseas empire; however, their individual characteristics and bureaucratic capacity as separate states became far more important than in the past. Tracing the contours and institutions of each of these ambiguously autonomous entities became the major task of the end of the decade, necessitating (somewhat ironically) a huge influx of French specialists into the region to lend expertise to the "decolonization" project. The population of French citizens in Niger jumped from 681 in 1945 to 3,040 in 1956 and eventually to 5,000 in 1964 (Lefebvre 2015, Annexe V, 467–70).

In the newly autonomous Niger, one of the first orders of business was to conduct the first systematic demographic study. Trained staff was borrowed from the Statistics Service of Côte d'Ivoire, analysis was done in Paris by the Institut National de la Statistique et des Études Économiques (INSEE), and the cost of the study was covered through French development funds. The result of this "Mission Démographique du Niger" appeared in 1962. The problematic study was not a census; rather, it sampled select villages in six zones marked off as homogenous in terms of ethnicity, population density, and agropastoral patterns. Population figures were then extrapolated in light of presumed village size and density within the region—a circular proposition given how little information on density was actually available (République du Niger 1962, 21). As much a study of agricultural budgets as of population, it focused exclusively on the agricultural zone and built on information conceptualized with the household as the unit of analysis and data collected through male heads of household. Still, given limited manpower and resources, an approach through sampling made sense and yielded data that was far more useful than any previous population estimate.

Despite its myriad flaws, the study revealed that the ratio of dependent members of a household to active members was high even for Africa and was rapidly becoming unworkable: roughly ninety-four dependents per one hundred active members (République du Niger 1962, 21). Sterility was quite common and very high in some regions, particularly near Lake Chad; 13 percent of women between the ages of forty-five and sixty surveyed had never given birth despite a very high rate of marriage (41). Male labor migration was quite common but varied by region and ethnicity (53–54). However, some oddities of the data appeared to undermine its credibility. The population pyramid, in particular, was intriguingly distorted: the age group of girls between ten and fifteen was startlingly underrepresented (19). Male household heads had evidently reported all females to be either unmarried prepubescent children (under ten) or married women (over fifteen). It was as if there was no such thing as an adolescent girl.

The first study of the nomadic populations was carried out between 1962 and 1964, once again with assistance from French technical experts from INSEE. This study focused on the more highly frequented northwest portion of Niger in a zone spilling out slightly over the borders of the *cercle de Tahoua*. By targeting a limited number of water holes where nomads were concentrated during the dry season, the researchers were able to question nomads of various ethnicities and status groups (Tuareg, Peul, Arab), both free ("true" Tuareg) and of presumptive slave ancestry (Bella); nomadic (Peul Bororo/Bella *nomades*) and fixed (Peul Farfarou, Bella *sédentaires*). It's difficult to know how these distinctions were made or the degree to which they matched the informants' self-perceptions (Loftsdóttir 2007).

Once again, adolescent girls were almost invisible in the count, and the sex ratio was skewed markedly toward men (République du Niger 1966, 76–78). A very large proportion of the male population was not married (roughly a third overall), in contrast with the very high proportion of married women (71% of Tuareg women, 89% of Peul); in general, men married much later than women (which contributed to the visibility of "boys" and the invisibility of "girls") (81). Men from among the Bella or former slave populations of the Tuareg made up a striking proportion of the men who had not achieved fully adult status through marriage (81, 115). Presumably many of the "wives" of freeborn men were effectively former slaves whose equivalence to freeborn wives would be ambiguous. One effect would be a reduction in the numbers of marriageable women available to Bella men.

The problem of infertility emerged forcefully—21 percent of Peul and 27 percent of Tuareg women had never had a child. Focusing exclusively on women over age fifty, sterility could exceed 25 percent among particular subgroups. Among "Farfarou" Peul women (relatively settled) over age fifty, 26 percent had never had a child. Among nomadic Bella women over age fifty, 29 percent had never had a child (95–96). These rates were extremely high for Africa in general and came close to those found in the infertility belt from Gabon to the Congo that had so interested Anne Retel-Laurentin.

In these studies, the variability of birth rates in different subpopulations was striking. Even in this very early study it was becoming clear that "free" Tuareg with an estimated Total Fertility Rate (TFR) of 1.15 would be demographically swamped in time by Bella with a TFR of 2.4 among nomads and 3.5 among the more settled. Peul and Tuareg who continued to be nomadic had significantly lower birth rates than their more sedentary counterparts (République du Niger 1966, 91) and much lower birth rates than the populations studied in the 1960 sample of sedentary groups (where TFRs ranged from a low of 4.1 near Lake Chad to a high of 5.96 in the farm regions surrounding the capital) (42). The interests of purely nomadic populations would inevitably attract less attention than those of the already far more populous sedentary populations over time, with snowballing effects as a result of differing investment in health and educational infrastructures.

Demographers under the auspices of the United Nations Economic Commission for Africa converged in Cairo in late 1962 to discuss the challenges and the urgency of collecting good data. Their recommendations emphasized the problem not simply of estimating population size in general but also of assessing population distribution and rates of growth. Some parts of Africa, they felt, appeared underpopulated and might benefit from a larger concentration of inhabitants to spur markets, diversify production, and improve socioeconomic life generally. But others appeared to have a larger population concentration than the habitat and land could perhaps support. Populations across the continent were growing rapidly as a result of improving birth rates and diminishing death rates. Population growth, some began to argue, would make it much harder to meet the cost of investing in and sustaining infrastructure, even in underpopulated countries (CEAF B 0057552/2 "Le Caire, Rapport 1962").

Tensions between French statisticians and the UN emerged not long after the requests for systematic demographic data for African countries became insistent. With limited resources, France favored the kinds of contained sampling techniques used in the 1962 and 1966 studies of Niger in order to gain insight into specific problems rather than a nationwide census. Training centers and advisers from the French INSEE had different models and approaches than the advisers sent by the UN (and in particular by the Food and Agriculture Organization), which frustrated local bureaucrats attempting to carry out the wishes of different national, bilateral, and international agencies. At the same time, the *chefs de service* within the French-speaking countries complained that their staff tended to leave the public sector for better pay with international organizations, a pattern that would only become more acute with time (CAEF B 0057552/3 "Rapport de Monsieur Ficatier" 1964).

Debates over how to interpret the data rapidly became highly politicized. If one read the data as showing a need to reduce population growth rates in order to keep pace with the growing demand for services, the best way forward in Africa would be to make contraception legal and available, following the lead of the United Kingdom (1930), United States (1965), and France (1965). Highly influential demographers and politicians in the United States made the case that high birth rates and high dependency ratios would impede the improvement of living standards (UNPD 2003, 13; Coale and Hoover 1958). The US government put more and more emphasis on the importance of population control to development, placing its resources and experts at the disposal of African countries in particular. By 1962, the UN had turned systematically to focusing on population as a major policy question, and by the close of the decade governments were expected to take responsibility for providing family planning services and information. A host of different specialized agencies began assisting in meeting this new "obligation" (UNPD 2003, 15).[1]

With the tensions and competitions of the Cold War, the United States imagined sizeable poor populations to be likely breeding grounds for communism; the decolonization period in Niger, as in many other colonial spaces, was darkened by European and American fears of a politics of redistribution incarnated in populist socialist or communist parties. This was not entirely unfounded. French intervention in the electoral process at the time of the referendum had driven Sawaba underground, forcing it to turn the tensions of the Cold War to its advantage by turning east for training and resources (van Walraven 2013, 397–510). A socialist-inflected uprising that attracted the growing underemployed urban underclass simmered from 1958 to 1966. Population control in poorer countries thus became seen as a matter of US national security. Under Kennedy, the United States Agency for International Development (USAID) became the institutional locus for humanitarian interventions with a strategic focus, featuring population-control measures as a major priority. By the 1960s, the United States had launched its "inundation strategy" to provide contraceptive access around the world (Patil 2008).

The Meanings of Contraception

Debates about contraception in Muslim contexts had begun earlier than is often recognized and focused less on "population" as a whole than on the quality of life of couples and their children (Atighetchi 1994). As early as 1937, the mufti of Egypt ruled that contraception was permissible among married couples if both spouses consented. In particular circumstances, a husband or a wife could unilaterally decide to prevent pregnancy: for a man, fear that he might produce an abnormal son because of poor life conditions; for a woman, if she wanted to prevent pregnancy too soon after giving birth. The Superior Islamic Council of Algeria declared in 1968 that family planning was legal with the consent of the individuals and to preserve the health of the mother and her future sons. And a congress in Rabat entitled "Islam and Birth Control" determined in 1971 that family planning was licit for married couples with the free consent of both spouses, so long as its purpose was to improve the quality of life rather than to reduce numbers (Atighetchi 1994, 721–22). In many ways, it was easier to make an Islamic argument justifying contraceptive techniques and even abortion for married couples than it was within the Christian tradition, in which the original texts were indifferent to questions of contraception.

However, arguments about population control were another matter altogether. By the 1970s, debates about the nature of development and the function of contraception were heated. The complexity of positions and players is visible in the reports of the 1971 African Conference on Population, held in Ghana under the auspices of UNESCO. At that point, the Economic Commission for Africa issued its own report, noting that only seven sub-Saharan African countries appeared to have an official population policy to check growth through family planning. Yet, in a different report, the commission appeared to take a more cautious approach, emphasizing population "redistribution" rather than population control (CAEF B 0057553 Conférence Africaine 1971). At the plenary session on policy and planning, the open discussion revealed the resistance of some representatives to the emphasis on family planning alone; some renewed a call for better maternal and infant health care, others noted the changing status of women, and some foregrounded economic concerns. The summary of the debate also noted that lowering sterility rates should be a priority, not simply lowering fertility. In short, there were clearly two camps: those who felt that the high population growth rates were a problem and others who emphasized the inequity in the "considerable gap between developed countries and developing countries." Although the persistent problem of underfertility emerged occasionally, it was rarely given a great deal of emphasis.

Newly independent nations in Africa struggled to find ways to address the challenge that population growth represented given their limited resources. Inevitably, many turned toward international institutions, bilateral arrangements with particular governments, and nongovernmental organizations such as Christian missions for assistance. Still, the challenge remained how to prioritize among broad primary health care, emergency relief, maternal and infant health, and the infectious diseases that contributed to mortality.

Government Medical Workers and Keeping
Pace with a Rising Population

Student theses written by young women studying at the national school for public health, the École Nationale de Santé Publique (ENSP), reveal the pressures that government medical personnel encountered in the face of an extremely rapidly growing population. The school was established after decolonization to complement the medical training institutions of Dakar. There were still very few educated women in rural areas, and the cultural gap between elite ENSP graduates and rural populations was considerable even in the late 1970s. Maliki Mariama and Moussa Rabi observed in their field study of problems facing young *sage-femmes* in the region of Madaoua (southern Tahoua), "[The *sage-femme*] is a health agent for obstetrics, a confidante, a role model, a midwife, and a childcare instructor all at once" (Maliki and Moussa 1980, 5). They emphasized that the range of duties assigned to a *sage-femme* was enormous and the expectations unrealistically high.

As the most highly trained member of her team at the PMI (Prévention Maternelle et Infantile), the *sage-femme* managed two nurses, an assistant social worker, two *matrones*, one general workman, a cook, a woman to pound grain, and the two chauffeurs. In addition to handling deliveries, she oversaw preventive prenatal care, educational activities related to nutrition and hygiene, well-baby visits, lessons on how to make weaning foods, vaccinations, the maintenance of the staff and building, and of course the ever-increasing production of reports and statistics. In addition, in order to maintain good relations with the community, she participated in "the activities of the Association of [Nigérienne] Women [AFN], wedding ceremonies, naming ceremonies, condolence visits to the families of those who die, and all the major arrondissement events [generally displays of support for the government]" (Maliki and Moussa 1980, 17–18).

Yet despite the *sage-femme*'s enormous burden, it is clear that it was almost impossible to meet the expectations of the rural women who knew very little about the range of administrative and health matters for which she was responsible and who found the experience of the maternity set-ting could be alienating. If she was respected by the population in general, "some women go so far as to follow her to her house abusing her verbally because of the episiotomies done on their girls or because they accuse her of taking all the prescribed medicines for herself" (21). A great many found the experience of the maternity unpleasant, even when they felt the *sage-femme* was well liked, because "the nurses and workers yell at us and especially at our *entourage*" (30).

For her part, the *sage-femme* felt that the women giving birth did not make her task easy; some refused a vaginal exam or insisted on injections rather than pills. Clearly, the numbers of women treated far exceeded what she alone could handle, and she had to hand many off to the nurses and other maternity staff as well as the visiting interns rather than attend to them directly. The students made two rather useful suggestions at the close of the memoir: ENSP students be required to study the national languages because language issues seriously impede the work, and efforts should be made to ensure that rural women understand the nature of the workload of the *sage-femme* (33–34). The *sage-femme* offered a piece of advice to other aspiring *sage-femmes*: "above all else, be patient, understanding toward the women giving birth and most of all to know how to respect professional confidentiality" (26). The *sage-femme* was, above all else, an intermediary in the sensitive and intimate domain of fertility and infertility.

The ENSP students in the field quickly learned that the *sage-femme* could not conceivably reach every patient. Despite the failed experiments with the use of *matrones* in both the colonial medical system and in SIM medical settings, the maternal and infant health system could not func-tion without them; the *sage-femme* in Madoua oversaw the work of two within her facility. Despite having access to a dispensary with a maternity since 1971, many rural women still did not benefit from the presence of a *sage-femme*. From their unstructured interviews with seventeen traditional birth attendants in rural areas, with thirty maternity patients, and with the *sage-femme* at the medical maternity facility in Keita, Fatoumata Mounkaila and Hamsatou Oumarou discovered positive dimensions of such *matrones'* practices, such as the use of an indigenous antiseptic soap (Mounkaila and Oumarou 1980, 34–35).

On the other hand, the two students discovered a considerable num-ber of practices they found troubling: food taboos reducing women's con-sumption of protein, forcible feeding and drinking during labor that could slow delivery and cause vomiting, discouraging women from actively push-ing even when fully dilated, and cutting an unduly long umbilical stump. Numerous practices could lead to infection: spitting chewed kola nut onto the umbilical cord, maneuvering the fetus with bare hands, treating the perineum with petrol, and having the woman sit on a rock or mound of sand. Other practices could cause hemorrhaging either during or after birth, such as pushing on the woman's uterus to promote the expulsion of the placenta. In general, traditional birth attendants did nothing to treat hemorrhaging, seeing it as a valuable form of cleansing (37–39).

SIM missionaries also found themselves constrained to find ways to build on village-level expertise, with similarly mixed results. One internal memo reveals dismay at how little impact the training of *matrones* had had on their actual practice in delivering babies. An evaluation of the village health project done in 1988 reported that "although [the *matrones*] can explain verbally what is involved in a normal delivery, in practice, they only go to the home of the woman delivering after she delivers, in order to cut the umbilical cord. Often, they take nothing more than a razor blade with them (and that not even a clean one)" (SIM SRG SR 28 Enns 1988).

The External Push for Population Control

Clearly, the gap between what the growing population needed in the way of health care and actual government capacity—even with the contribu-tions of missionaries and external aid—was enormous. Inevitably, Niger's government faced the question of whether to actively promote contracep-tion. The context for debating the question of reproductive control was very different in Niger and most of the developing world than it had been in the United States or France. The growth of access to contraception in much of the non-Western world was not prompted by arguments about women's rights to their bodies or even by the kinds of eugenic concerns frankly es-poused by upper-class white US feminists such as Margaret Sanger. If, in the United States, the 1970s saw the expansion of reproductive rights (*Roe v. Wade* 1973), highly visible efforts on the part of women and blacks to gain entrée into politics (Shirley Chisholm), and the emergence of fora for femi-nist debate that would include questions of sexuality (*Ms.* magazine), in the Sahel discussion of contraception and reproductive rights occurred against a very different backdrop.

In the Global South, externally driven arguments about the economic necessity of controlling female bodies in the service of the modernization of developing states prevailed. Together, the US government and the United Nations Fund for Population Activities (UNFPA) worked vigorously and openly to fund and execute efforts to control population growth in the developing world from 1969 to 1985.[2] Implicitly, the problem of underdevelopment derived from a lack of self-control, a disregard for technology, and an incapacity to plan for the future. Partly in response to the blame-the-victim analysis implied in modernization theory, theorists such as Walter Rodney and Emmanuel Wallerstein tended to focus instead on the global terms of trade, military technologies, transportation patterns, and the nature of industrial order rather than on "overpopulation" as the problem.

With the introduction of population-level arguments and the encouragement of wide availability of contraception to unmarried Muslims, contraception became widely perceived as a Western intrusion that would invite promiscuity. Attitudes against contraception began to harden as the external push to control population increasingly became associated with Western imperialism and an unfair preference for Israel over the Arab world. It was in that increasingly heated context that, in 1984, Pakistan proscribed all family planning on moral grounds (Atighetchi 1994, 722–23).

These currents and countercurrents were further complicated by increasing global concern about environmental issues. The notion that the Sahel was a space of particular fragility or danger had not really been in evidence until the great Sahel drought was well underway. The drought began in 1968, in a period of relative prosperity; there was no particular reason to read it as the harbinger of environmental disaster. By the time the crisis had begun to recede in the mid-1970s, the context for understanding drought had radically shifted. Suitable interventions were understood to be international rather than national in scale, in part because the drought had not been a respecter of national boundaries. Funding and expertise seemed to reside more or less "naturally" in the domain of external agencies such as USAID and France's Fonds d'investissements pour le Developpement Economique (FIDES). If the United States and supranational institutions were increasingly seen as *authoritative* in interpreting problems and presenting solutions, African governments were nevertheless understood to be *accountable* for the success or failure of those interventions, rendering them vulnerable to critique from both within and without. The fiction of African governmental accountability also created an atmosphere of nonaccountability in the metropolitan sites of finance and scientific "expertise," feeding the staggering accumulation of debt in African countries borrowing to fund the infrastructure of a "modern" nation.

By the time of the UN International Women's Year of 1975—the moment when open discussion of reproductive rights emerged globally—the Sahel had been radically reimagined in the West as a site of environmental fragility and overpopulation, a site in need of assertive interventions from the outside. African governments (and governments of many nonaligned nations) thus found themselves having to take a position on the issues of population and environment in the absence of a fully developed feminist movement with any articulated position on the issues of birth control, population policy, or environment. In Niger, contraception was not even legal in 1975, much less the subject of active promotion. Nevertheless, fertility reduction in the postindependence era became a key instrument in the toolbox of approaches applied to remedy perceived environmental decline in the "south" (Connelly 2008).

This intrusive context gave rise, at least at the outset, to a counterhegemonic impulse. By the time of the World Population Conference in Bucharest in 1974, developing nations felt empowered to contend that, in fact, "development is the best contraceptive" and to push for greater investment in stimuli to economic development rather than in contraception and sterilization programs. Certainly, the reasoning that only development would generate conditions suitable to reproductive restraint was as logical as the converse, that reproductive control would generate economic development. The two positions were mirror images of one another. Joseph Chamie notes that while most African authorities shifted from a position of indifference toward population growth or even a policy of promotion of population growth in the early 1970s, by the mid-1980s most were anxious about the implications of the rapid growth of their populations for the possibility of meeting needs in health, education, and employment (1988). By the mid-1980s, states such as Niger were far more likely to have adopted the neo-Malthusian frame of reference, not necessarily for reasons of environment but because of the fiscal drain of meeting the expectations of a growing population as African exports lost value and as international financial institutions become ever more exigent.

General Seyni Kountché came into power just as the UN Decade for Women was in the planning stages. The first order of business for Kountché after the coup d'état of 1974 was to generate an apparently civilian framework through which the military government could operate, one that would operationalize and lend legitimacy to military rule. He immediately transformed the PPN Party's women's wing, the Union des Femmes du Niger (UFN), into a government-sponsored structure to be known as the Association des Femmes du Niger (AFN) with branches throughout the country. Introducing a women's association under his control would facilitate relations with external actors at the United Nations, who expected Niger to send representation to the upcoming UN International Conference on Women inaugurating the International Decade for Women.

His government also established a government-controlled Islamic association (AIN) and a nominally "traditional" horizontal network of youth associations attached to simply constructed cultural centers (Samariya). The age-grade workgroups through which unmarried youth had once been initiated into sexuality and restraint were now repurposed for the development of the nation. The Samariya may also have been institutionalized in an effort to co-opt the energies of potential Sawaba sympathizers (van Walraven 2013, 304, 844). The fourth pillar of his regime, the Association des Chefs Traditionnels (ACT), institutionalized and channeled the power of the chiefs through whom France had previously governed indirectly. Labor unions were carefully managed through a single recognized trade union.

Kountché also established an institution for national planning that could generate the kind of data regarded as relevant by external organizations. The 1977 census was accordingly one of the first major efforts of the military regime of Kountché. This census was performed by the Direction de la Statistique et de l'Information within the new Ministère du Plan. The census depended on support from the UNFPA, with considerably less input from the French than the preceding studies. The effort called for enormous personnel (3,700 census takers, 329 *controleurs*, 56 supervisors, 7 regional directors, 360 chauffeurs, and 170 nomadic guides) (République du Niger 1985, i). The analysis of the data required another 84 trained individuals—in this instance, almost entirely Nigerien. In some ways, the census could be regarded as a kind of public works project at a moment when an infusion of cash across the country was urgently needed. As a demographic study, on the other hand, it left a great deal to be desired.

The technical expertise required for devising, organizing, and carrying out such a study was simply not yet in place. The data, in the end, was difficult to interpret because of a host of anomalies. Census takers working in regional capitals, not knowing what to do with the gender ratio skewed toward men they found in their data, tried to "correct" the figures to make overall numbers of men and women come closer to matching (République du Niger 1985, 27). This "correction" compounded the confusion, generating other discrepancies further down the line between rural and urban figures and between age sets (and therefore generations). Once again, the central quandary resulted from the social invisibility of adolescent girls. The data showed the numbers of women contracting in the age set from ten to fourteen and then swelling relative to men in the age sets from fifteen to thirty-four, only to settle lower than men once again at thirty-five to thirty-nine (République du Niger 1985, 53).

This pattern of "aging" nubile girls is not uncommon in the reporting of ages of children across much of Africa; in this instance, it gave rise to a kind of epistemological panic attack among the census takers that further muddied the already very confused waters. Now that the data had been contaminated, it would be hard to say whether in fact the excess of women in rural areas was balanced by a larger number of men who had migrated to urban centers, for example. Strangely, the data collection did not include the kind of information that would be necessary to study population dynamics; for example, no effort was made to determine fertility or mortality rates. It is as if the census takers had been instructed to steer clear of the question of population growth. Still, the data confirmed the "problem" of a very high dependency ratio that was increasingly seen to hinder development; those under the age of fifteen made up on the order of 46 percent of the population (62).

The Decade for Women as Seen from Niger

The UN-sponsored International Decade for Women from 1975 to 1985—which energized women across the globe by offering a platform to make visible women's concerns—fell at a relatively inauspicious moment for women in the Sahel. Given their more immediately pressing concerns about political instability, food security, and the absence of even the most basic health care, Niger's women were unlikely to embrace an assertive feminist movement based on the model of the autonomous liberal subject. Nor would it be likely that women in the Sahel would foreground women's rights to contraception and abortion in light of their preoccupations with subfertility.

At the outset of the International Decade for Women, Niger still operated more or less under the legal regime left in place at the time of independence from French rule. Because France had, in the interwar years, developed a deep fear of "race suicide," abortion and contraception were illegal in France from 1920 until 1967; indeed, it was illegal to even discuss contraception much less use it (which is not to say that French women didn't find ways around the law). France therefore bequeathed to her colonies a legal apparatus designed to promote population growth.

Initially, the women's movement in Niger was, as was common in many African countries, simply ancillary to the single party in power. In the early years of independence, the Union des Femmes du Niger under Hamani Diori had made a variety of demands that by and large accentuated the interests of married urban educated women seeking salaried labor in the formal sector. The group made no real effort to promote women's interests in specifically reproductive terms. Diori's UFN paraded independent single women in the foreground as emblems of modernity; however, it is not clear that the notion of women as autonomous citizens with rights apart from those of wives and mothers had any real purchase.

The shift from the Diori to the Kountché regime coincided with the initiation of the Decade for Women and might well have presented women in Niger with an opportunity to seize on the potential energy of the global women's movement. However, Kountché's carefully orchestrated "associationism" deployed the Samarya, the AIN, the ACT, and the reconfigured women's association (AFN) to emphasize Islamic values, rural needs, and a military asceticism. While it is commonplace for scholars to lament the passing of the UFN for the Association des Femmes du Niger under Kountché with the claim that the UFN was more radical, the AFN more co-opted, in reality neither association made particularly radical assertions in the interests of women as a whole (Djibo 2001, 116).

Kountché used the occasion of the UN events to launch the AFN and to channel its message. His newly formed AFN raised for the first time the questions of sex education and contraception (Djibo 2001, 115). It seems that Kountché himself found the issue of population growth worrisome; it was he, after all, who uttered the (in)famous pronouncement to Niger's women: "Pardon me, sisters, but you lay eggs excessively [*vous pondez trop*]" (Locoh and Makdessi 1996, 15). Women are depicted regularly in the region as "hens" whose capacity to produce eggs (*pondre*) is part of their value in marriage. But the conceptual line between domesticated reproduction and mindless spawning (also *pondre*) could become, as in this formulation, very thin.

Kountché's strenuous co-optation of Islam in the same moment tended to reduce rather than expand women's rights. For example, under the auspices of the World Muslim League, restrictions were imposed on women's international freedom of movement. Women had to seek the written approval of a husband or father to travel overseas (Djibo 2001, 158). Kountché's relationship to Islam did not strengthen women's bargaining power in marriage.

An interview with one of the women engaged in the gradual introduction of contraception in Niger offers a sense for the degree to which family planning was launched through male doctors and politicians rather than female activists. Madame D., a member of the AFN, had been raised by a widow in the Zinder region. She would go to school in the day and then come home and do door-to-door peddling for her mother to make ends meet. One day, she related to me, a French male doctor asked her why she was always asking for a job, and she started crying and explained everything. At that point, he felt sorry for her so he let her work for the dispensary registering people as they came in. They saw that she was a very hard worker, so as time went on she managed to get an equivalency for the brevet (roughly middle school completion). She kept getting training until she eventually was a specialist in pharmacy stock management. She would get regular training on the uses of the drugs. As a result, she was a very early adopter of contraception in the mid-1970s:

> MADAME D: It started with us! We were the first ones to introduce
> contraceptives! I had two babies close together and the doctor said, look
> you need to space them better. So from that time on, after the second
> birth, I used the pill. I spaced them all at least three years and ended up
> with five children. As for my own daughters, they each have three.
>
> BC: Did you tell your husband [a teacher], did he agree?
>
> MADAME D: No! I've never talked about it with him.
>
> BC: Didn't he wonder how you were spacing the children!?
>
> MADAME D: No, people back then didn't think that way, they just knew
> sometimes the babies come in two years, sometimes three, they didn't
> think about it. (Madame D. Niamey June 2, 2014)

When contraception was first introduced, then, it was through a very small number of urban women, many of whom worked in medical settings. Madame D. and a few other women were the first to try the pill and to make it available to other married women gradually through personal networks. Madame D. takes pride in her role in this, although she did not regard herself as an activist at the time.

Having created these associations, Kountché found himself caught between the genuine demands of women related to greater marital security and the expectations of the male representatives of the Islamic society and the chiefly class related to patriarchal control. Women used the AFN to push for (1) restrictions on men's ability to unilaterally dissolve a marriage through repudiation, (2) a higher marriage age for girls, (3) a cap on bride wealth, and (4) debate on marital property, polygyny, child support, and child custody (Kang 2015, 50). Their demands crystallized around the drafting of a notional family code that was to become an enduring emblem of women's thwarted activism, reviled by those who feared women's autonomy and upheld by those celebrating women's rights.

This first round of discussion of a family code in 1977 ended in a stalemate; women's demands appeared to be incompatible with the interests and views of the Muslim leaders and traditional chiefs on whom Kountché depended to run the government, and the proposed code was buried but never entirely forgotten (Kang 2015, 47–56). While the much-discussed code did not broach contraception per se, the specter of the introduction of French-style civil law as the *default* for all citizens combined with an *option* to claim Muslim or customary status appeared to some protesters to undermine the specifically Islamic character of Niger as a nation. Perhaps more importantly, it would also have undermined the authority of both Islamic leaders and traditional chiefs who oversaw the regulation of family matters of considerable economic import—namely, disputes over land and inheritance regulated by Islamized customary law.

However, Kountché took a more than merely instrumental interest in the problems of women and in particular in the conditions facing schoolgirls and single women. His Samariya structure provided a safe haven for the divorcées and widows relying on sexual favors to survive, women who had long served as scapegoats for drought in the region. By co-opting them alongside unmarried young men into the service of the state, building wells and schools, he provided a space in which they could earn a kind of legitimacy and citizenship (B. Cooper 1995). His regime pursued court cases in which male teachers who sexually harassed their female students and got them pregnant would be humiliated and punished, and he brought attention to the pressures on girls to become prostitutes in the context of drought through the state-controlled newspaper *Le Sahel*. No regime before or since has so systematically pursued protections for unmarried women.

But at the same time, Kountché's repressive regime was unforgiving of girls who were perceived to have committed infanticide. In the context of the Great Drought such cases attracted a great deal of attention and alarm. In her 1978 study of 120 male and female delinquents incarcerated in Niamey, Daniel Poitou found that after theft (by far the largest cause of incarceration), infanticide and rape were the next most common causes for the incarceration of youths. The case of a seventeen-year-old Zarma girl from a farming village in Dosso offers a glimpse of the kinds of ambiguous cases in the public eye under Kountché.

"M" lived with her extended family in her father's concession. No one in her family had been to school, and all depended on mixed agropastoral farming. Married and sent away at ten to a farmer in a neighboring village, she was sent back to her parents after two years. The couple had never had sexual relations because she was too fearful and he became angry with her. He migrated to Ghana in search of work, and she hadn't heard from him or received support in five years. She fell pregnant by an unmarried young man her own age in what seems to have been a casual relationship. She tried to hide the pregnancy, but soon everyone knew. She was arrested on suspicion that she had taken some kind of "medicine" to cause a miscarriage. M. claimed to have given birth to a stillborn baby in the company of her mother. Nevertheless, the younger brother of the village chief denounced her to the deputy district administrator in charge for fear that if he did not, his brother would be sent to prison for failing to report the "crime" (Poitou 1978, Case 3, 70). The case is suggestive of the array of strategies rural populations pursued to survive drought: marrying girls off to shed dependents, engaging in casual sex for favors, migrating in search of work. It also exposes the climate of fear under the authoritarian regime of Kountché as well as the presumption that any unmarried woman who claimed to have had a miscarriage had probably committed a crime.

In the wake of yet another severe drought in 1984, and with the analysis of the flawed but telling 1977 census in hand, Kountché signaled in 1985 his concern that there was a misfit between the population growth rate and Niger's production and land base (CEPED 14512 "Communication du Niger," 111). The *ministre du plan* hosted a national seminar on population and development in July 1986 as the first stage in developing a national population plan. Out of fifty-one participants, only six were women, of whom only three were Nigerien: a representative of the AFN (Mme. Zaratou Adamou), a representative from the Ministère de l'Interieur (Mme. Barry Bibata), and Mme. Halima Maidouka from the Ministère de la Santé Publique et des Affaires Sociales. The proceedings were meticulously reported in *Le Sahel*, which foregrounded the challenges of an exploding population and the importance of controlling population growth. In her presentation, Halima Maidouka argued that high fertility, close birth spacing, and multiple births contributed to the high infant mortality rate. She asserted that the optimal childbearing years would be from twenty to thirty-five; Niger could substantially reduce its infant mortality simply by delaying the age of first pregnancy (and implicitly marriage) and encouraging spacing (ANN C3351 "Séminaire National" 1986, 67).

Another presenter, Abba Moussa Issoufou, noted the ambiguity of the age of marriage in a setting in which it is puberty, not age, that is invoked when establishing nubility. Furthermore, the legislation in place required a married woman to obtain authorization from her husband to acquire contraception (ANN C3351 "Séminaire National" 1986, 169). He attributed the high numbers of abortions and infanticides in urban centers, and the high morbidity in childbirth of young brides in rural settings, to the lack of access to contraception (170).

The most intriguing presentation was made by the representative from the state-sanctioned Islamic association, Alkassoum Albahaki. In his talk, entitled "Islam and Family Planning," he asserted that contraception was not forbidden in Islam although it was only legal for those who were married. He also argued that abortion in the early stages of pregnancy was permissible in certain cases, for example, if medical opinion held that a pregnancy endangered a nursing infant. It would also be permissible to save the mother's life at any stage of pregnancy (ANN C3351 "Séminaire National" 1986, 176). If the presentation was not a broad endorsement of all women's rights to contraception and abortion, it certainly opened the way to consider whether Islamic arguments could be made to support them.

Legalizing Contraception versus Gaining Access

No legislative action resulted from these very modest suggestions until 1988, when the colonial-era anticontraception legislation was finally repealed. Even so, initially women could only gain access to contraception with the explicit approval of their husbands; single women could not gain access at all. Only with the gradual creation of health centers for women and children was access—in theory—available to all women whether married or not and without masculine approval. With the death of Kountché and his replacement by Ali Seybou, the late 1980s saw a remarkable opening toward reproductive health concerns.

During my first research in Niger, as Ali Saibou came to power, the change in atmosphere was palpable. The national women's association (AFN) was active throughout the country, conveying the implications of the new legislation to women in both urban and rural settings. In an interview in which I asked one AFN member, Hajjiya Agaani, what these workshops across the Maradi region were all about, she explained:

> It was so that we could enlighten [*wayo*] women about issues related to childbirth. Like, if they are there, what they can do to have more [children]; and like if they have had a lot of children, how can they raise the awareness of others [about how to succeed]. And things like, childbirth, they shouldn't have a little girl marry who isn't ready. Going off and having a baby that way, the baby dies and so does the mother. Sometimes you have a mother, but the baby dies, sometimes you have a baby, but the mother dies. And also, if a person is grown, but is getting old, really it isn't necessary to keep on giving birth, it's time to pull back. And like, if some people, like if you have a baby, you should wait a year or two or three before you have another baby. All that is what we did, raising their awareness. And once we have raised their awareness, then some of them can go into their homes, and the ones that don't know, little by little they will also raise their awareness. (Hajjiya Agaani, Maradi, April 12, 1989)

The AFN women engaged in this consciousness-raising were postmenopausal older women, generally well regarded in their communities. Many in Maradi were respected for having accomplished the pilgrimage to Mecca. They were not highly educated, but they were far more likely than urban Zarma-speaking women from Niamey to reach women in this region in which population growth was the highest in the country.

In retrospect, the ambitions of the Ali Seybou regime and the AFN seem quite bold and the dynamism of the moment full of promise, at least from the vantage point of reproductive control. Hajjiya Ta Mai Raga elaborated on their mandate:

> They [the national office of the AFN and by extension the Ali Seybou regime] had instructed us to have fewer children because there were so many children. Right. That we should have fewer births, and that way, our fields that we farm, that feed us, that way they would be enough—because if there are too many

children there aren't enough fields. No fields, no food. That's just trouble. And your child, you want to buy him something, if there are too many, you don't have enough money to buy them things that are healthy and make them strong. (Hajjiya Ta Mai Raga, Maradi, February 18, 1989)

At that time, the discussion of contraception did not yet provoke a great deal of heat. The women at the head of the effort had been trained in Europe, and funding was provided by United Nations Population Fund (UNPF).

Elsewhere in the Sahel, similar shifts were occurring. Pierre Pradervand, a Swiss development worker, recounted that when he first attempted to show a film about family planning in Burkina Faso in the early 1970s, the reaction was explosive: "At one moment during the film, two pen-drawn outlines of a teenage boy and girl standing naked next to each other appeared on the screen. The deep roar that went up from the crowd was unlike anything I had ever heard in my life. I really feared that the local 'prefet' would have me thrown in jail for disturbing the public order! It was clear that a powerful taboo had been violated." However, when he came back in the 1990s to Saye, he found that "men and women of all ages freely joked about sexual issues and family planning, in a good humoured, yet never superficial manner." Family planning was generally agreed to be a good innovation, although birth spacing was far more accepted than the notion of stopping births (Pradervand 1992). Twenty years of debate had altered popular perception of family planning significantly and perhaps only briefly recast what was and was not shameful to discuss publicly.

In 2014 I asked one of the key figures in the promotion of contraception, the founder of the Association des Sage-Femmes du Niger (ASFN), what had gone wrong—why had this promising beginning to discussions of family planning devolved into the current ongoing struggle between "feminists" and "Islamists"? Her response, which was echoed in the remarks of a number of other women of her generation, was that so long as women's issues were under the Ministry of Health, no one paid very much attention. It was only when Ali Saibou decided to create a ministry specifically for women's affairs that the tone of the debates shifted.[3] Instead of being perceived as an issue of the health of the population as a whole, birth control came to be seen as catering to the caprices of women who were insufficiently Muslim (Hajjiya Rakiya Kanta, Association des Sage-Femmes du Niger, Niamey, June 4, 2014).

Despite his gestures toward relaxing the rigidity of military rule and devising of seemingly democratic institutions, Ali Saibou's regime became increasingly unpopular because of pressures on the part of the World Bank to reduce funding for education. Students protested the release of an austerity plan that would make draconian cuts to education. Clashes with police and security forces led to the deaths of three students in February 1990. In the civilian coup d'état that ensued, the pillars of Saibou's "movement," including the AFN, became tainted by their association with an authoritarian regime.

Paradoxically, the democratization movement that swept across West Africa in the early 1990s contributed to the undermining of this fragile opening toward the availability of contraception for women and the open discussion of family size preferences. Nigerien women from a host of different backgrounds after 1990 were able to seize on the opening up of civil society institutions. Human rights abuses in particular could now be openly addressed, a relatively free media environment developed, and networks of citizens could initiate civil society groups based on their own priorities. That opening should in theory have made substantive debate of women's interests more possible; after all, there are now dozens of women's organizations and NGOs taking up questions of women's rights as human rights, traditional practices that are harmful to women's health, reproductive rights, and children's rights. But by the same token, the democratic transition fractured women's interests into a veritable myriad of women's groups organized around religion, profession, development philosophy, and funding sources.

Since 1990, a host of Islamist groups has emerged to assert the primacy of women's role as mothers and to counter even the most modest efforts to promote women's legal, medical, and social interests. Some are inspired by the Salafist Izala movement that entered into Niger via Nigeria in the 1980s. Others are Sufi counter-reform groups such as the short-lived Awaliyya (see Masquelier 2009). However, the position of devout Muslim women relative to women's rights as human rights can be quite complex. For example, the deeply rooted and theologically informed Tijaniyya Ibrahimiyya under "Mama Kiota" offers great promise for the support of the economic needs of women (see Barnes 2009). A longer Sahelian tradition of women's Islamic scholarship also gave rise to the popular radio sermons of Malama A'ishatu Hamani Zarmakoy Dancandu, who argued for women's education in both Islamic and secular schools (Alidou 2011).

Simultaneous with the explosion of civil society groups, international donors began to invest heavily in AIDS awareness campaigns in Africa in the early 1990s. It became not only possible but urgent to begin speaking openly about sexuality, largely from a masculine vantage point. As a result, today there is a broad familiarity with condom use among younger men and their partners—the ostensible goal being the prevention of the transmission of HIV. One result of the timing of this democratic opening against the backdrop of the AIDS epidemic is that in the minds of many Nigeriens, contraception is associated with sexually transmitted disease and illicit sexuality, and it is the prerogative of men.

Female Islamists have been quite vocal in religious associations opposing any change to the legal status quo affecting women (Masquelier 2012). Women leaders of secular associations promoting human rights approaches to women's issues are bitter about what they perceive to be the underhanded approach of the women representing the women's wings of Islamist groups. "Those women are just spies," I heard again and again, "they are just puppets of the conservative male Muslim leaders." Women supporting protections for women have begun to express to me the sentiment that the strategy of seeking progress through Islamic arguments has failed. If Muslim leaders are not willing to assist them in arriving publicly at an Islamic compromise, they will have no recourse but to turn to purely secular arguments (B. Cooper 2015).

As a result of this war of attrition, it is no longer even possible to raise the issue of female contraception as relevant to anything other than birth spacing for married women. The notion that a woman might choose to delay childbearing, to opt out altogether, or to prevent a pregnancy outside of marriage has been altogether effaced from public debate. Any open discussion of the Islamic justification for abortion, such as occurred under Kountché, seems a distant memory, despite the acceptance of abortion in numerous other Muslim-majority countries. In this atmosphere of hostility, and despite the gradual construction of a more robust health infrastructure in Niger, the adoption of contraception has been glacial in Niger outside the capital.

The problem has not simply been the practical challenges to getting access but also the many rumors and fears that concern women's reproductive health. Contending with such rumors was a major theme in the training of health practitioners as soon as contraception was legalized in Niger (AMSP Direction de la Planification Familiale 1989). The mistrust of Western institutions and of their motivations in the medical domain in the Sahel has been profound. That mistrust has regularly been articulated around the fear of infertility, as the polio vaccination crisis of 2003 reveals (Chen 2004). The evisceration of the hard-won public primary health care infrastructure developed under Kountché and Saibou, under structural adjustment programs, marked the powerlessness of African governments to protect their citizens; the empty dispensary had become a sign of the "ubiquitous absence" of the state (Masquelier 2001a). The conspicuous absence of infrastructure, argues Elisha Renne, has left many contemporary Africans with a "sense of government collusion or capitulation to the pressures of foreign powers" (Renne 1996, 133–34).

What was left in the wake of the neoliberal era was a handful of overtaxed extranational institutions (such as the SIM hospital at Galmi) handling cataclysmic care, a threadbare network of underresourced and understaffed state clinics for primary care and maternal and infant health (like Guescheme), and occasional expensive and noisy vertical "campaigns" by international organizations such as the Gates Foundation, WHO, and USAID focusing on polio eradication or AIDS awareness. Relative latecomers to the health infrastructure of Niger, Niger's maternal and infant health centers, known as PMI (Protection Maternelle et Infantile) were called on to bear the enormous burden of the nation's health needs for women and very small children. As a result of this health-care-on-the-cheap approach to public health policy, there has been a consistent linkage of vaccines and contraceptives in the experiences and imaginations of West Africans.

These episodic campaigns and the thin tissue of clinics have come to stand proxy for a genuinely broad and comprehensive primary health care system in much of the Sahel. Television, radio, and popular performance have all been marshaled ever more visibly and audibly to "sensitize" African populations toward the health priorities of national governments (intent on reducing the per capita cost of health care while shedding Africa's image as the site of starving babies) and of international donors (intent on reducing the perceived threat of African population growth and the spread of epidemic disease to the rest of the world) (Fairhead, Leach, and Small 2004, 6; Hartmann, Subramaniam, and Zerner 2005). Externally driven health priorities are immediately suspect in Niger for the very good reason that they are often wildly out of synch with local realities and needs.[4] The illogic of those interventions invites a fear that their hidden agenda is to undermine the fundamental Islamic values of Nigeriens.

Establishing "Muslim Values"

This skepticism about the meanings and intentions of purveyors of contraception and Western medicines produces such a noisy debate that it can be hard to draw discussion in more productive directions. The perception that contraception is inimical to Islam that is so common in Niger today flies in the face of earlier rulings of Muslim authorities both in other parts of the world and in Niger. Enduring debates in Niger also concern the appropriate age for girls to marry and their autonomy in decision making regarding marriage and divorce. But if there is a great deal of discord, preserving the values of Islam is a shared concern of the overwhelming majority of Nigeriens, no matter where they fall in debates about women's needs and rights. The problem is sorting out what those values are or should be.

Muslims in Niger today generally assume that the premium on girls' virginity prior to marriage across the Sahel and the preference for marrying girls off as they approach puberty are fundamentally Islamic. However, the lyrics of a song sung by "pagan" Hausa, recorded by Maurice Abadie in the 1920s, establish that virginity had long been celebrated in the region:

> Born of wedded parents, she will never be ashamed.
> Her father and mother must thank her
> For she has brought a happy outcome.
> Her bridegroom as well must thank her
> For she has remained a virgin for him.
> As soon as she sees him she is fearful
> For he is her superior. (Abadie 2010 [1927], 396 Annexe XIV)

Another common assumption is that it is Islam that dictates the early age of marriage for girls. But in speaking about whether a girl was ready to be married, women I have spoken with over the years referred not to age in any meaningful way but rather to the formation of breasts. It was the outward appearance of a girl that was noted first by her senior kin; menarche generally occurs at a later stage of development. It is likely that the first signs of puberty fluctuated with changing eating habits, periodic food scarcity, and the alterations to the activities of girls with urbanization. Girls in urban centers today are often far plumper than girls in rural settings. Overweight girls in particular tend to appear more physically mature than their peers, while overweight is also associated with early menarche age (Bralić et al. 2012). In other words, it is hard to know the marriage age of girls in calendar years either prior to or after the expansion of Islam or whether they were developed enough to bear children safely.

There can be an odd reticence in discussions of health crises in Africa regarding the silent explosion of "civilization diseases," including obesity and diabetes (Rothmaler 2012, 151). Eva Rothmaler has emphasized the striking nutritional decline as West Africans' diets have shifted away from the rich variety of native grains, fruits, and other plants toward foods that are regarded as "modern" and "clean" (and of course easier for overtaxed women to prepare). Traditional foods, when plentiful, are typically richer in proteins, fats, and minerals, and particularly in the iron so important in pregnancy than are the prestige foods eaten today (polished rice, corn and wheat flour, milk powder, Maggi cubes, canned goods, instant coffee, pasta, bread). They also include significantly less salt and sugar, and because they are less processed, they provide more dietary fiber (Rothmaler 2012).

Tracking the implications of these changes for the timing of menarche, the experience of pregnancy, and childbirth itself would be extremely interesting if there were sufficient data available. Because nubility or readiness for marriage was linked to visible signs such as the development of breasts rather than to age, changes in nutrition could have had an impact on when a girl was perceived to be ready to become a married "woman," possibly shifting the effective age of marriage upward (in times of nutritional stress) or downward (in times of relative abundance). However, any such shifts are unlikely to have been either unilineal or uniform across all populations and spaces. The rare nutritional studies focusing on adolescents (rather than on children under five) are suggestive of tremendous variation between urban and rural settings. The age of the onset of breast development as opposed to age at menarche can also confuse issues; in some settings, the onset of menarche can be quite delayed (Garnier, Simondon, and Benefice 2005). There are likely to have been bimodal patterns of change over time depending on whether girls were gaining in body fat (the typical urban pattern; see L. Jones et al. 2009) or losing in body fat (more typical of stressed rural populations; see Powloski 2002; Prentice et al. 2010). Urbanization exposed populations to new foods, to the seclusion practiced by Muslim elites, and to the education promoted by colonial administrators—with undoubtedly very mixed implications for the timing of marriage and sexual relations across time and space depending on education, eating habits, physical activity, and the availability of food.

Far more significant in terms of the implications of the expansion of Islam for marriage and fertility have surely been changes in sexuality within marriage. When I first began conducting research in Niger in the late 1980s, I spoke with many elderly women in Maradi about their marital histories bridging the late colonial and early independence periods. I discovered that women of that generation perceived sexual practices to have changed significantly over their lifetimes. I asked an elderly woman named A'i how many times she had given birth. She said six.

> A'I: Right, because once you wean a child, if I weaned him, then I'd wait another year, sometimes more.
>
> HAWA: Childbirth today isn't the same.
>
> A'I: People have more births now.
>
> BC: Because you wouldn't get pregnant again before weaning?
>
> A'I: I didn't give birth thoughtlessly [*ruwan ruwan*]. Nowadays—belly bursting right away, right after a birth you get pregnant all over again!? (A'i Kyau, Maradi, April 25, 1989)

Sexual restraint in marriage while nursing and for some time afterward had lost ground in her lifetime in ways she found shameful. In a conversation with another woman, I tried to learn more about the relationship between nursing and pregnancy.

> BC: I hear that in the past a woman wouldn't go to her husband if she was nursing a baby.
>
> HAJJIYA: Yes, not until you weaned the baby. Ah, but now, they won't agree to that!
>
> BC: Who, the men?
>
> HAJJIYA: Right, they won't agree to that. If you have done the forty days, that's it. Once you empty out your belly [of one pregnancy], every year you give birth, some [babies] stick around, some die—the babies. We [members of the national women's association AFN] have seen how worthless that is, it causes such suffering.
>
> BC: Do you talk about that [with husbands]?
>
> HAJJIYA: We don't say "only once the baby is weaned." Because they [the men] just say, "now we don't do it that way." Well, no matter what you say, they say, "Now is the time of Islam, and that was just a time of ignorance [*jahilci*], that business of 'only once you have weaned the child.'" (Hajjiya Ta Mai Raga, Maradi, February 18, 1989)

When I asked her to elaborate on why it was no longer possible to finish nursing a baby for two years before falling pregnant again, her response was blunt: "men today have no shame [*kunya*]."

To her, this failure on the part of men was a moral failing, revealing a lack of restraint and the decline of a traditional model of masculinity. The widespread adoption of Muslim identity had by the 1980s nullified the moral force behind conjugal abstinence while nursing. Women no longer had the means to counter the newer pattern of resumption of conjugal relations after only forty days (Cross and Barker 1993, 138). In many of these interviews, I sensed resentment at the presumption, verbalized under the Kountché regime, that it was the fault of *women* that there were "too many babies." And I sensed as well a hint of dismay that to object to constant childbearing would be to court an accusation of betraying Islam, of being an ignorant infidel.

As learning sexual restraint and sexual practices beyond intercourse through such institutions as the *samariya* and *tsarance* came to be seen by Muslims as immoral, the modest arsenal women could draw on to ensure marital restraint while nursing was undermined at the very same time that the "norm" of sexual resumption after forty days began to gain ground. The rejection of traditional patterns of nursing and weaning in favor of purportedly Islamic norms contributed to an invisible demographic earthquake. Shortened marital abstinence inevitably accelerated the fertility rate; a married woman's period of fecundity was thereby increased once early postpartum amenorrhea came to an end. While not all women would fall pregnant, many whose lactational amenorrhea (brought about by frequent and exclusive nursing) was brief for whatever reason almost certainly would. The decline of abstention while nursing was linked in the minds of my informants in the 1980s to a kind of undisciplined fertility; they did in fact see this abstinence as important to birth spacing and not simply to the purity of the milk.[5]

Those who fell pregnant would be constrained by the logic of the attribution of milk to the fetus to wean their nursing babies earlier than in the past. As women became more likely to fall pregnant while nursing, babies were more likely to be weaned before benefiting from mothers' milk for two years. But even more importantly, those children would need an alternative source of milk, which could only be provided by animal milk or, increasingly, reconstituted dried milk. In either case, the child's exposure to infections leading to gastroenteritis increased substantially. We have here the makings of an explosion in the birth rate combined with a steep rise in infant mortality. All this is invisible in the discussions of the demographers and the polemics of both feminists and Islamists.

These new conditions imperiled the health of small children, and they also increased maternal mortality. The decrease in birth spacing and increased exposure to pregnancy made it likely that a woman would not have sufficiently rested between pregnancies. She would become a high-risk grand multipare much earlier in her childbearing career than had been the case for her mother or grandmother. The only reliable way to counter these processes today would be to replace marital abstinence while nursing with the use of modern contraception.

However, thirty years later, most Muslim women I interviewed in Niamey had no collective memory of these earlier patterns of nursing and sexual restraint in marriage. I was surprised to find that a kind of amnesia had set in even among women who were in late middle age. The notion that it had once been normal to refrain from conjugal sex while nursing for two years struck many of them as astounding, so implausible that one woman challenged me to provide evidence of the practice. Among scholars of gender or demography in Africa, the decline of lengthy conjugal abstinence while nursing is so well known as to appear banal (Hunt 1988; 1999, 244, 279–80; Benefo 1995; Romaniuk 1980, 2011). But there is nothing banal about the deep-rooted assumption among Muslim women in Niger today that to adopt practices to prevent pregnancy while nursing would be to capitulate to the intrusive innovations of outsiders.

Notes

1. UNICEF, WHO, FAO, UNESCO, ILO, the World Bank, and USAID, and most directly of all, the United Nations Fund for Population Activities (UNFPA).

2. Although the United States supported UNFPA vigorously for many years, with the rise of the conservative right in the United States and the election of Ronald Reagan, the United States made an about-face. Under Reagan, the 1985 Kemp-Kasten Amendment barred US funding for any agency that "supports or participates in the management of a program of coercive abortion or sterilization" in the context of objections to China's "One Child" population control effort. Although reviews of UNFPA programs revealed that activities were not really in conflict with the amendment, Presidents Reagan and Bush suspended funding of UNFPA. Funding was restored under Barack Obama in 2009; however, Republican administrations have been consistently hostile toward UNFPA and family planning initiatives in general (Barot and Cohen 2015). In April 2017, under President Trump, the United States announced the suspension of support for UNFPA once again.

3. The health professionals who could promote family planning were all under the Ministry of Health, which was headed by a man. But the budget and planning was in the Ministry for Women's Affairs, which was the first to be headed by a woman. From that time on, there was constant fighting between the two ministries over staffing, budget, and strategy.

4. For a scathing indictment of the illogic driving the National Immunization Day program of the WHO, see Daniel Grodos (2008, 292–99).

5. Demographers debate whether postpartum abstinence or lactational abstinence can be seen as conscious forms of birth spacing in Africa and how to evaluate the significance of the variables of breastfeeding, amenorrhea, and abstinence; see Etienne van de Walle and Francine van de Walle (1989).

8

LET'S TALK ABOUT BASTARDS

It's a chilly day in January, and I'm visiting with the founder of an NGO promoting women's reproductive health. I am curious about problems related to rural girls' education and in particular why girls so rarely get to finish school before being married off.

> MADAME A: The parents say, "if she leaves her village to go to CEG [middle school] in a larger city, people will be angry, they will say, 'what will happen to her? Who will cover her?' The relatives will say, 'no, no we don't agree.'" So if someone presents himself to marry her they [the parents] will say yes, just to prevent her from leaving and going to Collège in another locality.
>
> BC: It seems as if there is almost a terror about bastards.
>
> MADAME A: Well, yes, that's just what I was telling you, it's shame [*la honte*], or rather it's fear [*la hantise*, dread or obsession] that if she leaves she might have an unwelcome pregnancy, there could be a rape, she might have temptations if her friend has a nice cloth and she wants one, someone will propose to her that she do something to get one, and she will say yes. That's why they marry off girl children: "good riddance!" [she says this with a hand washing gesture]. A girl is a problem, but a girl is also a guarantee of money [she makes a gesture suggestive of an eagerness for cash from the bride wealth]. (Madame A. (Niamey) January 3, 2013)

This parental perception that schooling and urban life promote immorality echoes the remarks made by a rural Takeita man in the late 1980s: "Our own daughters no longer ask our advice: they think they know all there is to know. They want to choose their own husbands and some don't want to marry at all—the towns and villages are full of bastards!" (Cross and Barker 1992, 142).

The anxiety about illegitimate children has endured, but it has been overshadowed by the related anxiety about women's sexuality. Struggle and debate in Niger over the elaboration of a secular family code, tendentiously nicknamed "the women's code," has raged more or less openly since 1975. Beginning in 2005, the government tried a different strategy, preparing a draft personal status code that would "put an end to legal pluralism and regulate family relations." But by 2010, after considerable resistance from conservative Islamic groups, the draft document was abandoned (UN CEDAW 2015, 7). While steady progress has been made in Niger in passing legislation to protect women from "tradition"—female genital cutting, for example, is now illegal—the passage and implementation of further legislation has been unimpressive. Little wonder, then, that any more ambitious program of legal reform regularly falters in the face of ever more carefully organized and orchestrated opposition couched in the name of Islam.[1]

While resistance to legal reform has often flared up over the question of whether women and men can be treated equally before the law, one might have expected the key debates to dwell on elements of the code that would have brought women's and men's rights in the realms of divorce and inheritance more in line with one another. These provisions do, of course, generate hostility. But interestingly, the most effective rhetorical rebuttal to the draft family code's provisions focused not on marriage or female inheritance but rather on *paternity* (Allio 2001). A provision in the draft to enable men to recognize illegitimate children was, according to protesters, tantamount to legalizing adultery. In fixing on this particular proposed provision of the draft code, Muslim groups focused popular anxiety on women's sexuality and the familiar problem of pregnancy outside of marriage. The underlying, but unspoken, issue is inheritance. On their father's death, would such children be eligible for part of his property, hence competing with the children of formal wives? The origin of the rejection of such children is not purely Islamic. Nor would any effort to protect them conversely be un-Islamic. To the contrary, one signal innovation of Islam was the protection of children, especially girl children, from infanticide. And yet rhetorically, in rejecting the personal status code in its entirety as "satanic" because it might render such children recognizable persons, activists opposing law reform have tended to argue that the notion of legitimizing children born outside of wedlock is a "Western" intrusion designed to authorize fornication (*zina*) and to undermine "our deepest Islamic values."

The longer history of the region suggests that local populations faced with the partially congruent and partially opposed moral systems of Islam and of the Bambara/Songhai cultural zone, have not fully succeeded in resolving the tensions between differing moral orders. If, in fact, in

Islam the child should be protected from infanticide, then the practices in place do not really reflect all the possible positions Islam might take toward these victims of moral indiscretion and societal rejection. In rejecting as "satanic" the provisions of the code that would protect these vulnerable children, Nigeriens punish the baby, for without support (family support, moral support, economic support) a woman's best solution to an unwanted child continues to be abortion, infanticide, or child abandonment. Yet one of the central innovations brought by Islam historically was the principle that no one could be punished for the crimes of another.

A counter-literature in Islam does exist, arguing not only that such children must be recognized and protected but also that Islam categorically prohibits punishing the child for the sin of the parent (Diouf 1998). One's predispositions regarding what is moral and acceptable in Islam are very much shaped by local concerns (WLUML 2006, 229–41). From well before the colonial-era expansion of Islam, the region in question rejected the humanity of illegitimate children. Focusing on the *zina* of the mother may simply be a way of deflecting attention from a deeper and more visceral ambivalence toward the monstrousness of the unrecognized child. The following comments of a Zarma *matrone* in Belende in an interview with Moumouni Adamou in 2000 are suggestive of just how profound such revulsion can be:

> If I am called to assist a girl who has gotten pregnant who knows how, that makes me feel very ashamed. I have even refused to respond, because I know that if the marabouts find out they will say that it is not the path to follow in the Koran . . . Even before hearing the first cries of the [bastard] baby people will run away because they say that anyone who hears it will go to hell . . . It's the head nurse who forces me to attend to them, he says that we don't have the right to discriminate that way. Still, it's a sin, it's the head nurse's sin, since he forces me to. (Olivier de Sardan, Moumouni, and Souley 2001, 31)

How and when a potential human (embryo, fetus, newborn, child, adolescent) becomes a recognized social person is at the heart of debates about contraception, abortion, infanticide, and child abandonment (Boltanski 2013; Lancy 2015). Success in family law reform in Niger would require contending directly with the question of the *personhood* of children born out of wedlock. Such children are physical prompts for the sensation of shame. Revulsion toward them and what they signify is part of the very fabric of social relations in Niger (cf. Livingston 2008). In this chapter, I will argue that many central social problems facing Niger today—child marriage, female illiteracy, infanticide, child abandonment, dangerous illicit abortions, and a high population growth rate relative to available government resources—have a single origin. They are, at heart, due to an unrecognized refusal of Nigeriens to address this unresolved moral problem: how to deal humanely with the seemingly monstrous illegitimate child. What would it take for an ethics of child protection to overcome the dehumanization that is attached to the visceral sensation of disgust? Let's talk about bastards.

"Clandestine Abortion" and the Nigerien Schoolgirl

Niger's abortion laws are extremely restrictive: abortion is only permissible with the agreement of a group of doctors to protect the health of the mother or if the fetus is determined to be highly likely to suffer from a serious "affliction" (Moussa 2012, 447). This does, of course, offer an avenue for women who have the awareness, the means, and the confidence to seek out a health professional who will attest to a medically approved abortion that would be technically legal. Certainly, some women do turn to health professionals for assistance with unwanted pregnancies—but so far as I can tell, only illicitly. Interestingly, to the degree that it can be known given that it is necessarily secretive, the profile of women who attempt to abort a pregnancy appears to be slightly different from that of the young women incarcerated for infanticide. From observations of women admitted to hospitals for complications due to abortion, public health specialists in Niger argue that clandestine abortion tends to be the recourse of the schoolgirl who has a boyfriend and who hopes to evade ejection from school and the rejection of family. A 2007 study by Salamatou Abdou of girls in major high schools in Niamey suggests that their reasons for seeking an abortion are similar to those of women who commit infanticide. The most commonly cited reason is to protect their honor (*sauver l'honneur*) in a context in which the male partner refuses to recognize paternity and dignify the pregnancy with the prospect of marriage (Abdou 2007, 32 Tableau no. 5).

The educational structures in Niger are characterized by a stark disproportion between boys and girls, differences that become ever more acute at more advanced levels of schooling. By the time girls reach high school, they may find that they are outnumbered by boys by close to two and sometimes three to one (Abdou 2007, 24, 26). They are vulnerable to assault by their peers, but, sadly, they are also quite prone to pressure to exchange sexual favors with men who work for the state (largely teachers) for gifts of cash or for passing grades (Maman 2003, 38). Despite a good grasp of the health risks of poorly performed abortions, over half (58%) of the 488 female students in Abdou's study knew someone who had had an abortion (Abdou 2007, 33). About half (52%) said they had never received any kind of education about abortion, which is to say that none of them were aware that medically approved abortion is actually a possibility. Only 18 percent of the young women indicated that girls seek abortions from health professionals. The others stated that girls attempt to abort on their own (22%) or by seeking assistance from a traditional healer (19%) or a Muslim scholar (7%). Most attempt to provoke a miscarriage by taking something toxic. The line between abortion and suicide is, consequently, rather slender. Many attempted abortions lead to hospitalization, although it is difficult to know how many do not, or how many attempts succeed in prompting a miscarriage or a death deemed an accident or a suicide. The recognized risks due to clandestine abortions, and a history of health services rejecting young women seeking postabortion care, prompted the inclusion of a requirement that health professionals treat women for complications for abortion in the 2006 reproductive health law (Moussa 2012, 447 Article 16).

Studies of unwed mothers, abortion, and infanticide all confirm the absence of effective sexual education in Niger. The attitudes toward sexuality characteristic of the Islamist women's organizations in Niger today are not conducive to open discussion of sexuality. "Islamic" training for girls does not address sexuality directly. When I asked Madame N., the head of one of the major Koranic institutions for women in Niamey, how her students are specifically prepared for womanhood, she responded that the Koran teaches about the dignity of humans and how to attain it. It is for all Muslims—not for men or for women:

MADAME N: There are five fundamental things Islam requires [ticking them off on her fingers]: the protection and respect of life including human life, the protection and care of material things necessary to life, the protection and respect for family life . . .

BC: What does that mean exactly?

MADAME N: The bastard [enfant naturel] can never inherit because there is no marriage; the father should recognize him, but that's it. The child belongs to the mother. [Counting on her fourth finger] Then religious training is necessary to protect religion itself. There was one more thing on the list . . . [she pondered a moment but couldn't recall the fifth].[2]
What really matters is honor—that is what defines a person as human, it's what distinguishes humans from animals.

HAJJIYA: Once, when I was in France, it was the French embassy that took us, they asked us "what is the most striking difference to you, either good or bad?" And I told them "men and women out in the open sucking one another on the street!" It was bestial! It was disgusting!
(Madame N., Hajjiya, Buzu, and A. Z., Union de Femmes Musulmanes du Niger, Niamey, June 18, 2014)

Instruction in sexuality in such a context simply informs girls to "be careful" around men, to veil, and to obey their parents. Girls frequently enter puberty with very little comprehension of the most basic elements of reproductive health, including menstruation, ovulation, the functioning of contraception, and so on.

In the late 1980s, under Kountché and Saibou, an effort was made in Nigerien schools to develop materials suitable for introducing concepts related to population issues at lower grades in science classes and a familiarity with family planning in higher grades. With support from the United Nations Population Fund and UNESCO, the initiative drew on materials and experiences of health specialists in Togo, Benin, Mali, Burkina Faso (formerly Upper Volta), and Côte d'Ivoire, all of which were evidently well ahead of Niger in this domain. The general economic crisis in the region meant that the project became more expensive than expected, as the relevant staff pushed for per diems and other forms of compensation to counterbalance their lack of reliable salary. This hampered the project's ability to complete the "sociocultural" baseline study. The political situation under Saibou deteriorated just as the materials were being tested. Strikes by students disrupted the follow-up and evaluation of the project. At the time of the democratic transition, the materials had barely been developed and introduced, much less tested (AMSP UNESCO/FNUP/MENR 1993).

The expansion of "education in family life" continued gradually, occasioning an assessment study of reproductive health programs in 2000. By then, the materials had been tested and (in principle) distributed, teachers had been trained, and inspectors had been able to observe the outcome. Not surprisingly, this study found, this educational innovation was handicapped by the contentious political climate in which it had been introduced, the economic crisis, and in particular by strong negative reactions among the newly vocal and organized Islamist groups. The author of the evaluation, Dr. Boubacar Diallo, explained the difficulties in implementation: "Certain issues are deeply shameful and marked by religious concerns—sexuality or contraception among unmarried people. This generates a lack of fit between the aspirations of the population and particular laws. This explains why, for example, the family code has not been adopted and why the law limiting the use of contraception to married couples (N° 88-019 du 7 avril 1988) still hasn't been amended to take into account the needs of young people; it is why although CEDAW has been signed it hasn't been applied" (AMSP FNUP/RNMS Diallo 2000, 23). Diallo's study occurred at a moment when state education was in crisis. In the late 1990s, as part of a response to structural adjustment mandates, experienced teachers were replaced with far less educated contractual teachers, hastening a decline in public confidence in the state schools. Parents turned increasingly to private schools, which in addition to purportedly higher standards were willing to accept paying students who had failed more than once. Significantly, unlike the perennially striking public schools, private schools could be counted on to hold classes regularly, a matter of importance to working parents. In rural areas, where there are fewer educational opportunities, the numbers of state schools and teachers increased, but the quality of education declined precipitously as measured in student failure rates in the finishing exams. Under the circumstances, it made less and less sense to send children, particularly girl children, to school at all. Parents who could afford to do so increasingly sent their children to private Franco-Islamic schools, with negative implications for their exposure to sexual education (AMSP FNUP/RNMS Diallo 2000, 23).

During my field research in May and June 2014, I interviewed dozens of female students in high schools and nursing schools in Niamey. Young women in this sample, who skewed toward relatively successful students and students whose parents work in the urban formal sector, should have been more familiar with "education in family life" than the average Nigerien. Certainly, functionary women (like many parents in the United States) assume that their children are adequately exposed to sex education through schooling and the media. While in principle, my informants all should have learned various modules of the new sexuality and population curriculum (known as Earth and Life Science and as Family Economy), it was clear that many students who had gone to religious private schools (whether Catholic or Islamic) had not been exposed to it at all and that students from public schools had retained very little of the information. The girls appear to have reasoned that such things are only necessary for married women—and they were not married.

One of Hadiza Moussa's informants expressed how uncomfortable teachers are with addressing sexuality in the curriculum: "I never succeeded in handling the issue of sexuality comfortably with my students. In Earth and Life Sciences there is a chapter on human reproduction but I never linger over certain elements related to sexuality. A lot of things are presented through dictation and are copied into notebooks rather than explained" (Moussa 2012, 137). Few of the girls I interviewed had a sense for what they might do to prevent pregnancy. They expressed almost universally a reluctance to talk about sexuality with their mothers, and what they knew about sexuality and family planning they had learned from their "entourage"—extended family, neighbors, and school friends. Even the daughter of a *sage-femme* knew nothing about her period until it came; it had to be explained to her by an older friend. The girl explained that "among Zarma it's taboo" to talk about sexuality and the body. So, she never spoke about such things with her mother (S.S. Lycée CLAB, Niamey, May 25, 2014). By contrast, another student had learned from her maternal aunt, remarking "among us, Hausa people explain things, but not everyone." To the degree that students knew much about "protection," they associated it with HIV/AIDS and condoms.

And yet all the same informants—every single one—personally knew a girl who had become pregnant before marriage, and all of them knew of someone who had been accused of infanticide. "Niamey is a big village," as the common saying goes. Every new acquaintance is the occasion for a sometimes lengthy discussion that does not end until the interlocutors have established how they are related to one another through kinship, schooling, or geography. It is impossible not to be aware of the danger of premarital pregnancy, and yet it is evidently equally impossible to talk about how to prevent it.

Child Abandonment and the Girl-Mother

While infanticide and botched abortions are particularly striking consequences of the absence of effective sex education for adolescents, the increasingly visible problem of child abandonment is clearly a related phenomenon. The need for state and NGO services to care for abandoned children is by all accounts growing. Public perception in Niamey is that children are abandoned when they are illegitimate and are the subject of shame and social rejection. While poverty is closely associated in their minds with child abandonment, it is difficult to distinguish the quality of being poor from the social condition of being unrecognized (Aougui 2008, 31). Niamey's residents assume in advance that such children will be depraved and delinquent. It is not entirely clear that such children are understood to be capable of moral behavior (34). Tragically, the proposed solutions to this problem tend to focus on anything other than social recognition for such children. Thus, Aougui Rassiratou found in her study of child abandonment that populations she interviewed felt people should be taught more about the ills of child abandonment and that the state should punish their mothers, find income-generating activities for unwed mothers, encourage education, promote abstinence, and reduce the cost of marriage (35). The sense that such children need to be embraced as full members of society by everyone—not just the parents of the *fille-mère* or "girl-mother"—does not appear to be among the solutions imagined by the people of Niamey.

Not all illegitimate infants are abandoned. A 2006 study, by Aichatou Tounkara Issoufou of forty "girl-mothers" (unmarried women under the age of eighteen) raising their own children in the neighborhoods of Gaweye and Kirikissoye, found that most had some schooling (almost a third had finished high school), more than three-quarters lived with their parents, and all said that the father recognized the child (Issoufou 2006, 41 Tableau 3, 42 Tableau 6). Whereas the parents of girls driven to infanticide tended to be farmers, these young women's parents had far more diverse sources of income and a higher degree of education. Often the child resided either with the father or his kin, or the father provided some kind of support (Issoufou 2006, 50 Tableau 21). Strikingly, fathers provide no food according to this study, which may account for why in a very poor household a mother might be constrained to abandon the child (51 Tableau 24). In well over half the cases (57%), both partners regarded the pregnancy as desirable (59). The couples may have been sweethearts who hoped to pressure their parents into allowing them to marry. Nevertheless, more than a quarter of the babies of the young women in the sample had eventually died.

Attempts by women to gain recognition of their babies through legal means reveal a more desperate story. In a study of eighty-five young women between fourteen and twenty years old who had initiated legal efforts to establish the paternity of their children between 2000 and 2003, Hadiza Mamane found that while many of them had some schooling (60%), most of them did not claim to have become pregnant because of love or "destiny," as in Issoufou's study, but rather through "negligence" (Mamane

2003, 24 Tableau 6). A quite striking 30 percent of these young women claimed that their partner was a state functionary, while another 23.3 percent claimed that their partner was a *commerçant*—a trader (38 Tableau 14). And equally strikingly, 70 percent of these young women had received gifts—overwhelmingly in the form of cash—from their partner (39 Tableaux 16 and 17).

Whether or not the author is correct in characterizing this exchange of sex for gifts as a kind of clandestine prostitution, it is clear that material conditions contribute to young women engaging in sex with relatively wealthy (and therefore probably married) men (2003, 53–54). Most of the young women characterized their life circumstances as poor and attributed their situation to the implications of the nonrecognition of the child (Mamane 2003, 46 Tableau 28). The study further reveals that only girls from relatively well-off and influential families actually succeed in pressuring the father to recognize the paternity of the child. The girls who most need the support of the father and recognition of the child, in other words, are precisely the ones least likely to succeed in getting it.

An encounter in the poorer neighborhood of Banifondou II provides a glimpse of this kind of relatively vulnerable young mother. In a chaotic and run-down compound of Zarma-speaking women, where seven or eight children were splashing noisily in the wash water, the woman head of the household, Sa'a, was busy dressing a grandchild. She scowled at the saucy young pregnant woman sauntering out of the compound with a cluster of girlfriends. I asked Sa'a what happens to a girl if she gets pregnant before she gets married. Sa'a talked about her daughter, Rafika, the pregnant girl we had just seen. That girl had been wandering about with her boyfriend, so Sa'a insisted that the young man marry her. Then Rafika fell pregnant, at which point her boyfriend lost all interest in her. He claims the child is not his (Sa'a Ta Wainiya, Niamey, January 10, 2014).

This case reveals the degree to which the problem of sorting these issues out falls to older women, as does the care of such babies. In a later interchange, after Rafika had given birth to a baby girl, I asked Sa'a whether she had encouraged her daughter to use contraception.

SA'A: Why would a woman who isn't married use contraception?!

HAWA: You can see how easily she gets pregnant! You have to talk to her about it! (Sa'a Ta Wainiya, Niamey, June 10, 2014)

The reticence about speaking directly about sexuality and contraception extends to a context such as this.

Testing Paternity

One of the most intriguing developments in Niger of late has been the potential of DNA testing to force the hand of men who refuse to take responsibility for their illegitimate children. The issue is extremely complex legally, but even where the legal implications of determining biological paternity are ambiguous, the moral obligation it can introduce is entirely new. In the past, there was never a way to establish a moral rather than legal obligation on the part of men. Technically, within local readings of Islamic legal precepts, a man is automatically responsible for the children produced by his wives; he is under no obligation to support any of his children born outside of marriage.

Not fully understanding the implications of this, I asked a magistrate whether women ever use DNA tests to secure recognition of their children. She responded that no, they are too expensive. At which point Hawa observed that actually she has two cases in which DNA tests are an element (Magistrate B. A., Niamey, June 11, 2014). The Association des Femmes Juristes du Niger (AFJN) pays for the test to be done, and if the outcome supports the woman's paternity claim, the man is pushed to pay the expense of the test as part of the unofficial settlement. Hawa later told me that in the case of the lycée student she was assisting, the paternity test came out positive, and his family must pay for the naming ceremony. Evidently, the girl's widowed mother was a domestic worker, and when she fell sick one day she asked her sixteen-year-old daughter to cover for her. The girl was raped by the son of the homeowner. When confronted, the boy's mother protested, "He's not even in lycée; how could he have gotten her pregnant?!"

Most of the public debates in Niger about illegitimacy systematically evade the reality of rape and the vulnerability of relatively poor and unconnected young women to abuse. They also leave unaddressed the sexual double standard by which it is perfectly acceptable for a man, but not for a woman, to have sex outside of marriage. In a case such as this, the child will not inherit from the father's side, but the public knowledge that he is indisputably the father because of the naming ceremony appears to have created a new potential to push for child support, if not full legal recognition conferring inheritance rights.

Whether the father recognizes him or not, such a child remains in local Islamic reasoning a bastard. If the pregnancy resulted from sexual abuse, to reveal that abuse would simply increase the shame of the pregnancy. In some parts of Niger, particularly Hausa-speaking regions, families may not be eager to establish the biological paternity of an illegitimate child, prefer-ring instead to absorb it quietly into the maternal family. Establishing bio-logical paternity does not necessarily confer clear advantages to the mother of a baby, and it opens the door to ambiguity about who has custody and who benefits from the child's labor and (if a girl) bridewealth. As a result, not all families would want to press the biological father's family to perform the naming ceremony. As one woman put it, "You know, sometimes the mother's family won't agree to that. They will say, just because you have done a naming ceremony doesn't mean the baby is yours" (Ta Konni, Nia-mey, January 11, 2014).

When a woman (or girl) is raped, the general attitude is that it should be ignored or hidden. When I pushed another woman in the legal profes-sion to talk about rape cases, she was deeply uncomfortable. She explained that this is a "taboo issue" and that there are many different kinds of rape, some of them in the family: "That is why incest victims don't speak up, be-cause of shame, it is a very delicate issue. There is not any attention to the rapist, it is the girl herself who is marked for life [*indexée à vie*]. She rarely wants to speak out in court. To make public this kind of abuse is to create social rupture that can never be undone" (Madame S., Niamey, January 4, 2013). While in theory a rape or incest victim has the right to abortion, in practice such cases never arise.

Paradoxes of Legitimacy: The Problem of the Sexually Active Child Bride

Despite the prominence of depictions of rampant female sexuality in Ni-ger's popular press and political debate, on the whole the notion of ado-lescent sex per se as a "problem" is absent. This is very different from, for example, the United States. The problems of infanticide, botched abortions, and abandoned children are not, by and large, constructed in Niger as prob-lems of *adolescent* sex. They are problems of *sex outside of marriage*. The solution to sexual profligacy is to guarantee that almost all young women will engage in unprotected adolescent sex by marrying them very young in a context in which contraception is very little used. This reality is disguised by a bit of linguistic sleight of hand. A married girl of fifteen who has a child is a woman/wife—usually the same word is used for both (so in French, *femme*). But an unmarried girl of fifteen who has a child is a "girl-mother" or *fille-mère*. It is only the unmarried fifteen-year-old who is indexed as be-ing a child.

Thus, two potential solutions are defined in advance as unavailable. One would be to provide reproductive health services and education so that young women, whether married or not, would not suffer from unwanted pregnancies before their bodies are fully developed. The other would be to ensure that young women are guaranteed social recognition, education, and access to the means to earn an income. Should they become pregnant (married or not), they will then have the means to care for the child. Instead, in Niger, significant proportions of young women face marriage from between the ages of fifteen and eighteen without any form of birth control and no useful sexual education. They almost universally drop out of school.

The fear that unmarried young women will become pregnant prompts girls' guardians to marry them off very young. In the most recent demographic study of Niger, over three-quarters of women between twenty and twenty-four had been married by the time they were eighteen (Institut National de la Statistique 2013, 4). The absence of a practical recognition of the sexual needs of unmarried teens generates countervailing forces that are detrimental to the health of teens, whether married or not. Unprotected sex among adolescent girls in Niger occurs overwhelmingly in the context of marriage. But that does not make it any less dangerous to their health or problematic for their capacity to attain an adequate education and earning potential. While the percentages of girls getting married and giving birth by age fifteen appears to be declining with successive cohorts, girls in rural areas are married routinely at thirteen or fourteen and often commence unprotected marital sex immediately. Girls married early also tend to have less schooling; in the same survey, women who had no schooling began their sexual lives on average at fifteen to sixteen, whereas women with a secondary school education began at about twenty-one (INS 2013, 4; further data analysis courtesy of Bill Winfrey, Avenir Health).

An interview with two young women from Ader in their twenties provides a glimpse into how such early marriages can be experienced. Chatting in her friend's house in Lazaret, the more loquacious of the two observed humorously that she was maybe twelve when she was sent to her new marital home. She had taken her wedding cloth and cut it up to make clothes for her dolls, which made her husband so angry that he beat her. Eventually, it was clear that she was not ready to be a wife yet, so Hajjiya, her co-wife, took her under her wing and began to teach her the things she would need to know to be a wife. When she had her first period, she thought she was bleeding from a wound, so she shut herself in the washroom and stayed in a tub of water crying for a long time. Eventually Hajjiya came and said, "Hey, what's wrong with you?" It was only then that she learned anything about her own body.

At that point her friend, Rabi, chimed in with her own story. She knew nothing about pregnancy when she was married as a girl. She was worried and upset thinking that she had a bad stomachache. She went to talk to her senior co-wife and said, "Look, I have something inside me that is pushing!" That was when she discovered that she was pregnant. Somewhat stupidly I asked, "Didn't you notice that you hadn't had your period?" She replied that she had not yet had her first period when she became pregnant; she didn't even know what menstruation was (Rabi and Indo, Niamey, January 9, 2014).

Young girls are often as much the "bride" of their mothers-in-law as they are of their husbands. Commenting bitterly on the marriage her ex-husband's family has arranged for her young daughter, a woman from Filingue named Mariama explained to me that her daughter would have to clean, winnow grain, pound it, cook it, carry it to the fields, and get water and wood and then deal with the millet for the dinner meal. All this is clearly not an appealing prospect from Mariama's vantage point. The couple will have children right away. There is no talk of family planning.

> BC: What did people in Filingue say during the debate about raising the age of schooling for girls to sixteen?
>
> MARIAMA: They said, "The government didn't give birth to those children, the government didn't feed them, so the government can't decide when they go to school." They were very much against it.
>
> BC: Will your daughter send her own children to school?
>
> MARIAMA: She sure will! I have told her she has to, and if they can't afford it in the village they are to come to live with me! (Mariama, Niamey, June 10, 2014)

State efforts to encourage parents to keep their daughters in school and to marry them off later, at sixteen to eighteen, can prompt visceral reactions among populations in some regions, particularly to the east in Maradi and Zinder. Such interventions are often seen as interfering with parental prerogatives and local mores. Islamists both promote such reactions and use them to justify retaining the status quo.

In a tense interview with Mallama O. of the Association des Femmes Musulmanes du Niger, who is known for her radio sermons and her madrassa for women, her reaction when I raised the question of marriage age was hostile:

> BC: What do you say to someone who says that it is okay to marry a girl at nine?
>
> MALLAMA O.: I tell them that yes, the Prophet had a wife who was nine, but he was a prophet, are you a prophet? I will marry my own daughter to a man if he is as pure and virtuous as the Prophet, but not before you bring him to me. You know, there was a woman government minister who was pushing for raising the marriage age, and they brought a case to court over a marriage of a girl who was under age, and the day the decision went down there were seven marriages all at once in Maradi, all of girls who were eleven, because people said, "The government didn't give birth to them, the government doesn't feed them, it's not the government's business." So you make things worse when you try to make changes like that. (Mallama O., Niamey, June 12, 2014)

This oft-repeated phrase, "the government didn't feed them," has become a kind of shorthand for the general sentiment that parents must take on the burden of social reproduction with little or no help from the government and that as a consequence the government has not earned the right to intervene in family matters.

What's Behind Maternal Morbidity and Mortality?

As a result of early marriage and long childbearing careers, maternal mortality is very high in Niger at 553 deaths per 100,000 live births in 2015.[3] There has been very encouraging improvement since the 2006 introduction of free maternal and infant care (WHO 2014, 54).[4] Maternal morbidity is also high, but it is far less carefully documented. Fistula, one of the more dire consequences of a problematic delivery, varies regionally. Data from the hospitals to which serious gynecological problems are referred reveal some important patterns. The Maternité Tassigui in Tahoua handled sixty-two fistula cases in 2014—7 percent of its cases overall. Of those cases, two concerned girls under the age of fifteen. Many more concerned women between fifteen and twenty-four and between twenty-five and thirty-four (twenty-five and twenty cases, respectively). The Maternité Centrale in Zinder handled 119 cases in the same period, 5.76 percent of its cases. By contrast, the Maternité Issaka Gazoby in Niamey only handled one case, representing 0.17 percent of its cases (République du Niger 2015, 276, 278).

In collecting the career history of *sage-femme* Mme. M. in Niamey, I gained a sense for how differently medical practitioners experience women's reproductive problems depending on where they are working. Her first posting was at the Maternité Centrale in Zinder, a very difficult post. They had many patients and not enough staff; "it was one emergency after another," and they had a lot of fistula cases. "The girls would be so young and so small! And they would be in labor so long before they even came in! There is a whole pavilion just for these women" (Madame M., Niamey, May 28, 2014).

After that she was at a polyclinic in Niamey that served many more Peul and Gourmantché women. She found that difficult as well: the women were circumcised and during labor they would get terrible perineal tears where the genital tissue had scarred. "You would have to stitch it up and you couldn't use anesthesia for it because that would harden the flesh and made it even more difficult to suture, which would in turn make it take even longer so that by the time you were halfway done the drug had worn off and in the end it was worse." They learned to do the stitches as quickly as they could. But it would be repeated with every single birth, so the same woman would have scar after scar. And sometimes it would cause damage to the urinary tract, which would be extremely painful for the women. There were a few who were infibulated and had to be cut just to give birth.

She said after two years doing that she never wanted to be in a hospital again. She much prefers the neighborhood maternity setting in Niamey where she works now. Her seniority means she doesn't have to handle emergency cases anymore. Those are referred to the major maternity hospitals. This means that the *sage-femmes* at the referral hospitals are likely to be among the least experienced.

Fistula is less likely, therefore, to appear to be a serious problem to women in Niamey, who no longer practice genital cutting and who tend to marry later. On the other hand, women from underserved regions must come to a major center such as Niamey to seek treatment. Age at first pregnancy among the NGO Dimol's fistula clients in 2007 was clearly related to fistula—over a third of the women were under twenty (Salamatou, Idrissa, and Tchemogo 2008). Of those who had succeeded in having surgery, multiple surgeries were required to repair the tear. Surgeries are not always successful. In 2007, 186 women had had the actual opening repaired. Of those, 112 were able to urinate normally, 74 still suffered from incontinence, and eight women had not healed at all (23). While the causes of fistula are complex—it can affect both relatively young mothers and grand multiparas—strong interventions from all sides to reduce unprotected sex among women under twenty would unquestionably reduce the incidence. Unfortunately, the Western preoccupation with fistula—one problem among many from the vantage point of women and doctors in Niger—has generated what Alison Heller characterizes as a toxic political scramble among politicians, NGOs, funders, and government health workers to capitalize on the potential income and stature fistula activism can generate (Heller 2014, 2019; Heller and Hannig 2017). The unseemly scramble feeds the popular distaste for Western donors' apparent prurience and meddling.

Setting aside for a moment the question of age at first exposure to pregnancy, even in the capital Niamey, young women appear to have little notion of how they might effectively space their births once they have begun having children. I didn't get the sense from any of the twenty high school girls I interviewed that they were aware that effective nursing can be an important element in successful birth spacing. Only one could account for how her own parents achieved the birth spacing in her family. Only three—one of whom was from Burkina Faso—had spoken with their mothers about contraception. Half had talked with an auntie or an older sister about childbirth in general. Typically, the birth spacing in their own families was three to five years, and most of them came from families of about five living children.

Interestingly, many of the girls had considered already how many children they thought would be ideal. None of them said, as is common among less educated rural women, "however many Allah gives me."[5] These girls tended to want four to five children. They had a sense that they have the ability to decide how many children they would have. I had the same experience speaking with modestly educated young Buzu women I interviewed in the context of a well-visit clinic across the river in Harobanda. All but one of those women was married, and all were already using contraception and appeared to feel no embarrassment talking about it; one advantage of "formerly captive" ethnicity is that shame-related comportments can be less constraining. The sense among married women that the means exist to regulate their own fertility should they choose to do so appears to be fairly well developed in Niamey today. Whether young married women are in a position to actually gain access to that contraception is, of course, another question. The situation of unmarried adolescents, however, is a great deal less encouraging.

Bad Faith in Contemporary Debate: Marriage, Schooling, and Population

In an effort to understand the perspective of the Islamist women who have actively thwarted efforts to raise the age at which girls leave school, I visited the madrassa of Madame N. The owner of a well-stocked and efficient pharmacy, she also runs a school nearby targeting women of all ages. Like Mallama O., she is a representative of the vocal Union des Femmes Musulmanes du Niger (UFMN). When I arrived for our appointment, Madame N. met me and Hawa at the door of her modest, unmarked school. She was roughly sixty years old and dressed modestly, but elegantly, as most Niamey functionary women would dress. The hovering summer camp students in blue hijab uniforms made way as she cordially ushered us in to meet the other women from the UFMN she had assembled to meet with me.

The women included a young woman in charge of instruction at the school who remained silent throughout the free-wheeling discussion, an older Fulani woman I will refer to as Hajjiya of perhaps seventy years of age who was veiled in the manner typical twenty years ago, a clearly poorer woman who simply identified herself as "Buzu" wearing a cheap black hijab, and a self-declared sociologist of perhaps thirty years of age sporting the latest hijab style. I will refer to her as Madame A. Z. After I described my historical project, Hajjiya asked me for an example of what I meant by saying that childbirth has a history. This was a pleasant surprise; relatively few people expressed an interest in the *historical* dimension of my work, turning readily to political concerns instead. I offered as examples the shift in marital abstinence from roughly two years to forty days and some of the bodily changes that might have affected childbirth and marriage as diets shift.

Hajjiya said she had never heard of extended marital abstinence in the past. She noted that perhaps it hadn't applied to her family, which she stated had been part of the "Islamic empire," meaning the state created by Usman 'dan Fodio. I pointed out that in any case until quite recently not everyone was Muslim; for example, there had been many Arna (Hausa-speaking non-Muslims) at the time of colonization. None of them were familiar with that word. In this setting, debates are not really between Muslims and non-Muslims. They are among Muslims themselves. The assumption in Niamey, reinforced by the regular assertion in discussions of Niger that 95 percent of the population is Muslim, tends to be that everyone is and always has been Muslim.

Hajjiya had been a *sage-femme* before she retired. Reflecting on this notion that there might be a history to both religion and childbirth, she noted, a little defensively, that such a long abstinence made a kind of sense.

> BC: Absolutely, it made for good birth spacing!
>
> HAJJIYA: So then you are saying that the close birth spacing is caused by Islam?
>
> BC: No, I'm saying that the shift to forty days is a factor, and the fact that men don't withdraw is a factor, and the fact that women don't use contraception is a factor, and the fact that they don't always nurse sufficiently is another. (Madame N., Hajjiya, Buzu, and A. Z., Niamey, June 18, 2014)

Redirecting the conversation toward their perspectives, I asked them to tell me about their own birth experiences. Buzu listed all her birth experiences, which included five years between the first two, and then three years, and then finally one year. "All that was from Allah," she declared. "There was no need for contraception! That spacing was from God!"

I remarked dryly, "Well Allah looked out for you; I'm not sure Allah looks out for the girl who has a baby and falls pregnant immediately." The retired *sage-femme* Hajjiya chuckled. It dawned on me that these women did not necessarily agree about everything. The younger Madame A. Z. insisted on sociological specificity. "They don't get pregnant immediately. Only from the end of the forty days." Okay, I conceded, after forty days. But in the face of this apparent rejection of contraception even for married women, I ventured provocatively, "The nursing baby, if his mother falls pregnant right away, and as a result weans him, that baby will die." They were silent for a moment. At length Madame N. said, "Well that child who dies was destined to die; birth spacing or family planning can't change destiny." I acknowledged with good humor that we were not going to agree and that it was fine to disagree. That concession seemed to defuse the tension, and we went on to have a friendly debate.

I described my not entirely successful efforts to sort out whether marriage and childbirth had shifted to a younger age and whether some of the childbirth problems women have today might also be a result of that shift.

> BC: The women I talk to often tell me that that delivery now is "harder."
>
> MADAME N.: Maybe the reason it is harder to give birth is what people take into their bodies, including all the poisons in the injections they get.
>
> BC: A lot of people talk about changes in what women eat.

MADAME A. Z.: There is no proof that having children young is a problem! There are lots of older women with fistula! Anyway there aren't that many young women with fistula. Who ever sees a fistula case outside of Dimol? (Madame N., Hajjiya, Buzu, and A. Z., Niamey, June 18, 2014)

At this apparent non sequitur, the two women trained in medicine, Madame N. and Hajjiya, retreated from the discussion. Hawa remained studiously silent. They did not appear to want to engage in a direct debate about fistula. Media representation of "the scourge of fistula" in Niger tends to focus on very young girls; it is true that such coverage might give the impression that great numbers of girls are married off as young as nine and that those girls make up the majority of fistula patients when in reality many are older women who have had numerous births. Evidently with those media images in mind, Madame A. Z. went on to insist that actually, girls are married at fifteen, not at thirteen. "Where are all these thirteen-year-olds they are talking about?" she exclaimed. "The reason parents do this is that school today is simply a site of debauchery—girls learn about sex in ways that aren't suitable! They become loose and sexually active, and as a result there are long lines of such girls seeking the pill at the Comprehensive Health Centers!"

I was openly amused at that claim, since I certainly hadn't seen long lines of young girls looking for contraception anywhere I had gone, and I had become painfully aware of how little sex education they actually receive. Observing my reaction at that point, others in the room came to her support. In their view, there was a serious problem of young girls becoming prostitutes in bars and on the street, and no one seemed interested in protecting those girls. They protested that outsiders are only interested in this imaginary "child bride."

Certainly, some young women wander the streets near the National Assembly building late at night hoping to turn a trick with one of Niamey's wealthier men cruising in a fancy car. Still, relatively few bar girls or streetwalkers in Niamey are from the immediate region, and most appear to be in their late teens or early twenties. Some are Peul or Tuareg women or women from neighboring countries working with greater anonymity than they could at home. Some of the local women are possibly divorcées, not very young girls. Far more prevalent than the bar girl phenomenon is the practice of schoolgirls accepting gifts and services of all kinds from men who pursue them in or near the schoolyard. Such gifts can range from favorable grades, to school fees, to cash for makeup and jewelry.

Sometimes sexual relations become part of the exchange. The streetwalker and bar girl have become rhetorical stand-ins for transactional sex more broadly.

Madame N. outlined for me with admirable clarity how they see the contemporary problem. As Muslims, they are forced to choose between two evils. One would be having a daughter who becomes "debauched." The other would be marrying her relatively young. Given this choice, it is clear to them that the lesser evil is marrying the girls at fifteen or so. At least then she won't lose her honor, they insisted. Hajjiya elaborated, "She won't be reduced to an animal." It's not that marriage so young is a good thing, they argued, it's that given how terrible the schools are, it's the lesser of two evils. I asked how schooling had changed, and they insisted that in the past there was a sound "moral education," that it taught people not to lie or steal, and that it didn't offend propriety. The students came away with something positive. Now they are taught about sex and come away debauched. The girls are neither housewives nor well educated, and they roam the streets shamelessly. The women's clarity sharpened my understanding of how differently they and I perceive the contemporary dilemma.

I would have said the two undesirables were young girls becoming pregnant before they are physically ready, on the one hand, and openly recognizing that sexual activity (including transactional sex among young teens) may call for access to contraception, on the other. Neither is ideal; few parents would be enthusiastic about girls under eighteen putting themselves at risk of pregnancy for gifts of cash and clothing. But an early pregnancy is both physically dangerous and educationally disastrous. For me, marriage does not solve the problem; the girls are still pregnant too young, and either way they are unlikely to continue in school. In its own way, marriage can be a form of transactional sex, as Engels so unromantically observed (Engels 1909 [1884]).

It became clear to me that the knot at the core of our disagreement concerned whether young married women could continue to go to school. Early marriage might not be so objectionable to *me* were it not for the dual consequences of early childbearing and withdrawal from education. Obviously, it is difficult to establish whether a girl has *chosen* to marry if she is deemed too young to make prudent decisions of her own, so the question of autonomy remains. Their notion was that parents should have the right to marry off their daughters in their best interests and that it should have no bearing on the question of education.

"These debauched girls, really," the Zarma sociologist exclaimed, "if they get pregnant, and then they have an abortion—sometimes they will do it at nine months! That girl will go to hell." Mme N. said that, setting aside the hereafter, a girl who aborts a baby will never be able to face herself later in life, and she will never be able to face the father of the child. So, in preventing abortion, they are protecting the girl from herself. Madame A. Z. proclaimed indignantly, "No one is protecting the rights of married women! There should be a law that lets women continue to go to school once they marry. That way they could satisfy their natural sexual needs in marriage and finish school."

But here's the rub. In fact, there is nothing in the existing regulations to prevent a married girl from continuing with her schooling. Some, in fact, do continue. Given how unimpressive the civil registry system in Niger is, it would be virtually impossible in any case to enforce any rule that barred married girls from attending school. In practice, married girls are pulled out of school by their husbands. UFMN members who protest that "no one is looking out for the rights of married women" are engaging in a bit of prevarication. UFMN rejected legislation supporting all girls—whether married or not—in their quest to continue schooling up to age sixteen. I was very struck by the bad faith on their part; they aren't really interested in married women going to school. What they resent is the perceived attempt of secularists to prevent them from marrying off their daughters young *by encouraging them to remain in school.* Everyone knows, implicitly, that with only rare exceptions, if she is in school, a young woman is not married and vice versa.

To be fair, however, for their part, actors promoting female literacy and better school completion rates for girls are often engaged in a variety of bad faith as well. There is broad agreement that a higher literacy rate among women in Niger will be necessary for living standards to improve, for democracy to function effectively, and for the economy to flourish. But another reason for promoting women's education is that globally, female literacy is inversely correlated with fertility, particularly for women who continue beyond primary school. Increasing education rates for girls is typically argued to be the single most effective way to reduce the birth rate. A central tenet of World Bank policy, particularly from the mid-1990s, has been that improving girls' schooling rates will contribute to economic development by delaying marriage, reducing fertility and therefore population growth, and enhancing employment (Heward 1999, 1–14). Smaller populations and family sizes will free up resources that can then be used to jump-start the economy, an effect optimistically known as the "demographic dividend."

While scholars have debated the realism of the "education as contraception" approach, the assumption of a link is a more or less open secret in the international aid and NGO world. However, from the vantage point of parents in countries like Niger, schooling girls comes at a high opportunity cost. Women value the labor of their daughters and daughters-in-law at home, and they may believe that money expended on girls' education would yield a better return in terms of eventual wage employment if spent on boys. The high social cost of shame as a result of premarital pregnancy also weighs heavily in families' perceptions of the worth of female education (Wynd 1999).

The goal of outsiders in promoting girls' education is generally not simply to better women's lives; it is to slow the growth of the population. That goal has been pursued with insufficient attention to other factors shaping women's health and well-being, including the devastating effects of structural adjustment. In general, it is true that girls who succeed in passing secondary school entrance exams are more likely to stay in school and are therefore likely to be married later. My interviews suggest that it is also true that they are more likely to take an interest in eventually controlling their own family size. The virtue of promoting girls' education is that one need not directly confront resistance to birth control. However, this open secret feeds the general mistrust that Nigeriens feel toward the unspoken agendas of outsiders.

Frankly Addressing the Reality of Adolescent Sexuality

Texts that promote women's reproductive health in West Africa tend to begin with the assumption that the most productive approach will be to support women's rights within an Islamic framework (B. Cooper 2015). Abdel Rahim Omran's *Family Planning in the Legacy of Islam* was framed with a host of prefaces from Islamic authorities attesting to its value, depth of research, and theological accuracy. The book clearly targeted Islamic public opinion throughout the world. Omran's work has been particularly important in efforts to influence fertility behavior of Muslims in Africa (Omran 1984) and did little to advance the scholarly understanding of sexuality in Islam, which had already been treated with considerable subtlety by the medical historian B. F. Musallam (1983). Rather, Omran brought to the discussion his credibility as a Muslim medical professional attesting to the legitimacy, within Islam, of adopting contraceptive practices.

Omran's treatment of family planning emphasizes the compassionate and forward-looking qualities of the Islamic approach to contraception: "It is quite evident that Islam sanctions family planning and that the companions of the Prophet practiced birth control even when the Muslim nation was in a stage of rapid growth and expansion. Birth spacing is indisputable in Islam and is in great harmony with African cultures and tradition. Family planning is not only sanctioned, but actually encouraged, by Islam" (Omran 1984, 122–23). In support of this position, most discussions of family planning in Islam begin by setting out the Islamic understanding of the family and go on to argue that the Prophet permitted *al-azl* (withdrawal) so that men could avoid producing offspring beyond their means, putting their nursing wives and children at risk, or degrading the beauty of their partners. The stance in such texts is that Islamic withdrawal is acceptable and therefore, by analogy, other forms of birth control short of sterilization benefit society in general and women in particular.

The argument leaves unspecified which women in fact "benefit" from this Islamic sanction. For married women, *al-azl* comes up most consistently in the context of breastfeeding. In order to enable a woman to live up to the expectation that she nurse her infant for a full two years, so the argument goes, withdrawal was historically used to prevent a new pregnancy that might compromise her ability to nurse. Only a married woman nursing a child benefited from the right of her husband to practice withdrawal within this logic. However, the hadith related to *al-azl* did not concern wives but rather slave women. The rationale for withdrawal with a slave woman was to avoid the Islamic prohibition on the sale of a concubine who had borne a child to her master. Withdrawal was a means of preserving a man's (and by extension his legitimate children's) wealth. It was only in bearing a child that a concubine could earn a degree of security and status. Freeborn women, by contrast, might seek to enforce their rights as wives to limit men's right to withdrawal, leading to considerable legal debate about whether a man required his wife's consent to practice *al-azl*.

There is absolutely nothing in any of the Islamic debates about the permissibility of contraception that applies to an unmarried woman or to sex between an unmarried freeborn man and a woman who is not a slave. In other words, sexual activity and withdrawal are legitimate only between married partners and between masters and their slaves. While Musallam's historical discussion of the logic of sexuality in Islam makes all this relatively clear, others writing to influence perceptions of "family planning" tend to gloss over the emergence of *al-azl* in the context of slavery and do not underscore the ways in which the Islamic logic surrounding it is patriarchal in rationale and execution.

The question of premarital sexuality remains deeply problematic. A graphic text created for UNFPA-funded youth clubs in Senegal as part of "Family Life Education" (FLE or EVF in French) is entitled "The Risks Tied to Sexual Behaviour Among Adolescents." Schoolgirl Bineta has a sexual relationship with her cousin Moussa. Despite the dismay of Moussa's male friend, Moussa declines to protect himself from STIs by making use of condoms. The discussion between the young men does not feature the potential pregnancy Bineta might face. Five months later, Bineta confides her fear that she is pregnant to her friend Fatou, who is more knowledgeable about the dangers of adolescent sexuality because she has just returned from a Family Life Education summer camp (UNFPA n.d.). Fatou advises Bineta not to "try to do anything that can worsen your condition" (meaning seek an abortion) and goes with Bineta to the doctor associated with the youth counseling center.

When a test confirms that Bineta is three months pregnant, the woman doctor rejects Bineta's unarticulated desire for an abortion, saying that it is illegal and "moreover it is dangerous for you. You can become sterile after this operation." The doctor acknowledges that while childbirth for a young woman who is not fully mature is difficult, she implies (falsely) that all forms of abortion are more risky still. Potential genetic problems due to the fact that Bineta's partner is a cousin are not mentioned at all. The most this female doctor has to offer Bineta is advice to seek psychological counseling and the continuation of her pregnancy. When Bineta announces her pregnancy to her parents, they fear the shame to the family and express regret that they hadn't broached "family life education" with her earlier. Bineta's mother and father had been too uncomfortable to raise the subject with her, each leaving it to the other to raise.

Conspicuously absent in the *bande dessinée* is any attempt to provide Bineta with counseling on contraception. Later we learn in following the two young men that what FLE consists of is debates in which religious exhortations to remain abstinent until marriage are countered by a grudging suggestion that if one can't abstain, one should use a condom. Sex is presented as a profound danger to be avoided at all cost. We are left hoping that

Moussa will take up the challenge of assisting Bineta in raising the baby. Nothing in the text offers much hope that a frank and positive assessment of adolescent sexuality is likely to occur in the context of "family life education," although FLE is presumably a bit more useful than the exhortation to remain abstinent by the religious leader depicted in the text. But nowhere is female contraception addressed; abortion is inaccurately portrayed as universally more dangerous than childbirth.

In real life, a young woman of Bineta's family background in a city such as Dakar or Niamey would probably arrange for a clandestine abortion at home or in a private clinic, which is why the text insists several times that she imperils her future fertility if she pursues an abortion. Thus, although this text attempts to enter into a productive but noncombative dialogue with Islamic notions of sexuality, the approach taken does not seem particularly promising. Young men discuss condoms and STIs; young women must endure pregnancy (B. Cooper 2015).

Conclusion

While a far more effective argument could be made for recognizing the needs of sexually active Muslims, both married and unmarried, than has been made so far in Muslim West Africa, it seems to me that a very compelling case can also be made for social reform in the name of protecting children. Such an approach might open the way for a rather different debate about how to combat a range of serious problems facing Niger as a whole, not simply Niger's women. Adolescent sexuality, both outside of marriage and inside, contributes to high rates of maternal morbidity and mortality, the tenacity of infanticide, growing child abandonment, low female literacy rates, and botched abortions. Any serious evaluation of its negative consequences cries out for a reappraisal of the rejection of the bastard child head on.

As Kamran Hashemi has pointed out, the concept that children possess rights is not new within Islamic law. As a result, Muslim states have generally signed the Convention on the Rights of the Child although with a variety of reservations surrounding the notion of maturity, the question of adoption, and the thorny issue of legitimacy (Hashemi 2007). The Convention on the Rights of the Child never provokes much political uproar in Niger, despite the host of interesting questions it raises that are, in a sense, prolegomena to any genuine debate about women's rights. Similarly,

Karima Bennoune has persuasively argued that the International Covenant on Economic, Social and Cultural Rights (ICESCR) implies a variety of important protections to women and their children. Yet, it has not prompted the controversy or the crippling reservations so typical of the Convention on the Elimination of All Forms of Discrimination against Women (Bennoune 2005). The ICESCR convention opens the way for a discussion of some of the key areas in which illegitimate children and their mothers are disadvantaged economically.

However, such discussions must attend to the affective and ontological dimensions of the issue: if the visceral experience of shame drives so much of sexual, family, and legal life in Niger, Nigeriens must face their *sentiments* toward illegitimate children. Are there ways to humanize bastards, to render them into social persons? Are there ways to embrace the full personhood of nubile girls to protect them from the consequences of early pregnancy—whether in marriage or outside? While it is worthwhile to look to other Muslim societies for models of legal arrangements and arguments, it may be far more important to open the way to new modes of ethical sentiment about vulnerable children and child-mothers. The development panacea of "sensibilization" might then actually begin to refer less to cognitive issues and return to the far more powerful domain of feeling.

Notes

1. In the most recent round of struggles, Islamist groups prompted the abandonment in 2011 of efforts to specify provisions within Muslim personal status law relating to marriage, divorce, paternity, and inheritance.

2. Traditionally, the final obligation would be the protection of reason or mind.

3. For the purpose of comparison, the appalling continental high is to be found in Sierra Leone (1,360) and the continental low in Cape Verde (42). Niger has been spared the ravages of the AIDS epidemic by and large, which has affected maternal mortality in southern and eastern Africa far more significantly. At the more privileged end of the spectrum, France has a very respectable 8 maternal deaths per 100,000 live births, and the United States a much less respectable 14. WHO 2015, Annex 7.

4. In the 2006 Demographic and Health Survey, Niger's maternal mortality rate in the period from 1996–2006 was higher, at 648 (INS and Macro International 2007).

5. Desired fertility is notoriously difficult to measure; nevertheless, there are consistent patterns in differences between women of different regions, schooling levels, and socioeconomic condition. Women in Zinder and Maradi regularly show far higher desired fertility (8.2 and 8.0 respectively) than women in Niamey and Agadez (5.0 and 5.4 respectively); women who have secondary schooling or above have far lower desired

fertility (4.7) than women without education (7.8); women in the uppermost economic quintile economically desire fewer (5.9) than women in the lowest quintile (7.9). Since schooling and higher incomes are concentrated in cities such as Niamey, such preferences translate into significantly different patterns across ethnic groups. Hausa speakers typically show higher desired outcomes than Zarma speakers. INS 2014, Erratum, December 2, 2014, Table 7.6 Taux de fécondité desirée.

9

CONTEMPORARY SEXUALITY AND
CHILDBIRTH

[Welcome to] Niamey, our common courtyard . . .
Every family's got a story
In mine there's 12 children
I know their mother because everybody's together
But I don't know their daddy

Niamey, our common courtyard
So my neighbour, he's got 4 wives and 16 kids but
Whenever he leaves the house you hear him go, "Thank God!!!"

Here's our shared courtyard
My own mama, she is still waiting for my daddy's return—but what daddy?
A man who took off, claiming he was going to rescue us all?

Niamey, our common courtyard
Then there's our sisters: out of shame when they fall pregnant they brave an
       abortion
Some of 'em go to all the trouble of 9 months of pregnancy
And then later you find the dead baby wrapped up and thrown in the gutter
(Jhonel 2014, 13–14)

A S WE HAVE SEEN, UNMARRIED WOMEN WHO ARE at risk of pregnancy
generate tremendous anxiety; they disrupt the equivalence of "woman"
and "wife," and their fecundity threatens a social order in which property and social position are established through an identifiable patriline.
Childbearing is both a woman's greatest accomplishment and a source of
pain and sorrow. For married women the problem of managing fertility—
their own and their daughters'—can be extremely difficult. Slammer Jhonel, whose song is quoted above, captures the public intimacy of the city
of Niamey, the frustrations of young men whose fathers fail to live up to

the ideal of the Muslim male provider, and the perils of childbearing for women both young and old.[1] Women must prove themselves fertile quickly in marriage and therefore fear infertility more than almost anything else. On the other hand, if they show a lack of control in their childbearing—if it is unrestrained—they will be derided by other women as animal-like. Repeated close births can be exhausting, yet women have relatively little control over the birth intervals in contexts where the use of contraception is furtive and abortion is illegal. The task of raising numerous children with inadequate resources falls, in the end, to them.

Achieving appropriate birth spacing and a successful reproductive career has become, I argue, more difficult with the decline of abstinence while nursing. The challenge of keeping babies conceived close together healthy makes motherhood harder. The impulse to rely on exclusive breastfeeding as a contraceptive threatens the health of both babies and their nursing mothers. Mothers are treated as both the source of the problem of infant mortality and the solution to it. Questions related to access to health services, the ability to nurse "properly," the timing of pregnancy and weaning, and the uses of contraception are all entangled. Although this chapter focuses on the dilemmas of married women, implicit throughout is the question Jhonel's slam raises: Where are the men? Where is *their* shame?

Having begun with a rap by a young man, I will now draw on women's songs from across the Sahel to illustrate some major themes related to the challenges of womanhood today. By setting them alongside ethnographic observations, I hope to draw to the surface some of the paradoxes of contemporary reproduction in Niger. Not least among them is the coexistence of an anxiety about what to do with illegitimate children and an urgency to resolve the problem of infertility. I will circle through the reproductive life course beginning with infertility, through childbirth, to the challenges of birth spacing, the twin conundrums of legal contraception and illegal abortion, to return finally to the figure of the child-mother and the ironies of a setting in which there are both too many illegitimate children and too many childless wives.

The Challenge of Conjoining Reproductive Success with Reproductive Restraint

"The cry of the laughing dove can't keep the millet from maturing. The one who hasn't given birth, I say Allah cleared her of blame long ago Asawari" (song sung in Hausa by Hawa Almajira in Maradi, March 15, 1989).

While it is generally not appropriate to speak openly about sexual matters in the Sahel, anything, as René Luneau observed, can be sung (Luneau 2010 [1981], 12). Women's songs often reflect on motherhood; through them women praise, shame, or console one another. The song above, sung by a childless elderly woman in her nineties named Hajjiya Algaje, links infertility and piety, suggesting that God forgives the infertile, whatever others might say. Infertile women who never experience menstruation are known in Zarma as *annabi woyey* (wives of the prophet). Such women may compensate for their infertility by centering their lives around religious devotion and koranic studies (Moussa 2012, 186). Hajjiya's greatest joy was the son she fostered, who supported her in old age and sent her on pilgrimage to Mecca (B. Cooper 2001).

But simply marrying and producing children is no guarantee of happiness either, as a Bambara song collected in Mali in the early independence era laments:

In the bush
I would transform myself into a doe
In the bush.
Being married,
That is sorrow.
Being unmarried,
That is sorrow.
I would change myself into a bird
In the bush.
Having a child,
That is sorrow.
Having no child,
That is sorrow.
I would become a doe
In the bush.
(Luneau 2010, 124)

The socially approved condition of women prior to menopause is to be married and either pregnant or capable of becoming pregnant. And yet excessive pregnancy is also inappropriate. Women's reproductive struggles in Niger today are aptly captured in the title of Hadiza Moussa's rich anthropological study of fertility management in Niamey: women are caught between the "the absence of children and the refusal to have them" (Moussa 2012). Moussa's study focuses, rightly, more on the circumstances of Niger's enormous majority of married women than on the relatively small numbers of sexually active unmarried women who haunted the preceding chapter. Understanding the realities of married women's lives requires observing the dynamics within households, particularly within multigenerational and polygynous households.

A family compound in the neighborhood of Yantalla—a rabbit warren of narrow unpaved streets, clogged sewage canals, and cacophonous motor-bikes and donkey carts—offers such a setting. Three co-wives of a disabled mechanic share a common courtyard teeming with children. Their husband, too crippled with rheumatism to continue his trade, sells cigarettes from under a shed on the corner of their street. The fourth co-wife took off when he became ill, leaving the others to care for him and the children. Two of the remaining wives engage in little enterprises selling handmade shampoos and lotions as well as cooked foods. The more outgoing of the two, Mami, has six children: five boys and a teenaged girl named Dela who is evidently quite a handful. Dela, according to Mami, is enrolled in *école bis-ime*, running about doing who-knows-what rather than attending her classes. This was one of many occasions on which women expressed to me the enormous anxiety that raising girls produces.

Hawa and I spoke with Mami about her experiences with pregnancy and childbirth. She explained that there was one very difficult time when she fell pregnant right after giving birth. She had gone in for an ultrasound sometime near the forty days, and they told her she was pregnant. She broke down in tears right there. They said, "Don't cry, it will be all right, just go ahead and nurse this baby and go on with the pregnancy." But, she said, it wasn't okay; the baby was stillborn and the nursing infant died at nine months, so she lost both of them. That was when she started using contraception. I asked whether her husband had agreed to that, and she said, oh yes, of course. "Do the other co-wives also use contraception?" I wondered aloud. Perplexed at the question, she said she had no idea. They do what they do; she does what she does.

Her younger co-wife Aissa spoke little French or Hausa. Like Mami, she knew little about her body or childbirth when she was married. She had not been told what being pregnant was or what her period meant. All she knew was what she had overheard as a girl listening to older women gossiping. She knew that if a girl did not "wash," that meant that she had done something bad, something shameful. And so Aissa thought that when she stopped having her period and had no reason to perform ritual postmenstrual washing (in Arabic *ghusl*), she must have done something terribly wrong or that people would think she had done something wrong. Washing meant you were good, and not washing meant you were bad. Eventually, she came to understand that she was pregnant. Today she has all girls and one teen-aged boy, who is as much trouble to her as Dela is for Mami. He does not work, stays out all day in town, and then comes home and complains that there is no food. Her daughters are married. Unlike the boy, they help when they can. But they are off in their own households. She complains bitterly that their senior co-wife's sons do bring food, but they don't share any of it with their paternal half-siblings, only their maternal siblings. She hadn't had trouble with childbirth until she had her ninth child. She went in for a checkup and they told her she would need a caesarean. The medical staff called her husband in to get his approval, and he gave it. They told her she shouldn't have any more children and performed a tubal ligation.

The senior wife, surrounded by a host of scampering grandchildren, was elderly and unable to work. Her room seemed no more comfortable than her co-wives'; the gifts of her adult sons do not appear to have gone all that far, given how many small children she was looking after. She had little interest in talking; she was preoccupied with the tiny grandchild she was holding for whom they had recently done a naming ceremony. The four co-wives had all been very happily married to a man they loved, had been successful in childbirth, and their lives had been enviable until their husband fell ill. Without the small income-generating activities of the remaining two healthy wives and the contributions of adult children, the household with its many young children and two elderly dependents would have had very little means of support. On the other hand, successful children are the lifeline of the elderly; without them the senior wife would go hungry. It is impossible to predict which of one's children will prove to be burden or blessing (Cross and Barker 1993, 145).

This compound reveals the degree to which married women's introduction to contraception occurs in the context of poor birth experiences. Married women generally do not exert any control over their reproductive lives until something tragic occurs or until their own health is in jeopardy. Co-wives are reluctant to speak openly about their reproductive aspirations or concerns with one another; they are frequently competitors, not collaborators. Indeed, one of the popular "cures" for infertility in a couple is to introduce a fertile second wife into the household. The new bride's pregnancy will provoke "womb jealousy" in the first, awakening her fertility (Family

Care International 1998, 33). It is in this sense that polygamy might be said to "cause" high fertility even though, in theory, multiple wives should make it possible for women to "rest" between births by maintaining lengthy conjugal abstinence.

Often women have little sense that they have the right to make decisions about reproduction on their own. Women are expected to consult with their husbands to determine whether the men will agree to interventions into their fertility. Women defer to their husbands in such matters in part because men control most of the household income and are charged with determining whether the family can afford medical expenditures. As Armelle Andro notes, the reproductive lives of couples in the Sahelian region do not, in a sense, belong to them—"the relations between couples are constructed and overseen in a social manner" by the extended family, in particular that of the husband (quoted in Moussa 2012, 230). This broader therapy-managing group generally oversees women's health, including matters of reproduction (Janzen and Arkinstall 1982, 4–5).

When I interviewed nurses and *sage-femmes* in training, I asked each of them to relate a *cas pratique* (a practical case study) from their field experiences as interns, something that was memorable or struck them personally. Rahilatou's *cas pratique* in a rural clinic in Dogondoutchi concerned a parturient woman who needed special attention because she had had a prior caesarian section. A vaginal birth after a caesarian has to be done at a larger and better equipped obstetric center rather than the maternity in rural Dogondoutchi. The woman arrived at the maternity already in obstructed labor, but there was no ambulance prepared to take her to the referral facility. The maternity in a neighboring village had an ambulance that could take her the twenty-four kilometers to the reference maternity ward, but it had no gas. By the time the transport was secured, both the woman and the baby had died.

Hawa asked her how the father reacted. Rahilatou replied, "He didn't react; they just said 'It's the will of Allah.'" Hawa felt that this was less a story about poor services than a story of a failure of communication. The family needed to understand in advance the implications of the cesarean section so that they don't wait to go to the larger hospital, she emphasized. That has to be part of their plan for when labor starts. It isn't necessarily the fault of the smaller maternities. For Hawa, the solution was not always revamping the entire system when there are neither the funds nor the personnel to do that but rather improving the chain of communication and follow-up (Rahilatou I., Institut Pratique de Santé Publique, Niamey, May 31, 2014). This woman's therapy-managing group, which included her husband as well as others, had entered the pregnancy process in what appears at the outset to be a very passive manner, leaving what was a predictably dangerous labor to the will of God. Where Rahilatou felt that the husband was at fault, Hawa argued that it was the responsibility of medical staff to make sure each patient has a well-developed plan for delivery; the problem is communication. For my part, I wondered whether the paucity of family resources to pay for transport played a role. Often in a poor household the cash available is simply not sufficient to meet even urgent medical needs. It can be hard to know whether the failure to seek timely medical help in rural populations is due to ignorance or to the lack of sufficient funds to follow the recommendations given to them.

Another case illustrates the kinds of improvisational strategies rural medical staff have to pursue in light of the poverty of their clients. In Habsou's bittersweet *cas pratique* in a rural setting, a pregnant woman in labor came in with a serious blood pressure problem. The ideal solution would be to send her to the referral maternity center. Unfortunately, once she went there, her treatment would no longer be free; only the actual childbirth is covered by the state, not hospitalization and tests for other things. Her family didn't have the money. So rather than send her to the larger hospital, the *sage-femme* and the family decided to go forward with the birth on site. They treated the blood pressure with what they had on hand, which was magnesium, and fortunately all ended well. Habsou was impressed with the kinds of practical solutions such *sage-femmes* have to come up with on a daily basis; clearly it was a bit of an eye-opener for her (Habsou I., Institut Pratique de Santé Publique, May 31, 2014).

The Significance of Support from Maternal Kin

Because in marriages today the wife almost always lives in the place of her husband's choosing, most women do not have the support of women from their own families during pregnancy and only rarely during labor. Co-wives are often very reticent toward one another. As we learned the reproductive histories of women in different neighborhoods, it became clear to me and Hawa that having access to supportive and knowledgeable maternal kin matters tremendously.

Multiple generations across the family of Tanti reflect the gradual shifts in childbearing experiences and expectations among Zarma women. Tanti's grandmother had twelve children, of whom ten lived. Her mother had ten, of whom seven lived. She had seven, and five are still living. The steady progression toward smaller uterine groups is striking. Her preference for her own daughters is that they have no more than three. At the time that we spoke, one of her daughters was close to term with her second pregnancy and extremely distraught. After her first baby was born, she had been relying on Norplant to avoid becoming pregnant while nursing. One day she felt something in her uterus and she asked her mother, do you think it is a fibroid? So they went to get an ultrasound, and it turned out she was several months pregnant. She broke down in tears. Hawa and I puzzled over that one; how could she be pregnant? Perhaps Tanti's daughter had already been pregnant when the Norplant was inserted. At the time, she had only recently given birth. She and her husband probably had intercourse at the forty days but before she had the Norplant inserted. So now she was nursing and pregnant and miserable.

Tanti was very clear that, in her view, three is enough if you want to take good care of them. Everything costs money now, she declared—school, medical care, everything. Women like Tanti have had a tremendous influence on the younger women in their lives; they support them in their reproductive goals, provide advice, and see the goal of child rearing not as maximizing the number of births but rather maximizing the number raised to a successful adulthood (cf. Bledsoe 2002). Other women, like Sa'a in the preceding chapter, whose daughter Rafika appears difficult to control, were not successful at negotiating or mastering their own fertility. Despite her daughter's difficulties, the idea of using contraception was entirely alien to Sa'a. Many are like Mami and her co-wives, who came to control their fertility late in their marital lives as a result of major health crises.

Three patterns emerged out of our discussions with women in various neighborhoods of Niamey. Some women, often from rural backgrounds and relatively impoverished settings, received little or no reproductive training from kin prior to marriage. Their reproductive lives have been overseen by their in-laws; women dominated by their in-laws may not give birth with their mothers, may not feel empowered to consider birth spacing, and may feel that their own well-being is contingent on continually producing babies. They have little ability to impose postnatal abstinence within their marital homes. Economic considerations may take precedence over the mother's health.

Other women, whose maternal kin have been solicitous and have shared experiences and insights related to childbirth and child rearing, generally have slightly more education although not always. They can use their maternal kin to help them leverage better conditions in marriage. Women whose kin are on the lookout for their interests have their first babies near their maternal kin and are more likely to receive medical attention early when things go wrong. They are also likely to be supported in their desire to space or even to reduce their births.

Most women fall somewhere in between; they (or their husbands) take their reproductive health in hand because of a crisis in their lives. Women who learn as a result of a crisis can be tough and resilient, but their attitudes toward younger women can be mixed. They may protect their own daughters while retaining a proprietary attitude toward the fertility of their daughters-in-law.

But it is the women who struggle with reproductive problems alone who face some of the worst outcomes. A nurse trainee named Rahilatou saw particularly troubling cases in Gaya, where Dendi is spoken rather than Zarma. She related the *cas pratique* of a woman who came in who had delivered earlier at home. The placenta had not been expulsed. She was put on antibiotics, and the gynecologist managed to extract the placenta. The woman's cervix was green, and the placenta was deteriorating. The woman had not come in for prenatal care, and it appeared that the baby had been stillborn (Rahilatou I., Institut Pratique de Santé Publique, Niamey, May 31, 2014). This case may well have involved an infanticide; it is impossible to know. But the woman's failure to seek care prior to delivery and for so long after is, at the very least, suggestive of an aversion to approaching medical facilities. The language and cultural differences between her and the Zarma-speaking staff surely heightened her sense of alienation. She may also have been single or without resources to pay for travel; if the pregnancy was unwanted, she may have feared that going to a maternity clinic would make public a condition she preferred to keep out of sight. In Rahilatou's discussion of the case, there was no evidence of a therapy-managing group at all.

Experiencing Reproductive Health Care

Yannick Jaffré and J.-P. Olivier de Sardan's landmark 2003 study of hospitals in five major West African cities revealed starkly the failure of medical structures across West Africa to earn the trust of the citizenry (Jaffré and

Olivier de Sardan 2003). It has become clear that the reason West Africans sometimes do not avail themselves of biomedical care is not a failure to value or understand Western medicine but rather the inhospitable—even venal—treatment they receive in some settings. From the mid-1980s, structural adjustment programs eviscerated medical systems and state capacity throughout the region at the same time that population exploded (Turshen 1999). Modest but free medical care was replaced with "cost recovery" and privatization amid the collapse of state salaries. Cash-strapped medical staff extracted what they could from their patients or shifted costs to the private sector and NGOs. Resources, training, facilities, and medical ethics were all woefully inadequate to the needs of the populations of the region. While there has been improvement in both the domain of medical ethics and affordable service provision, a great deal remains to be done to ameliorate care across the Sahel.

Nurses and *sage-femmes* regularly expressed a sense of embattlement in our interviews; they feel that the failings of the medical system are unfairly laid at their doorstep, when they perform an extremely difficult job that they have chosen out of a sense of civic duty. This stress on the system not only affects the quality of the care but also causes burnout among the medical staff and complicates the training of students. Hadiza I. was shocked by what she saw as the poor treatment of women in the Ayerou clinic where she interned. She found one of the *sage-femmes* to be kind and polite to them, but the other was always rude. Dismayed that they made women pay for things like gloves, the bed, and prescriptions, Hadiza repeated an adage that many of the students had internalized: *la patiente bien accueillie est déjà à moitié guérie* (the well-treated patient is well on her way to healing). Hawa's response was gentle but chiding:

> HAWA: That is a really tough posting, because you know it is right near the refugee camp, right? And so you take a center that was working at capacity, and then you add all these women from the refugee camp and the women working there are overstressed, there aren't materials, and the crowds are much harder to manage. So, for example, there aren't enough gloves. The staff goes to the trouble to buy gloves themselves in the market, they call them *gants de soudure*, to make do until the next order comes in.[2] They pay out of their own pockets; they have to charge for them. It's better than sending their clients away to go find gloves themselves.
>
> BC: Mm hm! Is it legal to ask for payment for services that are otherwise meant to be free?

HAWA: The government has loosened things a little since 2005 [when free maternal and under-five care was introduced]. So long as they meet with the commune representatives and everyone is in agreement, they can raise the fees in some domains in order to cover the costs in others. (Hadiza I., Institut Pratique de Santé Publique, Niamey, May 31, 2014)

Hawa pointed out that she herself had encouraged the rural Malian women in that refugee camp to take advantage of the free maternal services in Niger, stretching the services even further. "You have to teach them how to wait in line," she remarked, "and if you communicate well they are very cooperative." As if to pursue this line of thinking, Hadiza I. elaborated that one time, a better-off local woman jumped the line; she insisted that they had to provide her contraception injection immediately or she would leave. The *sage-femme* kept politely saying, "No you need to wait outside in line; you will get your turn," but the woman kept barging into the examination room. The woman rebuked the *sage-femme*: "We pay you to come here and you refuse to do your job, you'll see!" And she stormed out with her entourage.

Even in a well-regarded maternity center in Niamey, a host of problems result from the poor financing of health, the limited educational background of the patients, and the sizeable cost-free but ineffective labor pool of student trainees and elderly *matrones* now dubbed *filles de salle* (cleaning women). Observing activities in the Maternité Poudrière, I came to wonder how much the patients actually understood about their options, and I was struck that so many, after giving birth numerous times, still appeared to know little about contraception or about how to nurse effectively. A great deal seemed to rest on chance or on the skill of untrained staff (cf. Abba, De Koninck, and Hamelin 2010).

Fieldnotes May 26, 2014
    Maternité Poudrière
    I am sitting in the family planning room during consultations. The very first woman came in for a refill on her pills. She hands over her card, which is specifically for this purpose to record the dates of the consultations, what was prescribed, and the date the woman needs to return for another round. The young sage-femme chides her, "you are very late! Why are you so late? You are supposed to come when you have one pill left, did you skip days?" She carefully goes over how to use the pill container. "You start here and then you follow the arrows up, and then down, and then up, and then back down, and when you have one left then it is time to come back for a refill." The passive and unresponsive woman, who is perhaps 24, with a baby on her back under

her hijab, does not inspire confidence. When the baby starts crying she and the sage-femme speed up the routine so she can escape.

Then another woman came in without a card and was sent off to get one. A third came in, older and more confident in need of a contraceptive injection. Without much ado the sage-femme filled out her card, and prepared her for the shot, which was very quick.

The woman who needed a card came back and they set to work getting her launched for the first time. The sage-femme pulled out a display case of contraceptive materials to explain the options.

"Ok, so there is the shot, which lasts three months. Then there is the six month Norplant. Then there is the three month Norplant. There is the IUD, which goes inside and can stay in as long as you want, a decade if you want. And there is the feminine condom [which she made no effort to explain]. And there is the pill [which she didn't trouble to explain either]. So what do you want?"

"I want the three month kind," the woman replied. By that point an older and more experienced sage-femme named Dije had come in and was watching. She intervened.

"Now all of them can work for three months, so that isn't an answer, you need to look at them and tell us which one you want."

"I want the three month one," repeated the woman, evidently meaning the three month Norplant.

"Ok," Dije said, "you need to understand that the government provides this to you for free, but it is not free, so if you come back in two days and tell us your husband refuses and that you have to take it out, that is a lot of money the government has thrown away. We don't like that, so if you want to do that you have to go home and make sure your husband agrees. The other things are not so much an issue, you can put the pills where they can't be found, but this one is expensive."

Ultimately they decided on the pill, and the sage-femme explained in detail to her how to use the first packet while nursing for the first month, and then explained that she would shift later to a different kind that was stronger once the baby was bigger.

Dije spoke at length to her about nursing, explaining that anything the mother consumes goes into the baby. So it was in this later consultation around family planning that all the advice about breastfeeding occurred and it wasn't clear to me that it would have happened at all if the woman hadn't come in to ask about contraception and if the more experienced sage-femme hadn't been in the room

After the woman left, the three of us chatted a little bit. I asked whether husbands often object to the Norplant. Dije said that they do, and when that happens they have to take it out. If the insertion point heals quickly the husband may not notice, but that can take several days. That's the advantage of the shots.

"But the shots are very strong," Dije elaborated. "We really don't like to give those to just anyone; the woman might be too 'small' and the dosage might mean she will have trouble getting pregnant later. Every woman is different." Clearly Dije's preference is for the pill despite the problems it presents in terms of follow-through. In this setting, if you end up pregnant while married it's not the end of the world. What could be the end of the world or at least the end of a marriage would be to fail to get pregnant quickly once a baby is weaned.

Barrier methods were irrelevant. The diaphragm was not even available, and the female condom was the source of ribald jokes. The problem with both, they explained, is that you can't actually use them without the man's cooperation. For married women, that cooperation is not always a given. In any case, women associate the condom with prostitution; it is not regarded as appropriate for a proper married woman. As one married woman exclaimed, on the suggestion on the part of a *sage-femme* that she and her husband use the condom in light of the problems she was having with hormonal contraceptives, "God protect us! We will never use those rubber things, those are for *gabdi* [loose independent women]" (Moussa 2012, 326).

The male condom has become common in urban Niger since the late 1990s as a result of HIV/AIDS interventions, prompting considerable anxiety about its moral implications and Western motives (Schoultz 1998, 241–49, 284–85). The AIDS epidemic generated resentment at the depiction of Africans as the source of contamination and sexual aberration and increasing demonization of sex workers and homosexuals across the region. Systematic repression of prostitutes across the border in northern Nigeria prompted a large influx of single women into Niger's border towns. In the early years, it was not entirely clear how the epidemic would affect Niger, but in tracking incidence from the first reported case in 1987 to 2000, the United Nations Population Fund (UNFPA) noted that seroprevalence in the general population went from 1.4 percent to 5 percent in Tahoua, with particularly high rates in towns like Konni on the Nigerian border. In studies among prostitutes, the seroprevalence rates could be very high.[3] Today the epidemic is concentrated in particular populations, and the prevalence in the general population is a comparatively low 0.4 percent. Among sex workers the rate is much higher at 17.3 percent (République du Niger CISLS 2014, 5). In 2013, close to ten thousand Nigeriens were on antiretroviral therapy, 63 percent of whom were women. The overwhelming majority of patients are over fifteen (94.6%) (Niger CISLS 2014, 16).

Niger has relied almost entirely on external funding to counter HIV/AIDS, which attracts more attention and resources than most other health problems in the country despite the relatively low prevalence rates. The high visibility of such external actors reinforces the perception that the open discussion of sexuality is brought in by outsiders. Nevertheless, that opening has made it more possible to discuss reproductive issues in general, including female genital cutting, in the context of AIDS prevention. Women in maternal health today are proud of the progress they have made in understanding the disease and treating patients respectfully.

The epidemic affects women disproportionately for a variety of reasons: male to female transmission is more likely than the reverse, women are more likely to engage in transactional sex in order to achieve the standard of living they aspire to, and polygamy by definition involves multiple concurrent sexual partners. As a simple mathematical matter, there are more women in polygynous marriages than men; therefore, more women than men are exposed to the risk such marriages entail.

But most importantly, the epidemic affects them because it leaves them widowed, infected, and caring for children and other dependents. They have little prospect or inclination to remarry in pursuit of male economic support. As a result, HIV-positive women are disproportionately represented in NGO support groups for widows. One dynamic middle-aged widow explained that she and her three co-wives had been in limbo for six years. When their husband, who had been a trader at the Marché Katako, died, his brothers refused to provide the widows with anything substantial enough to support all the children in the house. She has, by her reckoning, gotten a reputation as a troublemaker because she had the temerity to dispute the division of the inheritance. She says a woman isn't supposed to do that; she is supposed to stay silent because of "shame." There is an expression they use to describe a woman like her, she told me with a hint of defiance. They say she is a bird who opens wide its wings so you can smell the stench of her underarms.

Nursing and Weaning "Properly"

When I spoke with two women associated with the Islamist Izala movement, both emphasized nursing as a means of preventing pregnancy. They knew that if a woman nurses "properly" she reduces the likelihood of pregnancy. But how does a woman ensure that her nursing will be sufficient to prevent pregnancy? After all, conversely, if she falls pregnant she will not be able to nurse properly. With shifts in conjugal abstinence patterns, remedies to prevent pregnancy prior to the weaning of a baby became more important. Dominique Traoré noted a number of such remedies in the early 1960s, including an amulet to be put on the nursing baby to keep the mother from getting pregnant again and a string belt to be worn around the mother's waist until she is ready to wean the child (Traoré 1965).

Given the significance of nursing to women's birth spacing strategies, I spoke to women at considerable length about their approaches to nursing. From my interviews I am persuaded that women are right—a woman who nurses more or less exclusively for two years has a good likelihood of achieving good birth spacing (something close to three years). Many women I interviewed who had never used contraception had had very regularly spaced births. While World Health Organization recommendations would certainly approve of nursing for two years, ideally at six months a mother would introduce other foods into the baby's diet. Successful suppression of ovulation through *exclusive* breastfeeding beyond six months implies delayed introduction of those complementary foods, risking under-five undernutrition and vulnerability to disease. Not surprisingly, those same women's children tended to do well unless they were struck by a childhood illness.

So, what is "nursing properly" exactly? The more vigorously the baby sucks, the more likely it is that a woman will experience sustained lactational amenorrhea. Mothers will also do better if they don't fall ill themselves. Elderly women insisted that "milk draws milk," meaning both that it is important to keep nursing and that drinking milk protects a nursing mother's milk supply. But in general, I couldn't sort out whether "nursing properly" was a deliberate achievement or an accident of good fortune. Many women did feel that changes in nutrition were an important source of ill health generally and of reproductive problems in particular. This is a complex subject because nutrition affects the body of the pregnant woman, the fetus, and the nursing infant. Certainly there is a strong sense in Niger that sugar is a source of both moral and reproductive problems (Masquelier 1995).

One elderly Zarma woman had powerful convictions on the subject: "You have to eat millet that has been pounded by hand, not ground in a machine; eating all those Western products, macaroni, and rice, that is not good. You must avoid sugar, soda, and Maggi cubes. When you have *fura* [a millet smoothie of sorts] you should always add sour milk, every day. All these cold raw things they call 'salad' are foreign. I never eat them" (Tsofuwa ta Zarmaganda, Niamey, January 11, 2014). Her middle-aged daughter was amused by this litany of nutritional injunctions, but it was true that the older woman was the picture of wiry good health while her plump daughter on an urban functionary diet suffered from high blood pressure and has had a far less straightforward reproductive history. My hunch is that shifts in nutrition are indeed important to the history of pregnancy and nursing, but it would be difficult to prove. The typical size of the baby at birth may have fluctuated as well, affecting the experience of delivery. And of course, changes in diet could affect mothers' milk and weaning foods long after the birth of the child.

Since 1950 or so, dried milk, refined sugars, soda, dried noodles, and white rice have overtaken local diets. Julie Livingston found that this kind of shift in Botswana contributed to earlier onset of menarche, producing an existential experience of a quickening of the female life cycle: "pregnant children" became women earlier, and adult women felt "half-dead" from work and stress before their own mothers had (Livingston 2003). Similar processes in different locales would surely have quite different meanings (Jones et al. 2009; Bralić et al. 2012; Prentice et al. 2010). In Niger, earlier menarche would very likely have triggered a reduction in the age of marriage for girls and a heightened alarm over the sexual vulnerability of girls in public spaces, particularly schools. Some of the food taboos imposed on pregnant women in the past but increasingly discouraged today may also have had the effect of keeping the fetus small, facilitating delivery. The loss of sources of iron in the diet may, as well, have contributed to the anemia that is a common source of complications in pregnancy in Niger. With changes in diet, the size of babies at birth may have grown and the quality of women's milk may have declined. The data is simply not available to pursue these questions.

Changes in diet and nutrition over the long twentieth century, however, have probably not been uniformly experienced or unilineal in impact. Long stretches of drought and food shortage undoubtedly reduced both women's fertility and the survival of infants. Because such conditions come and go unpredictably, women's nutritional condition has probably always fluctuated, particularly in rural areas and particularly for women of low status. The introduction of cash cropping had mixed implications for consumption; cash could make it possible to purchase new foods, including vegetables and meat, but only if women could gain access to it. Women's access to cash to purchase foods has also been changeable depending on much broader socioeconomic processes, including the defeminization of agriculture and the growing practice of seclusion (Diarra and Monimart 2009). Today, income-generating activities are generally the solution preferred by women to improve their children's nutrition rather than the more nutrition-specific interventions preferred by donors (Nisbett et al. 2017).

But another leitmotif of interviews done in the 1980s was the degradation of the farmland. Reduced fallow periods as peanut farming expanded, populations grew, and yields declined have affected farmland across the Sahel. Another theme is the rapid decline in diversity of plant and animal life. The Sahel in the early twentieth century was still capable of yielding wild game, fish, and an abundance of nutritious wild tree products (Cross and Barker 1993). The variety of foods rural populations could eat declined, contributing to the erosion of nutrition across the board. Today, public health experts take a great interest in nutritional life histories because periodic food shortages may produce stunting that has longer-term implications for children's growth and their risk of cardio-metabolic diseases as adults (Said-Mohamed, Pettifor, and Norris 2018). African countries struggle with growing chronic disease burden (hypertension, obesity, and diabetes) as a result of major changes in diet at the same time that they contend with the infectious diseases characteristic of less developed economies; there has not really been an epidemiological "transition" so much as an expansion of health problems (including HIV/AIDS) without a pronounced demographic transition and without robust health systems. As a recent study noted, existing models used to predict change are based on the notions of demographic, epidemiological, and health transition that are inadequate to regions "where changing contexts of health, disease and mortality patterns are embedded in significant uncertainties" (Defo 2014). Little wonder, then, that women experience childbirth as "harder."

One thing that hasn't changed is the critiques of how women nurse and wean; these have been a regular theme through the history of the region from the beginning of the twentieth century. In the latest major round of critiques, at the time of the food crisis of 2005, once again women's weaning and feeding practices were offered to account for the seemingly sudden appearance of severe malnutrition among small children. The irony in that moment was that women brought their ill children into visibility because they sought access to the one innovation that appeared to actually produce results: PlumpyNut paste (B. Cooper 2007, 2009). They were, it turns out, quite attuned to the importance of providing nutritious food for children under five. It is in some ways easier to point to practices that are deemed to be "bad" than to determine how to actually nurse and wean "properly." Practices that are "bad" include withholding colostrum in the first days after the birth of the infant, giving infants medicinal teas, introducing foods that are difficult to digest too early, and failing to introduce solid foods early enough. Waiting for up to several days to nurse, which means the baby misses out on the immunity protection of colostrum, is uncommon outside the Hausa-speaking region near Maradi and among some Peul women.

In my interviews, I devoted a fair amount of attention to the question of how to wean. Some women had a great deal to say about what foods are good for weaning, but most recited in a rather rote manner various *bouilli* (boiled porridges) they had been instructed to cook in the context of assorted interventions delivered by Peace Corps nutritionists, missionary women, and NGOs. Their recitation did not inspire confidence in me that they were actually interested in the topic or capable of improvising in the absence of the many expensive and difficult-to-obtain ingredients they listed, such as powdered milk. I asked Hawa whether powdered milk referred to in the context of infant feeding wasn't too expensive for women. She said that when she was giving nutrition training years ago on a UNICEF program for weaning, she eventually stopped emphasizing adding milk powder to the *bouilli* because the women just don't do it. They put in sugar instead because it is cheap and their husbands will buy it. If you give them milk, they end up giving it to all the children in the house, so the baby doesn't get it. What actually works, she said, is telling them how to make baby food purée out of things like squash, potatoes, and carrots with only a pinch of salt so that the other children don't like it. You can also make the *bouilli* out of sorghum, which is easier to digest than millet.

So, what do women actually do, as opposed to say they do? A measure of the striking difference between what health trainers proclaim and what women actually do emerges by examining the practices of female medical professionals themselves. I learned a great deal about the kinds of therapeutic practices women in Niamey make use of during pregnancy, during nursing, and during weaning by talking to nurses, *sage-femmes*, and social workers about their own habits. All these relatively educated women spoke of using the infusions known as *bauri*; if they didn't, their in-laws and neighbors would see that failure as a kind of child abuse. If women trained in public health continue to use such infusions, it is a safe bet that other women do as well. Rigid adherence to "exclusive" breastfeeding is followed by very few women of any background.

These kinds of herb teas fall generically under the broad category of *icce*, meaning potent medicines derived from trees (leaves, roots, bark, seed). Women of particular ethnicities are seen to be experts on these therapeutic products; in Niamey, Dendi women are reputed to have good medicines. An elderly Zarma woman explained to me that *bauri* teas make the baby strong and protect it from the evil eye. In the past, a woman would collect the necessary materials herself; she would never buy them from a stranger. She would dry them out to save for later: *kasan ture, andogo, nunebaskagi, diringa,* and *kobesayi.* She would boil them with potash using four handfuls of the *icce* to make the tea for a girl, three for a boy. It would get progressively stronger each day (Gidan Kakan Hawa, Niamey, January 15, 2014).[4]

I visited the stall of a woman from Benin reputed to sell effective *bauri* infusions. Her bustling daughter explained that a woman would pay five thousand CFA (about nine dollars) in the morning to obtain *bauri* and that when she returned in the afternoon she would be given a clay cook pot full of the infusion. In preparing the infusion, they would use several *icce* together: *han kufa* bark to strengthen the body of the infant, 'kabe bark to give the baby appetite, *kan bugu/hannuwa biyar* leaves to make the baby grow, *dirgidirgi* to protect him from evil eye, *fegen danni* to counter the shivers babies get "when they become afraid," *na maari* or *yawo bargi* to treat dysentery, and *seke seke* seed pods to give strength. When she prepares the *bauri*, she places these bundles in a clay cook pot and boils them for two hours. When it is ready, she explains to the client how to give it to the baby. You wouldn't give it straight, she explains; you would dilute it with water: three measures for a boy, four measures for a girl. You would reduce the dilution each day—first you bring it to a boil, and then you dilute it. The nursing mother would also drink the same solution, diluted with milk, because milk draws milk. Similarly, there are decoctions women can drink to stop bleeding after giving birth and medicines for malaria and hemorrhoids (Mai Bauri, Niamey Marché Katako, January 23, 2014). Women consider that anything the nursing mother drinks is likely also to be passed through the milk to benefit the baby as well.

When women are successful in spacing their births well, weaning their children at the right time, and raising the child to adulthood, they attribute that success to the power of the *bauri* they have used. When things go badly, the tendency is to conclude that the medicines weren't the right ones or they weren't administered properly; no one I spoke to ever attributed the death of any baby to the use of *bauri*. One of the effects of the purifying drive of the Izala movement has been to characterize the use of these kinds of *icce* medicines as signs of *kafirci* (paganism); women should rely only on Allah. One devout woman explained to me that once she began being more observant, she threw away all the protective charms and gave up *bauri*. But later her little girl died. She is now considering returning to using *bauri* with her next baby, even though her community would disapprove.

The advice to nurse "exclusively" is counterintuitive to most women. Despite NGOs' regular association of infant mortality with the use of such infusions, I have not seen a systematic study that establishes a link. Often the assumption is that the infusions are made with dirty water; obviously, if the water supply is clean then that concern is mitigated. But these teas are boiled and then cooled before dilution; the danger they present by comparison with, say, an unclean baby bottle, seems minimal. *Bauri* use may reduce the period of lactational amenorrhea by potentially reducing the strength of the baby's suck if the child is "full," but the servings offered to children are not particularly large.

Of course, one of the most important ways a woman should protect the milk of the nursing baby is to ensure that she doesn't fall pregnant; the problem is circular. I encountered numerous nursing women who were distraught to discover that they were pregnant. One potential justification within Islam for the use of contraception is that it is more important to protect the nursing child, who is living, than the potential child, who is not (Atighetchi 1994, 720). The challenge in feeding the nursling, the mother, and the fetus at the same time is well known. In contexts of poor nutrition, competition between the three is even more desperate. The notion of "bad milk" may be a residue of a sense that nurslings of pregnant mothers often fall ill; the competition for nutrients privileges the fetus over the mother or the production of milk. Historically, the solution has been to wean the nursling as quickly as possible, which leads to equally calamitous results. But it does mean that both the mother and the fetus will be protected. The other solution would be to abort the fetus to protect the nursing infant and the mother. There is a ready Islamic justification for this reasoning, which is that the mother is urged to nurse the baby for about a year and a half.[5] To protect her ability to nurse, an abortion could arguably be the lesser of two evils.

The Shame of Giving Birth Like a Mouse

Prior to the mid-twentieth century, when women went to their father's and mothers' homes to give birth and remained there until ready to resume their sexual duties as wives, conjugal abstinence was lengthy. Even after a woman returned to her marital home, the social opprobrium on couples having sexual relations while nursing was considerable enough that husbands were likely to observe sexual restraint. Under such conditions, it was surely comparatively easy for women to sustain healthy spacing between their pregnancies: from three to four years (Schoultz 1998, 163–64).

Gradually the practice of women returning to their parents' homes declined and the timing of the resumption of sexual activity became less clear. A common marker became when the baby could walk. Among the herbal remedies Dominique Traoré records from the early 1960s are a variety of decoctions in which to bathe the child to hasten its ability to walk (Traoré, 1965, 514–15). In Muslim areas, eventually a period of forty days provided a religiously sanctioned marker. Returning to the maternal household by women and lengthy abstinence by men was increasingly marked as a sign of "paganism." Early resumption of marital sex became the mark of a Muslim man. As the norm of a forty-day abstention spread, women's ability to meet the social expectation of good spacing, which nevertheless endured, inevitably declined (Schoultz 1998, 166).

Despite a general consensus that the ideal birth spacing should be two to three years between children, the reality is much closer to one year (Family Care International 1998, 30). Today women are regularly informed by Muslim scholars that to refuse to have sex with their husband is a terrible sin and that it will result in their going to Hell (Moussa 2012, 143–46; Masquelier 2009, 261). Yet as one respondent to a survey on reproductive health remarked, with perhaps a hint of defensiveness, "Even God says two years of birth spacing is good" (Family Care International 1998, 30). This major shift occurred all across the Sahel, producing friction and resentment that women could perhaps only express in song, as in this particularly rich Diola song collected by Rokhaya Fall in Senegal in 1998:

A Call and Response Song: "The Torments of Labor"
Call: Oh, the signs of labor had started.

Response: *All I wanted was delivery.*
Call: Oh, the signs of labor had started.
Response: *All I wanted was delivery. . . .*
Call: So Aunt Sadiya arrives.
She says: "What's wrong with you, girl?"
I tell her: "I'm going to die."
She says: "But, if you die, people will say you're a witch."
Response: *All I wanted was delivery.*
Call: At long last, the baby was there.
I say to her: "I don't want this child."
My Aunt Sadiya is childless. So she says "I'll take it."
I tell her, "Before you take it, ask me why I don't want the child."
Response: *All I wanted was delivery.*
Call: When my labor started, I saw my husband leave his room dressed like a
    king.
He said he was going to a sacred ceremony [a marriage or a naming ceremony].
Response: *All I wanted was delivery.*
Call: Then when the child took his first steps,
Back came my husband, to solicit me, on his knees.
I knew it was starting all over again.
And later he would abandon me.
Response: *All I wanted was delivery.*
Call: If only I had thought this through before,
I would have gone to my father's,
So he could find a key
To lock up my private parts.
But my father didn't think of this either.
Response: *All I wanted was delivery.*
Call: Maybe, that way, I would have had four years of relief.
Response: *All I wanted was delivery.*
(Sutherland-Addy and Diaw 2005, 354)

While for husbands this amplified sexual access does not appear to have
led to a sense of shame in their interactions with other men, for women it
did. Among the sources of shame for women today are being pregnant while
nursing, having children at the breast and on the back at the same time, and
having children at the same time as their own daughters or daughters-in-
law (Family Care International 1998, 16, 25–26).

An expression captures nicely the shared image of proper birth spacing: *yara su imma juna* (Hausa) or *zankey I ma du ga hini care* (Zarma),
meaning that the older child should be able to carry the younger on his or
her back (Moussa 2012, 300). The image, which inspires a sigh of nostalgic

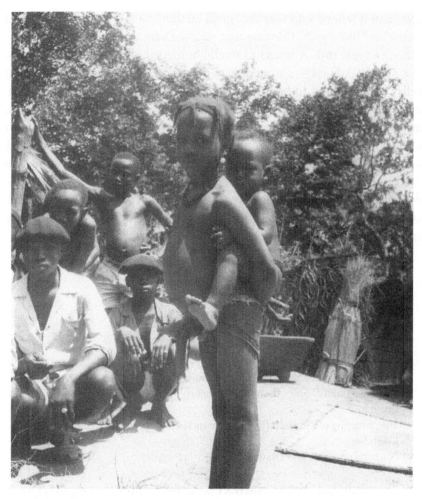

Zarma girl with her little brother in Niamey, 1957. Courtesy of Archives Nationales d'Outre-Mer.

satisfaction when evoked, is of a child of about four carrying a baby brother or sister on his back; the children care for one another.

There are specific expressions of mixed pity and contempt for a woman who regularly fails to achieve suitable birth spacing and timing. She is regarded as incapable of self-restraint, or perhaps even worse, as having a husband lacking in self-restraint who is "always between her legs." Her regular pregnancy makes visible that shameful lack of restraint. Of such a woman it will be said that she "gives birth like a mouse" or "like a black locust" or "like a goat" (Moussa 2012, 303–4; Doka and Monimart 2009, 141; Schoultz 1998, 163). A woman literally burdened with children (in Hausa *mace da goyo da ciki*—a woman with a baby on the back and a baby in the belly) is considered to be like a mindless animal, not like a rational human. Her children will be unkempt and short-lived (Moussa 2012, 306). The most contemptible overly fertile woman is an older woman whose sons are marrying and introducing young brides into the household. When such a mother-in-law continues to bear children excessively at the same time as her daughters-in-law, she violates important markers of generation and demonstrates her lack of capacity to feel shame. A Zarma insult song collected by Fatimata Mounkaila in Niamey in 1999 illustrates how intergenerational tensions might be expressed:[6]

> A Pounding Song: "My Backside"
> My strong black biceps—Insult her!
> Insult her! Insult her! Insult her!
> She makes more babies than the bean fodder plant,
> Insult her!
> She makes more babies than a female locust,
> Insult her! Insult her!
> She makes more babies than termites and mice,
> She makes more babies than a watermelon,
> Insult her!
> That cunning old woman [the mother-in-law],
> Insult her. . . .
> (Sutherland-Addy and Diaw 2005, 262)

The many indigenous practices designed to prevent pregnancy or to eliminate an unwanted pregnancy existed well before the advent of Western ideas about sexuality or the expansion of Islam in the nineteenth and twentieth centuries. Traoré's collection of African herbal remedies is rich in advice about how to avoid pregnancy: drink water in which a gold ring has been boiled, or drink water containing the urine of a ram (1965, 505). To prevent pregnancy and the shame of revealing a lack of restraint, married women wore a kauri shell on a string around the waist to avoid pregnancy, or a charm made by a Muslim specialist, or they drank *bauri* to encourage their milk so that they could prevent their periods from returning, or they counted the days from their periods, or they drank an infusion with pounded calabash or pottery shards to "enclose" the womb to protect it. A cooperative partner might practice withdrawal.

Contraception, then, is not a foreign or modern introduction into the region. Furthermore, such remedies were not primarily used in the context of *illicit* sexuality. Married women managed their reproductive lives to the degree that they could with the techniques available to them. Nor were women passive about attempting to improve their fertility. Alarmed by the absence of menstruation—one mark of fecundability—women also used emmenagogues of solutions of salt, ginger, henna, or neem leaves to "cleanse" their wombs in hopes of becoming pregnant. Of course, the distinction between encouraging the return of one's period and eliminating a potential pregnancy is slender, so long as the pregnancy is not yet visible (Moussa 2012, 307–13). Methods to provoke a miscarriage were well known; across the region, women were aware that drinking a tea from the roots of the indigo plant was an effective abortifacient (Abadie 2010 [1927], 209; Traoré 1965, 506; Cross and Barker 1993, 103). Whether married women occasionally attempted to rid themselves of an early pregnancy is difficult to know but certainly easy to imagine given the ridicule to which they and sometimes their partners could be subjected. The problem with inducing abortion with toxic substances, however, is that they would be likely to kill a nursing baby as well.

The alternative to eliminating a poorly timed pregnancy was to wean the nursing baby early and quickly. The conceptualization of the failure of restraint as producing "bad milk" rendered this solution necessary if a woman and her husband failed to show restraint. Unfortunately, as a solution it virtually guaranteed that the nursing baby would be poorly nourished with substitute milk, generally goat's milk, and shifted to solid foods earlier than would be normal. Today baby formulas are available to women in urban centers such as Niamey, but they are exceedingly expensive, and it is difficult to enforce quality control regulations (Sokol, Aguayo, and Clark 2007). It also requires the use of bottles and a clean water supply. Early and "abrupt" weaning has long been decried as the source of poor health outcomes among small children in Niger, but the connection between weaning, conceptions of piety and marriage, and shifting sexual norms has rarely been made. Early weaning might not save a woman from the ridicule that comes with being incapable of managing her procreation.

My presumption, therefore, is that married women are more likely today than in the past to entertain having an abortion because they are more likely than in the past to need one (see also Moumouni 2000), and it no longer requires consuming toxic substances. While the public outcry over abortion generally focuses on unmarried women, the reality is probably closer to these cases collected by Hadiza Moussa among married women. The first was a thirty-three-year-old married woman who sold snacks in Poudrière. The second was a thirty-three-year-old teacher with four children living in Balafon.

> I was on the pill but sometimes I forgot to take it. Even though I caught up by taking the ones I missed when I remembered, apparently that didn't resolve the problem since I got pregnant. At first I thought it was just that my period was late. But after two months I was dizzy and vomiting. That's when I decided to have an abortion. My baby is only 8 months old, it's too early to have another. (Moussa 2012, 337)

> At the dispensary, thanks to a friend I went to school with, they put me on Synto [Syntocinon, used to provoke uterine contractions in routine deliveries] for a day. First they gave me a shot. At the end of the day I bled profusely. That's how I lost my six week pregnancy. (Moussa 2012, 365)

The argument that abortion has become more necessary for married women would appall most Nigerien Muslims today, but it seems an inescapable outcome of the elimination of conjugal abstinence during nursing, the only infallible local form of contraception. The ridicule facing a woman who gives birth "like a mouse" has not disappeared, yet the means to avoid it have. Without a general recognition that abstinence must be replaced by contraception, married women are at increased risk of both pregnancy and ridicule than in the past. Not to mention financial strain.

Because Niger's abortion laws are so restrictive, discussing abortion is very sensitive. To the degree that it is visible, it becomes known in the context of medical complications due to an attempted abortion in a nonmedical setting, almost universally by an unmarried schoolgirl. Any medication or chemical with a pregnancy warning label may be tried. The potential materials that have entered the list has grown to include anything from antimalarial medications to toxic chemicals. In one recent case, a girl consumed battery acid. Obviously, some of these efforts lead to the death of the pregnant woman, in which case it may be difficult to distinguish from a suicide. However, many end up in the hospital; since 2006, by law medical professionals are obligated to treat them. Magistrate B. A. explained to me that most abortion charges begin because someone at a maternity clinic reports the case of a woman seeking postabortion care. Hawa offered as an example a case she encountered of a woman who had come in to one of the maternity clinics who had a strip of millet stalk stuck through her cervix. Evidently, she had gone to a traditional medicine seller, who had given her an herbal decoction she was to drink to soften and open her cervix. Then later she was to use a stick to do a kind of homespun curettage.

The magistrate said that schoolgirls are in the habit of taking something (probably black-market Syntocinon) to "open" the cervix, and then after bleeding at home they come in to a private clinic for curettage. One clinic reported this to the government because it seemed to the staff that an unusually high number of girls were coming in having "miscarried." The magistrate said, "Look, all these young girls are in nursing schools, they know how to do all these things, and so they do it for their friends!" She and Hawa were clearly appalled by this (Magistrate B. A., Niamey, June 11, 2014). Such medically assisted abortions, while clandestine, appear to be relatively safe in Niger; they don't make headlines at any rate. But the dangerous improvised and "traditional" methods that poorer and often single women use can make for grisly publicity. In 2012, a retired *matrone* in Dosso was allegedly approached by a pregnant widow for assistance in obtaining an abortion. In a jocular online "miscellaneous news" piece, one journalist referred to the *matrone* as a "sorceress." He reported: "The goal of the sorceress's intervention was just to break the water sack to provoke labor. But unfortunately the nail she used went through the soft head of the baby. Not surprisingly, three days later this 'nailed' woman suddenly went to the maternity where, upon inspection, the *sage-femmes* discovered the presence of a nail in her uterus. At first she hesitated, but eventually she made a confession implicating [the *matrone*] who she claims sank this nail into her" (Super User 2012).

Sensational news stories like this, which reveal the desperation of poor single women, blur the line between abortion and infanticide, medical technique and witchcraft. They also provoke disgust and abhorrence for abortion of any kind, even when medically necessary.

Mothers and Daughters

Professional women in a relatively well-equipped urban maternity related a variety of instances in which outraged Islamist husbands intervened to prevent appropriate care for their wives. The latitude of mothers to direct their own care or the care of their daughters can be very limited where insular attitudes among rigid Islamic purists intrude. Ader is reputed to be one of the most conservative regions of Niger. Hawa and I went to visit a very good-natured widow named Rabi from Ader, whose friend Furera was visiting as well. Rabi's mother had been married to a paternal cousin, and as a result Rabi had some very serious congenital vision problems. Two of her own little boys also have problems with their eyes; Hawa had noticed it right away. As we were chatting, Rabi's seventeen-year-old daughter Rashida came in and shed her hijab to reveal her school uniform of a skirt, a button-down shirt, and a pink necktie. She is in school to learn finance; she smiled shyly and went into the back to change and to pray.

Although Rabi was a widow, they were more comfortably off than some of the other widows we had encountered: there were more furnishings, and the house was abuzz with the comings and goings of young workers collecting Solani milk packets to sell. As we talked, Rabi revealed that there were plans afoot to marry this daughter to her father's brother's son. I asked, "Why is that; is it a matter of inheritance?" Her initial reply was, "It's to keep the family close. That way, see, if you lose your husband, your brother-in-law will take care of you because you are all related." Exasperated by Rabi's reluctance to call a spade a spade, her friend and neighbor Furera exclaimed, "Of course it is because of property; they want to keep it all together." Rashida eventually came back in to seek further information from Hawa about the eye problems she overheard us discussing. She too has poor night vision. Hawa explained why they had poor vision and stated that marrying Rashida to her cousin would lead to similar problems. "Speaking to you not as an adviser, but simply as a medically trained professional," Hawa said carefully, "you would want do a test early in a pregnancy to see whether there were any genetic anomalies." In other words, although Hawa did not say so explicitly, this would be a case in which a medically approved abortion might be recommended.

Genetic disorders are of increasing concern to the Niger government because of the high medical costs they can incur. Among the most significant of such disorders is sickle cell anemia. According to the minister of public health, between 18 percent and 22 percent of Niger's population carries the trait, which of course confers resistance to malaria. However, when the bearer carries two alleles (one from the mother and one from the father), the likelihood of severe infection or anemia is very high and requires careful preventive and therapeutic intervention (Maman 2014). It is in the context of sickle cell trait screening that genetic counseling has become available in Niger.[7] The disease can require very close monitoring of the patients. One of the women we interviewed who was training to become a nurse was doing so in part so that she would be able to care for her husband and two children, all of whom have the disease (Habsou I., IPSP, Niamey, May 31, 2014).

Other problems that arise from close intermarriage are hearing problems, poor bone formation, sterility, and paralysis of the feet. Preferential cousin marriage has long been practiced in Niger; a very sizeable proportion of my elderly informants in the late 1980s had been married into a cross cousin marriage in their first marriages. The advantage of such marriages is that when the bride goes to live with the groom, she may remain in the same village as her close kin. When she gives birth, her maternal kin are close at hand. The inheritance of land remains closely circumscribed within the extended family, reducing the fragmentation that can render farming concerns unviable. In principal, uncles care for the children of their orphaned brothers. The system has served Rabi well in the sense that she did appear to have some support from her brothers-in-law. But the disadvantages were also clear: the men of the family were anxious to marry Rashida to a cousin so that the cost of caring for Rabi's children would be compensated through the acquisition of a daughter-in-law. The wealth of the family would be contained, and the risk of this dependent girl becoming pregnant before marriage and producing another mouth to feed would be moderated. Furthermore, once she married, they could be relieved of the cost of her schooling.

On another occasion I asked Rabi, "Why not find another husband for her who isn't such a close relation, since you know that it causes eye troubles?" She said, "No we can't do that; it has been planned for a long time. We talked to the two [the prospective bride and groom] and talked sense into them and they have agreed." I asked, "If they didn't agree, would you do it?" She said, "Oh no, we don't do *armen dole* [forced marriage]." But of course they were putting great pressure on Rashida to marry the cousin, even when she appeared reluctant. The two are extremely close cousins (their fathers were twins), and the doctor as well had recommended against the marriage. When we ran into Rabi again five months later, Rashida had already been married to her cousin.

When I spoke to her friend Furera after a lengthy absence, she gave me the news that her own fifteen-year-old daughter was now married. Seeing my dismay, Furera somewhat defensively explained that it was the girl's decision. The groom has a new house with electricity, and since moving there her grades have improved, according to her mother. I pushed a bit, asking whether they were planning on having children right away. She said, "Oh no, she hasn't even started menstruating." According to her, the groom agreed to wait. I gave her a skeptical look, and she said that when she looks at her daughter she can tell that she still doesn't "know" about sex. "Why did you have her marry early rather than wait until she finished school?" I asked. "Well," she said, "sometimes a young person will get restless, and it will be harder for her to get married. It is better this way." He is in his thirties and is looking for a job with an NGO. In the meantime, he buys and sells cars for a living.

Were Furera's daughter to need contraception to increase her prospects for finishing school, Furera would be of limited assistance to her. When I asked her what she thought about family planning, Furera replied that her own teacher says that family planning is permissible in Islam and that the way to do it is to count from the beginning of your period fifteen days and abstain then or the man can withdraw. You can't use the pill. This was the only time a woman mentioned withdrawal without my introducing the subject first. Intrigued, I asked whether a lot of couples did this. Embarrassed, she replied, "All I know is that's what our teacher told us. If you don't want to get pregnant as a couple, then the thing to do is not to let the man's water enter into the woman's inside, because the eggs are in the man's water. So if they don't go in, how can you be pregnant?" Later she remarked that her teacher also taught the women not to hit their boys in the head, because you might kill the eggs, which are stored there. When I asked her friend Rabi about withdrawal, she said that it is haram (forbidden) but that her teacher had taught her how to count the days and abstain on the dangerous days. The likelihood that either woman understood the rhythm method well enough to explain it to a daughter seemed very low to me.

While it is possible that Furera's daughter was indeed happy to be married to a man twice her age, other "consensual" marriages that took place in families I had interviewed were not so happy. I had gone to visit a woman named Mai Talla in Boukoki to catch up on her news. Mai Talla reported with glee that the youngest of her daughters, who was fifteen, had just been married off to the son of her younger sister back in the village near Birnin Konni. Mai Talla took the chip out of her daughter's phone and replaced it with a new one before sending her off to the village so that she and her boyfriend in Niamey couldn't communicate.

MAI TALLA: In the village she is in her own house near the in-laws; she leaves her house every day to work for them.

BC: So will she work the fields?

MAI TALLA: [snorting] She doesn't know anything about farming! But they will teach her little by little.

BC: Do they have running water?

MAI TALLA: No.

(Mai Talla, Boukoki, June 9, 2014)

I predicted that she would run away as so many women I have interviewed over the years did when their first marriage was not of their choosing. Mai Talla said, "Well, I told her to be patient." I turned to Mai Talla's daughter-in-law, who was quietly listening close by, to ask whether she thought the girl would stay. She smiled and replied, "Someone who is used to Niamey!?" One strategy for such a girl would be to feign infertility through clandestine contraception use in the hope that she would provoke a divorce, as another of my informants had done when she was younger (see also Moussa 2012, 339).

The Paradox of Overfertility amid Infertility: The *Affair des Bébés*

Abinda wani ba ya so, shi wani ke nema
The very thing one person rejects, another is seeking
(Hausa proverb often invoked in context of unwanted pregnancies)

One of my informants in Maradi in 1989 explained to me why it was so painful for her when she lived as an adult woman in her paternal village. Having been divorced because she failed to produce children, she was known by everyone to be living in her father's house, not her husband's. Whenever there was a celebration, there were particular songs to which women who had given birth were invited to dance; infertile women could not participate. She was regularly insulted in such songs in a public manner. Other women threw celebratory events, but she was unable to reciprocate in any way by throwing a wedding or a naming ceremony of her own. "Where is the happiness in that?" she asked me. And so, she moved to Maradi where she survived as a *karuwa* (a "courtesan" woman who satisfies a host of domestic needs for one or several men in exchange for money and other rewards) but never succeeded in having a child of her own.

Women can be very cruel to one another, vaunting their own fertility and ridiculing others without children. The internal domestic hierarchy across the Sahel includes fertility as part of ranking, as a Bambara woman in Mali lamented in song:

> Slave, you are the slave of women
> Who have children,
> Kumbre, kumbre
> With those who don't have children
> You are the slave of those who do
> Kumbre, kumbre
> (Luneau 2010, 96)

Infertile women of all backgrounds, education levels, and economic conditions suffer a sense that they are incomplete and not fully adult. Even a wealthy man with several wives may find his household to be unhappy because of the infertility of one or more of his wives. To an outsider for whom adoption is one imaginable solution to the problem of childlessness, the paradox that there are so many babies and children who need homes and at the same time so many men and women who need children is quite striking. Why don't they just solve one another's problems through adoption?

Adoption as understood in the United States or France is anathema in Islam. In practice, everything related to family life in Niger is regulated in light of local understandings of Islamic juridical tradition. The foster child of a Muslim can never be equivalent in social and legal standing to legitimate biological children. The child will retain the name of a biological relative and can't partake of the inheritance of the foster parents. In economies in which individuals survive through farming and herding, exclusion from inheritance is no minor thing. Like illegitimate children, orphaned, abandoned, and fostered children may have no recourse but to become mendicant Koranic students. As a result, children who can't be supported are often essentially abandoned in order to "study the Koran" (Amedome 2010, 23). Niamey has an increasingly visible population of unsupervised children, who support themselves through begging, theft, or the exchange of sex for money or other kinds of support. Unsupervised children are referred to as "delinquents" as a kind of equivalent for "homeless." They are automatically in advance assumed to be criminal.

The rejection of full adoption within Islamic legal practice results from the emphasis on blood relations generated in legitimate marriages to the establishment of recognized personhood. Adoption disrupts the clarity about bloodlines, about prohibited degrees of relationship in marriage, and most importantly about who can and cannot inherit. By extension, the only forms of medically assisted reproduction permitted in most Islamic legal traditions today are artificial insemination of the wife using the husband's sperm and in vitro insemination using the eggs of the wife and the sperm of the husband. Surrogacy is not admissible; it is seen as equivalent to fornication. Men in an infertile marriage who hope to produce legitimate children may take another wife or pursue sperm-enhancing technologies. Because the husband generally controls decisions about health investment, infertile women are less likely to receive effective medical intervention than men, particularly if treatment requires an expensive trip to another country, as is often the case (Hörbst 2010; Family Care International 1998, 17, 31). Today, although access to infertility treatment through artificial insemination and IVF is included as a right within Niger's 2006 law on reproductive health, the technological capacity in Niger is very low and treatment does not necessarily produce the desired results (Moussa 2012, 124–25). As is true elsewhere in Africa, such technologies are generally approached in secrecy; while they are not technically illegal, they may run counter to the cultural and juridical logics to which these offspring and their parents will be governed in daily life (Bonnet and Duchesne 2016).

It is against this backdrop that the infamous baby scandal (*affaire des bébés*) has unfolded in Niger. Sometimes referred to as the Baby Factory Affair (*histoire des usines à bébé*) this ongoing scandal began with rumors about a number of well-known women in Niger who had managed to become pregnant after a long struggle with infertility. They had sought the medicine of a woman known as Happiness Ogundeji in an unremarkable village named Ilutitun in southeast Nigeria. These elite women claimed to have benefited from her traditional remedies and to have given birth in Nigeria (Thiénot 2015). Rumor gave way to judicial uproar in June 2014 with an announcement that twenty or so people, among them the wives of some well-known political figures (including notably the leader of the opposition and head of the Parliament, Hama Amadou), had been arrested in the dismantling of a transnational "baby trafficking ring" that had introduced babies into Niger from Nigeria via Benin. The central crime that the Nigerien women were accused of was *supposition d'enfant* or the false claim to be the biological and legal mothers of the children after feigning pregnancy. The women involved had each allegedly acquired twin babies that had been born in Nigeria and brought into Niger via Benin (*Jeune Afrique* 2014).

This tabloid-worthy story has only become more intriguing with time. Having allegedly participated in the pretense that his wife had given birth, Hama Amadou was faced with the prospect of DNA testing to establish whether he was, in fact, the father of the twins. Rather than be tested, which he claimed was contrary to Islam, he fled to France, leaving his wife still in detention pending a trial. This prompted a great deal of debate about whether DNA testing was contrary to Islam, whether it was in any case relevant in this instance, and what such testing might mean for establishing legitimacy more broadly. The possibility that the whole thing might be a conspiracy on the part of President Mohammadou Issoufou to discredit his main rival was also raised, generating its own flurry of debate.

It remains to be seen what the fate of the children will be. It is hard to tell from the coverage whether some of the birth mothers had been pregnant before they entered the "factory"; if so, they may have sought out the network in search of a better solution to an unwanted pregnancy than an illegal abortion, infanticide, or simply abandoning a baby. The network seems to be acting as a kind of fly-by-night adoption agency, whatever the biological and legal technicalities at issue.

Across the border in Burkina Faso, a pair of enterprising reporters interviewed an imam named Ismael Tiendregeogo for his thoughts on the matter. He pointed out that in Islam, the legitimacy of a woman's child is determined exclusively by the existence of a legal marriage. Biology, curiously, is irrelevant. Because doing a DNA test to establish paternity might undermine the sanctity of the private life of the married couple, it should not be used in this case. Muslims should never call into question the paternity of a child born in a legal marriage. It is important not to disrupt kinship ties; there is a *presumption* of paternity in favor of the child such that "every child born in a marriage has as father the husband of the mother" (Drabo and Toe 2014). This protective impulse within Islamic reasoning in the region obviously has some merit, long honored even when circumstances seem implausible through the notion of the "sleeping embryo" (B. Cooper 2010a).

However, for unmarried women, the resounding determination that DNA testing may establish *identity* but shouldn't be used to establish *paternity* in a legal sense is sobering (on the technical issues, see Shabana 2012). While Niger claims to be a secular state, Islamic legal reasoning has a grip on sexual and familial life. The state may occasionally pressure men to provide child support for illegitimate children, but it can't guarantee such children recognition in the context of descent and inheritance. As a result, men are rarely held accountable for the occasional difference between the ideal of the married male provider and the reality of unfettered masculine sexual prerogative outside of marriage.

Whatever the facts of the matter, the baby scandal highlights the ethical incoherence of reproductive life and paternity reckoning in Niger. On the one hand, bloodline is all—an adopted child cannot become equivalent to a biological child. On the other hand, biology is irrelevant—only the status of the marital relationship between a man and the woman giving birth is relevant. Men have great latitude in choosing sexual partners, seeking solutions to infertility, and opting to neglect or abandon their birth children. The situation for women is very different.

Hama Amadou returned to Niger in late 2015 to run as the candidate for the opposition coalition in the 2016 election, only to be arrested at the airport. The entanglement of this case with the election of 2016 has contributed to the confusion about how to understand the nature of the scandal. While awaiting trial, Amadou was given a medical release to return to France for unspecified treatment on March, 16, 2016, just a few days before the final round of the election, which was ultimately won by Mohammadou Issoufou. In the slow dénouement of the Baby Scandal, Amadou was sentenced *in absentia* to a year in prison on March 13, 2017 (Balima and McAllister 2017). In April 2018 he lost his appeal (Al Jazeera 2018). Meanwhile his wife, Hadiza Hama Amadou, whose name is rarely mentioned but who quietly endured the whole saga in Niger, completed her term in prison and was released on parole in December of 2017.

Notes

1. This is my colloquial translation of a portion of the title song in a collection by slammer Jhonel, popular in Niger today (Jhonel 2014). The title plays on the legal and domestic senses of *court* and *courtyard*.

2. The *soudure* is the hungry season prior to the harvest. The gloves from the market are emergency rations of a sort.

3. Dirkou (Agadez department) 27.90 percent in 1995; in Firji (Maradi department) 35 percent in 2000; and Komabangou (Tillabéry department) 50 percent in 2001. Consistent efforts under UNFPA, NGOs, and the PEPFAR initiative from 2008 have significantly improved the perception of the disease and the preventive options available.

4. Dominique Traoré also recorded Dendi, Bambara, and Hausa infusions intended to prevent wasting among infants, particularly on weaning, including a tea made from the leaves of the raidore or *cassia occidentalis* (1965, 511).

5. Gwarzo cites chapter 46 sura 15 of the Koran: "His mother bears him with hardship. And she brings him forth with hardship, and the bearing of him, and the weaning of him is thirty months" in the context of the acceptability of contraception, but the same sura could be used to argue for an obligation to nurse the baby, since this would not be to reduce progeny but to protect life (Gwarzo 2011, 150).

6. On insult songs in Zarma-Songhai culture, see Bornand (2005, 2012).

7. For a sensitive study of the implications of genetic testing and an awareness of sickle cell for immigrant women in France, see Bonnet (2009).

CONCLUSION

Traveling Companions and Entrustments in Contemporary Niger

NIGER'S EXTREMELY POOR MATERNAL AND INFANT HEALTH, ITS strikingly high population growth rate, and its tenaciously pronatal culture are neither natural nor inevitable; they have resulted from the peculiar position of Niger in the Sahel and within France's West African empire. I have attempted in this book to show how women's reproductive well-being has been consistently sidelined in favor of other priorities over the long twentieth century. The story begins immediately prior to the colonial period because so much depends on three critical changes introduced under French rule. The first was the slow and ambiguous decline of slavery, which shifted the burden of attracting wealth in people to biological reproduction in marriage. The collapse of the slave/free hierarchy also heightened the importance of shame to establishing social distinctions, for by definition those who have no shame are slaves. The second innovation was the introduction of a colonial medical culture focused on the military rather than the needs of women and children. Whereas in many other parts of Africa missions filled the vacuum in social services, in Niger the evangelical mission most engaged in the region did not take up reproductive health as a central concern. The final key change was the very rapid expansion of Islam as colonial institutions favored the legibility of Islamic religious culture over the myriad of indigenous political and cultural formations of the region.

My research was driven by a desire to understand a central paradox: Niger has an extremely high fertility rate, and yet at the same time it is the site of extraordinary anxiety about infertility. The history of childbirth in the region is also centrally a history of subfertility, both perceived and real. One of the women I interviewed in 1989 captured the deeper logic driving this concern to have children. She explained why her second marriage was better than her first, even though she did not choose her husband: "Well, there I was, I didn't want him, and they [her senior family members] said, 'Well we're doing it,' so there I was. And then *arziki* [prosperity, well-being] came! From the moment I gave birth, *arziki* entered [the marriage] you see? Back then, what did you need other than childbirth? That's where *arziki* is, real wealth, if you have a child, you have wealth, Safiya [my nickname]. Because one day that child will look after you" (Rigu, Maradi, October 11, 1989). The well-being derived from childbirth blessed her marriage and her life in a kind of virtuous cycle. In a context where there are precious few ways to invest, where the ecological, political, and economic environment is uncertain, investment in children makes enormous sense.

But producing children is also a kind of moral obligation to one's ancestors: humans come into the world burdened with a debt to their parents and grandparents. They have been entrusted with paying back that debt through childbirth; to fail to make good on that debt would be the ultimate source of shame. As the importance of successful childbearing has risen with the decline in slavery, the urgency to prove oneself fertile has also become acute. The emotional and existential experience of childbirth has gradually shifted; this book is in part a history of fear and shame. Marking social distinctions once slavery was no longer legal depended on performing the capacity to feel shame in highly gendered ways. Shame was at play in establishing the family standing of the freeborn and in insisting on the nonpersonhood of illegitimate children, particularly in patrilineal societies that practiced endogamy. The burden of both childbirth and sexual restraint fell most heavily on women. Fear of the shame brought to a family as a result of an illegitimate birth fed anxiety about the sexuality of young women. At the same time, the fear of the shame of failing to produce enough children compared to others fed demographic competition at multiple scales (between wives, between men, between ethnolinguistic and religious groups). These understandings of propriety and shame became entangled with perceptions about proper Muslim behavior during the rapid expansion of Islam under colonial rule.

I have also tried to piece together an account of how Niger came to have such an impoverished medical and educational infrastructure; this book is a history of absence. A leitmotif is the misfit between the ambitions of the French "civilizing mission" in West Africa and the number of personnel on the ground. Without sufficient personnel, the colonial administration could not even arrive at a credible count of the population under its control, much less promote population growth. Any investment in Niger had to come from the revenues derived from taxes. In an impecunious budget regime, there were simply never the funds to build a robust infrastructure (civil registry, rural extension, courts, schools, and most importantly medical facilities). Without schools, Niger couldn't produce graduates suited to medical school, so that what little medical infrastructure there was could not easily be staffed.

All these elements combined to produce the Niger that we see today. Girls are married when they reach puberty to shield them from the risks of the shame of pregnancy. Demographic competition takes on an Islamic allure as the period of conjugal abstinence after childbirth has fallen from two years to forty days. The infanticide practices that had eliminated babies that were regarded as asocial are now regarded as criminal, yet there is no solution to the problem of the babies themselves; they are still stigmatized as shameful and shameless nonpersons. Early marriage leads to early childbirth and rapid achievement of grand multipara status among women, both of which contribute to high maternal and infant mortality. Finally, the anxiety to produce children contributes to iatrogenic behaviors that aggravate the problem of infertility. The only way forward, I suggest, is to "talk about bastards." A society that focuses so much on shame can surely implicate men who marry off their daughters too young, impregnate unmarried women and abandon them, and punish children for the failings of others. Shame might also be assigned to older women who heap psychological abuse on their daughters-in-law, co-wives, and young daughters.

However, childbirth is above all a delight and a blessing; if I were to close this book without reweaving the themes in ways that capture the joyful anticipation of pregnancy and the beauty of childbirth in Niger, I would have done a terrible injustice to the complexity of the topic. Demographers have elaborated in ever more nuanced ways the elements that account for differences in fertility rates between different populations; these "proximate determinants of fertility" include many I have touched on in this book: age at first marriage, attitudes toward contraception, the length of postpartum infecundability (due to nursing, abstinence, or contraceptive use), the prevalence of induced abortion (or, in its absence, infanticide), the prevalence of miscarriage (or the popularity of emmenagogues), and rates of sterility as a result of scarring and sexually transmitted diseases. All these are important. However, there are also what I think of as the emotional determinants of fertility—"drivers" such as shame, fear, jealousy, and most importantly the pursuit of joy.

Most of my visits with women in Niger over many years have been full of laughter and pleasure; they were not by any means dismal, particularly if there was a baby to dandle, tickle, and tease. In the context of this book project, my interviews were also particularly pleasurable when I was able to speak at length with the *matrones*, whose pleasure in speaking about childbirth could be infectious. This came as a surprise to me, since these were the very women who had proven to be such a regular disappointment to the authors of the various archival documents on which I have relied: colonial medical officers, missionaries, and student interns. All these biomedical professionals expressed dismay that these older women could not reliably shoulder the immense and expensive burden of improving reproductive health in Niger.

It was not until I set aside my disappointment at the technical limitations of the traditional birth attendants of the region that it dawned on me that simply because I do not regard the burial of the placenta as a major event in the unfolding of a successful birth and a woman's future health does not mean that it is not a crucial part of childbirth for women and their families (Cooper forthcoming). The proper handling of the placenta continues to be a matter of great concern in much of West Africa, even among women who give birth in maternity wards. While the *sage-femme* will be called on to supervise the second stage of active labor and will return to check on the expulsion of the placenta, the *matrones* remain with the women, wash the baby, and most importantly, handle the placenta, which is washed, checked for integrity, and placed in a plastic bag to be turned over to the woman and her family.

What strikes me first of all about what I learned speaking to women in Niger about the placenta is the universality of its burial at home. Every woman of every ethnic background or religious persuasion I specifically asked had disposed of the placenta of each child through burial. Or, to be more precise, a handpicked older woman had buried it. When I pushed women who had recently given birth about how the placenta had been handled, they responded either in annoyance or embarrassment that they *themselves* had never done it; that is the work of older women who know how to do it properly. As I in turn coaxed more detail from such elderly informants, the beauty and resonance of these rituals began to emerge. Recall the lovely image of the axis-mundi recorded by Guy Nicolas in which the seed of the young bride's doum palm doll was buried in her new marital hut (G. Nicolas 1975, 256–57). The abundant doum palm tree provided the building material for the central pole of the hut; even in the absence of a "real" pole, the seed planted in the floor gave rise to a kind of potential central pole, an axis that would support her hut, her married life, and her ability to produce children.

In Hausa the word used to convey "birth" is *haifa*. The placenta is the *mahaifa*—the organ or site of birth. There is no easy way to distinguish the uterus from the placenta in Hausa—in effect, the placenta is conceived of as the womb. Accordingly, sometimes the word *mahaifa* is used to refer to the uterus, which complicates the issue of how to describe the placenta. If the placenta is the *site* of birth, then it must be in some sense *prior* to it. The afterbirth is at once the "second birth"—younger twin born after the older twin—and something much older, perhaps the spirit of someone who went before. The placenta seems to embody the entanglement of the human world and the world of those who have died and those who have not yet been born.

With the expansion of Islam, the practice has been reimagined as a form of human burial. Birthing practices and beliefs across Niger among sedentary populations today are broadly similar (Olivier de Sardan, Moumouni, and Souley 2001, 13). The careful handling of the placenta is typical; one reason may be that typically the birth is not announced until the placenta has been expelled—the danger is far from over until then. Aside from a breech birth, a retained placenta presents the greatest risk to the mother in the minds of most midwives. Accordingly, the placenta is anxiously anticipated and treated with great respect once it arrives. The following is a lengthy description of childbirth practices elicited from a Hausa woman in 2000:

> You take care of the placenta first, before washing the baby. When you have cut the umbilical cord, you wash the placenta, and you dig a hole for it. The hole should be as deep as the length of your forearm. We make a nest for it. If it's a boy, we make the hole to the north to the right. If it's a girl, it is on the left. We ask for a bit of a broken ceramic pot and some goat manure. After we've put in the placenta we place the pottery pieces on top and some goat manure, and then we close the hole. Then, someone waters it. If it's a boy you water it three times, for a girl four. Then we wash the baby, and we clean up the blood. We take a plastic teapot [used to wash before prayer] and we do the same ablutions to the baby as we would before praying. We make the call to prayer in its ear. And then we put it on the bed. Then we gather up the blood [from the sand on the floor] and there's a hole for it, we put the sand there. We do that with our hands, and we put water on the place and wash the floor. Then we cover it with fresh sand. Since the beginning of the world, that's how it's been done. (Olivier de Sardan, Moumouni, and Souley 2001, 15)

The modifications to practice here appear largely to concern the socialization of the infant into Islam. Placing pottery shards on top of the placenta rather than placing the placenta inside a pottery container echoes Muslim burial in which often a layer of wood or stones may be placed on top of the body to prevent direct contact between the body and the soil that will fill the grave. One of the beautiful expressions common among Muslims on learning of a death is "may the earth rest gently upon her." Intriguingly in such descriptions of a Muslim burial of sorts, the placement of seeds with the placenta continues to be a feature of the burial. Intrigued by the echoes of Muslim burial, I asked one elderly woman how Muslim scholars felt about this practice. She suggested that for the most part they see the burial of the placenta as a sign of respect and that sometimes a man might even say a prayer.

"Why would they agree to this?" I asked, puzzled by what appeared to me to be residues of a pre-Islamic practice in the ritual (such as the burial of cotton seeds with the placenta; cf. Last and Al-Hajj 1965). A classically Islamic answer might have been to explain that like fingernails or hair, the placenta is part of the mother and must be buried as a result. But that is not quite what she replied. "The placenta is like another person," she explained patiently, "you must treat it with respect. If you treat it badly, then later you will have trouble in your next childbirth." The principle of reciprocity, so prominent in social norms in Niger, applies to the relationship between the family and the placenta as well.

Hadiza Moussa argued that the concern to bury the placenta properly should be seen as a ritual of protection for the new mother. In effect, handling the "traveling companion" well is one way to prevent secondary infertility. The placenta should not be buried by a woman who has never had a child, who might somehow thereby communicate her own infertility, but by an older woman who has given birth. While a failure to bury the placenta properly is rarely offered to account for the infertility of anyone in particular, the perception that a woman can be rendered infertile if her placenta is "tied up" feeds fears of witchcraft: "The magic that attacks a person's fertility draws strength from a spirit of vengeance and a desire to thwart someone else. Vengeance may be sought by a co-wife, a jilted lover, an ex-spouse or a known or hidden competitor. The co-wife and jilted lover (or former spouse) carry in them a budding vengeance. To satisfy this vengeance he or she might 'tie up' the targeted woman's womb/placenta through magic charms" (Moussa 2012, 176–77). The association of thwarted fertility with a kind of malevolent "tying up" brings to mind an image of a closing off, a blockage of a flow—as if indeed the companion or baby could no longer traverse from one realm to another.

If the downside of all this is that a woman's fertility can be thwarted through malevolence by mishandling the placenta, the upside is that her fecundability can be regulated voluntarily as well. When I spoke to another elderly woman from the Zarma heartland about childbirth in her youth she explained that it used to be that a woman who had just given birth would take her own placenta and the attached umbilical cord before it was to be buried by the *matrone* and she would tie a number of knots in the cord, one for each year she wanted to rest before becoming pregnant again (Tsofuwa Ta Zarmaganda, Niamey, January 11, 2014). This account obviously reiterates the key theme of birth spacing I have emphasized, and it proves once again that women could be quite self-conscious about attempting to control their fertility in order to both protect the nursing infant and to preserve their own capacity to give birth subsequently. If there is a dark side to the belief that a womb can be "tied up" through maleficent occult practices, the brighter side is a sense that the placenta is a kind of mediator of birth whose comings and goings can be negotiated.

Interestingly, placenta burial practices have been adopted even by some highly educated coastal women who were not born in Niger. A woman whose family had arrived in Niger from Benin under colonial rule had herself become a reasonably successful white-collar worker, which was not quite typical of Hausa and Zarma women in Niamey. And yet, she too buried her placentas just like everyone else. "It's a nice practice" she remarked. "You put in seeds of all different kinds; that way you will have variety in your children, not just girls, not just boys."

Unlike other informants, she improvised by adding cowpeas to her seed repertoire. The logic of assemblage, of producing not simply multitudes of children but children with differing personalities and capacities, appears to be shared and ritually expressed today across all social barriers.

The earliest ethnographic references to planting seed with the placenta appear to me to be in Hausa contexts, where cotton was an important symbol of the threads that bind humans to one another and to the spirit world. However, as the practice has migrated, other seeds have entered in, predominantly grains. Only later was manure introduced. In some ways the contemporary practice, which has spread and been elaborated on among all ethnic groups in Niger, offers a lovely example of the profound intermingling of peoples, ideas, and practices of the region, the intercultural encounters or *brassage culturel* celebrated by Ousseina Alidou in her work *Engaging Modernity* (2005). If non-Muslim Hausa speakers brought with them a relatively recognizable burial practice, others appear to have elaborated on it, introducing (among other things) a shroud of sorts, the invocations proper to a Muslim burial, a multiplicity of kinds of seeds, and manure. There does not seem to be a single coherent and consistent set of beliefs at play other than an unarticulated sense that the spirit world, perhaps the world of ancestors as well, is the source of children. Somehow, the placenta mediates between these worlds and, if properly respected and wooed, it will guarantee a woman's success as a mother. But when pushed, women seem disinclined to overthink precisely how the placenta does the work of traveling companion or where it goes to get the child.

In his study of the illogic of neoliberal assumptions that mortgaging land is the best way to trigger development in Africa, Parker Shipton notes, "Patrimonial land is a sacred trust, or something like one—connecting the living with each other, with the dead and unborn, and with the places on the landscape where graves and buried placentas anchor their being" (Shipton 2009, 233). The most morally binding debts may be intergenerational, indeed transgenerational. These debts are a form of "entrustment." These are not necessarily reciprocal debts—you pay me, I pay you back. Rather, they are likely to be serial. These debts may be passed from one generation to the next, as "a favor expected to be passed on to someone else, and to keep moving" (17). Such debts mark the contours of social life: delayed marriage payments, the school fees of older children repaid by paying the fees of their younger siblings, the borrowing of animals to be repaid with the next generation of offspring, and the fostering of children across generations. In a sense, humans are born in debt and will pass debt to their children, who will pay it as they can and pass it along to theirs. That is what it is to be human.

The placenta could be thought of as the essential broker and embodiment of the most sacred of these entrustments—the transit between the permeable worlds of the living and dead through the permeable bodies of women. The family owes it to the placenta to treat it with respect. In an unarticulated intergenerational agreement, the unborn (perhaps spirits, perhaps ancestors) will be ushered into the world of the living through the mediation of the placenta as its "twin," "mother," "brother," or "traveling companion." The practice of burying the placenta will undoubtedly continue despite the reservations of a few Muslim scholars because of this sense of debt or entrustment. To fail to produce children is in a sense to die permanently oneself and to disappoint the trust of one's ancestors and in-laws. Without children, there will be no one to repay the debt with which each of us is born, and there will be no one who owes a debt to us in turn. Anything that threatens fertility threatens far more than an individual; the argument that reproductive concerns are private can be difficult to articulate in Niger. Being a human is fundamentally relational, not intrinsic to the individual. The beauty of the placenta burial ritual is the beauty of the cosmos—the intertwined worlds of the living and the dead, humans and plants, ancestors and infants. When a woman succeeds in producing another child, planting another placenta, she takes on some of the beauty of that anchored and yet mobile universe. This is a source of great joy and pride. Fertility is not simply an attribute of the individual; it is a blessing produced and sustained (God willing) by and for families, across generations and through the mediation between this world and that of ancestors or spirits and babies.

WORKS CITED

Published Texts

Abadie, Maurice. (1927) 2010. *La colonie du Niger*. Paris: L'Harmattan.

Abba, Aissa, Maria De Koninck, and Anne-Marie Hamelin. 2010. "Rehausser le taux d'allaitement maternel exclusif dans la communauté urbaine de Niamey, au Niger: Propositions des professionnels de la santé." *Global Health Promotion* 17 (2): 62–71.

Abdalla, Ismail Hussein. 1981. *Islamic Medicine and Its Influence on Traditional Hausa Practitioners in Northern Nigeria*. Madison: University of Wisconsin.

Abdou Assane, Zeinabou. 2017. "A la recherche d'une explication juridique de la gestation pour le compte d'autrui au Niger." *Revue CAMES sciences juridiques et politiques* 1: 155–71.

Ag Erless, Mohamed. 2010. *La grossesse et le suivi de l'accouchement chez les Touaregs Kel-Adagh (Kidal, Mali)*. Paris: L'Harmattan.

Alidou, Ousseina. 2005. *Engaging Modernity: Muslim Women and the Politics of Agency*. Madison: University of Wisconsin.

———. 2011. "Rethinking Marginality and Agency in Postcolonial Niger: A Social Biography of a Sufi Woman Scholar." In *Gender and Islam in Africa; Rights, Sexuality and Law*, edited by Margot Badran, 41–68. Stanford, CA: Stanford University Press.

Al Jazeera. 2018. "Former Niger PM Hama Amadou Loses Appeal in Baby Smuggling Case." April 12, 2018. Accessed December 17, 2018. https://www.aljazeera.com/news/2018/04/niger-pm-hama-amadou-loses-appeal-baby-smuggling-case-180412072554871.html.

Alpern, Stanley B. 2008. "Exotic Plants of Western Africa: Where They Came From and When." *History in Africa* 35: 63–102.

Andersen, Margaret Cook. 2015. *Regeneration through Empire: French Pronatalists and Colonial Settlement in the Third Republic*. Lincoln: University of Nebraska Press.

Appadurai, Arjun. 2006. *Fear of Small Numbers: An Essay in the Geography of Anger*. Durham, NC: Duke University Press.

Atighetchi, Dariusch. 1994. "The Position of Islamic Tradition on Contraception." *Medicine and Law* 13: 717–25.

Audouin-Dubreuil, Ariane. 2004. *La croisière noire: Sur la trace des explorateurs du XIXe siècle*. Paris: La Société de Géographie.

Azevedo, Mario. 2017. *Historical Perspectives on the State of Health and Health Systems in Africa*. Vol. 1. Basingstoke, UK: Palgrave Macmillan.

Bado, Jean-Paul. 2011. *Eugène Jamot 1879–1937: Le médecin de la maladie du sommeil ou trypanosomiase*. Paris: Karthala.

Baldus, Bernd. 1977. "Responses to Dependence in a Servile Group: The Machube of Northern Benin." In *Slavery in Africa: Historical and Anthropological Perspectives*, edited by Suzanne Miers and Igor Kopytoff, 435–60. Madison: University of Wisconsin Press.

Balima, Boureima, and Edward McAllister. 2017. "Niger Sentences Exiled Politician in Baby-Trafficking Case." Reuters, March 14. Accessed December 17, 2018. https://af.reuters.com/article/africaTech/idAFKBN16L0OP-OZATP.

Bargery, G. P. 1934. *A Hausa-English Dictionary and English-Hausa Vocabulary*. London: Oxford University Press. Available in a searchable online version at http://maguzawa.dyndns.ws/.

Barnes, Shailly. 2009. "Religion, Social Capital and Development in the Sahel: The Niass Tijaniyya in Niger." *Journal of International Affairs* 62 (2): 209–21.

Baroin, Catherine. 1985. *Anarchie et cohésion sociale chez les Toubou. Les Daza Késerda (Niger)*. Paris: Maison des Sciences de l'Homme.

Barona, Joseph L. 2010. *The Problem of Nutrition: Experimental Science, Public Health, and Economy in Europe, 1914–1945*. Brussels: P. I. E. Peter Lang.

Barot, Sneha, and Susan A. Cohen. 2015. "The Global Gag Rule and Fights over Funding UNFPA: The Issues that Won't Go Away." *Guttmacher Policy Review* 18 (2): 27–33.

Barreteau, Daniel. 1995. "La mort et la parole chez les Mofu-Gudur (Cameroun)." In *Death and Funeral Rites in the Lake Chad Basin*, edited by Catherine Baroin, Daniel Barreteau, and Charlotte von Graffenried, 243–71. Paris: ORSTOM.

Barry, Boubacar. 1998. *Senegambia and the Atlantic Slave Trade*. Cambridge: Cambridge University Press.

Barth, Heinrich. 1857. *Travels and Discoveries in North and Central Africa: Being a Journal of an Expedition Undertaken Under the Auspices of H. B. M.'s Government, in the Years 1849–1855*. 3 vols. New York: Harper and Brothers.

Barthélémy, Pascale. 2010. *Africaines et diplômées à l'époque coloniale (1918–1957)*. Rennes: Presses Universitaires de Rennes.

Basilico, Matthew, Jonathan Weigel, Anjali Motgi, Jacob Bor, and Salmaan Keshavjee. 2013. "Health for All? Competing Theories and Geopolitics." In *Reimagining Global Health: An Introduction*, edited by Paul Farmer, Jim Yong Kin, Arthur Kleinman, and Matthew Basilico, 74–110. Berkeley: University of California Press.

Belloncle, Guy. 1980. *Femmes et développement en Afrique sahélienne: L'expérience nigérienne d'animation féminine, 1966–1976*. Dakar: Nouvelles Éditions africaines.

Benefo, K. D. 1995. "The Determinants of the Duration of Postpartum Sexual Abstinence in West Africa: A Multilevel Analysis." *Demography* 32: 139–57.

Bennoune, Karima. 2005. "The International Covenant on Economic, Social and Cultural Rights as a Tool for Combating Discrimination Against Women: General Observations and a Case Study on Algeria." *International Social Science Journal* 184: 251–369.

Benoist, Joseph-Roger de. 1987. *Église et pouvoir colonial au Soudan français: Administrateurs et missionaires dans la Boucle du Niger (1885–1945)*. Paris: Karthala.

Bernus, Edmond. 1981. *Touaregs nigériens: Unité culturelle et diversité régionale d'un peuple pasteur*. Paris: ORSTOM.

Berry, Sara. 1992. "Hegemony on a Shoestring: Indirect Rule and Access to Agricultural Land." *Africa: Journal of the International Institute* 62 (3): 327–55.

Bertillon, Jacques, ed. 1900. *Commission international charge de réviser la nomenclature des causes de décès*. Paris: Chaix.

Bivens, Mary. 2007. *Telling Stories, Making Histories: Women, Words, and Islam in Nineteenth-Century Hausaland and the Sokoto Caliphate*. Portsmouth, NH: Heinemann.

Bledsoe, Caroline H. 2002. *Contingent Lives: Fertility, Time, and Aging in West Africa.* Chicago, IL: University of Chicago Press.

Boddy, Janice. 1989. *Wombs and Alien Spirits: Women, Men, and the Zar Cult in Northern Sudan.* Madison: University of Wisconsin Press.

Boltanski, Luc. 2013. *The Foetal Condition: A Sociology of Engendering and Abortion.* Translated by Catherine Porter. Cambridge: Polity.

Bongaarts, John, Odile Frank, and Rob Lesthaeghe. 1984. "The Proximate Determinants of Fertility in Sub-Saharan Africa." *Population and Development Review* 10 (3): 511–37.

Bonnecase, Vincent. 2011. *Pauvreté au Sahel: Du savoir colonial à la mesure international.* Paris: Karthala.

Bonnet, Doris. 2009. *Repenser l'hérédité.* Paris: Éditions des archives contemporaines.

Bonnet, Doris, and Véronique Duchesne, eds. 2016. *Procréation médicale et mondialisation: Expériences africaines.* Paris: L'Harmattan.

Bonnichon, Philippe de, Pierre Geny, and Jean Nemo. 2012. *Présences françaises d'outre-mer.* Paris: Karthala.

Bordat, Stephanie Willman, and Saida Kouzzi. 2009. *Legal Empowerment of Unwed Mothers: Experiences of Moroccan NGOs.* IDLO Legal Empowerment Working Paper No. 14. Accessed December 17, 2018. https://namati.org/resources/legal-empowerment-of -unwed-mothers-experiences-of-moroccan-ngos/.

Bornand, Sandra. 2005. "Insultes rituelles entre coépouses. Étude du marcanda (Zarma, Niger)." *Ethnographiques.org*, Numéro 7 (avril). Accessed August 2, 2016. http://www .ethnographiques.org/2005/Bornand.

———. 2012. "Voix de femmes songhay-zarma du Niger: Entre normes et transgressions." *Cahiers "Mondes anciens"* 3: 1–18. Accessed October 1, 2016. https://doi.org/10.4000 /mondesanciens.675.

———. 2017. "'La mort vaut mieux que la honte' ou le concept de hààwi chez les Zarma du Niger." In *Le langage de l'émotion: Variations linguistiques et culturelles*, edited by Pascal Boyeldieu and Nicole Tersis, 165–92. Leuven: Peeters.

Bousquet, G.-H. 1950. "L'Islam et la limitation volontaire des naissances." *Population* 5 (1): 121–28.

Boutrais, Jean. 1994. "Pour une nouvelle cartographie des Peuls." *Cahiers d'études africaines*, no. 133–35, 137–46.

Bouvenet, Gaston-Jean, and Paul Hutin. 1955. *Recueil annoté des textes de droit pénal (code pénal, lois, décrets, arrêtés généraux) applicables en Afrique Occidentale Française.* Paris: Éditions de l'Union française.

Boyd, Jean, and Beverly B. Mack. 1997. *Collected Works of Nana Asma'u, Daughter of Usman 'dan Fodiyo (1793–1864).* East Lansing: Michigan State University Press.

Bralić, I., H. Tahirović, D. Matanić, O. Vrdoljak, S. Stojanović-Spehar, V. Kovacić, and S. Blazeković-Milaković. 2012. "Association of Early Menarche Age and Overweight/ Obesity." *Journal of Pediatric Endocrinal Metabolism* 25 (1–2): 57–62.

Brett-Smith, Sarah C. 1982. "Symbolic Blood: Cloths for Excised Women." *RES: Anthropology and Aesthetics* 3 (Spring): 15–31.

———. 1983. "The Poisonous Child." *RES: Anthropology and Aesthetics* 6 (Autumn): 47–64.

———. 2014. *The Silence of the Women: Bamana Mud Cloths.* Milan: 5 Continents Editions.

Brock, J. F., and M. Autret. 1952. *Kwashiorkor in Africa.* Geneva: World Health Organization.

Brown, Lester, and Erik Eckhom. 1974. *By Bread Alone.* New York: Praeger.

Buekens, Pierre, Siân Curtis, and Silvia Alayón. 2003. "Demographic and Health Surveys: Caesarean Section Rates in Sub-Saharan Africa," *British Medical Journal* 326 (7381): 136.

Burns, Emily. 2014. "More than Clinical Waste? Placenta Rituals Among Australian Home-Birthing Women." *Journal of Perinatal Education* 23 (1): 41–49.

Burrill, Emily S. 2015. *States of Marriage: Gender, Justice and Rights in Colonial Mali.* Athens: Ohio University Press.

Burton, June K. 2007. *Napoleon and the Woman Question: Discourses of the Other Sex in French Education, Medicine and Medical Law.* Lubbock: Texas Tech University Press.

Cabut, Sandrine. 2006. "Niger: Un faux vaccin contre la méningite a tué 2500 personnes au Niger en 1995." *Quotidien*, January 28, 2006. http://www.liberation.fr/week-end /2006/01/28/un-marche-juteux-mais-dangereux_28069.

Cahn, Naomi. 2009. "Accidental Incest: Drawing the Line—or the Curtain?—For Reproductive Technology." *Harvard Journal of Law and Gender* 32: 59–107.

Caillié, René. 1830a. *Journal d'un voyage à Temboctou et à Jenné dans l'Afrique centrale: Précédé d'observations faites chez les Maures Braknas, les Nalous et d'autres peuples; avec une carte itinéraire et des remarques géographiques par M. Jomard.* 3 vols. Paris: Imprimerie Royale.

———. 1830b. *Travels through Central Africa to Timbuctoo: And Across the Great Desert, to Morocco, Performed in the Years 1824–28, with M. Jomard.* 2 vols. London: H. Colburn and R. Bentley.

Caldwell, John C. 1977. "Economic Rationality of High Fertility: An Investigation Illustrated with Nigerian Survey Data." *Population Studies* 31: 5–27.

———. 2005. "Sub-Saharan Africa." *Encyclopedia of Women and Islamic Cultures: Family, Body, Sexuality and Health* 3: 347–49.

Carde, Jules. 1927. *Instructions sur le fonctionnement de l'assistance médicale indigène, gouvernement général de l'Afrique Occidentale Française.* Gorée: Imprimerie du Gouvernement Général.

Carpenter, Kenneth. 2003a. "A Short History of Nutritional Science: Part 1 (1785–1885)." *Journal of Nutrition* 133: 638–45.

———. 2003b. "A Short History of Nutritional Science: Part 2 (1885–1912)." *Journal of Nutrition* 133: 975–84.

———. 2003c. "A Short History of Nutritional Science: Part 3 (1912–1944)." *Journal of Nutrition* 133: 638–45.

———. 2003d. "A Short History of Nutritional Science: Part 4 (1945–1985)." *Journal of Nutrition* 133: 3331–42.

Chamie, Joseph. 1988. "Les positions et politiques gouvernementales en matière de fécondité et de planification familiale." In *Population et sociétés en Afrique au sud du Sahara*, edited by Dominique Tabutin, 167–90. Paris: L'Harmattan.

Chen, Cecilia. 2004. "Rebellion against the Polio Vaccine in Nigeria: Implications for Humanitarian Policy." *African Health Sciences* 4 (3): 205–7.

Children and Youth in History. n.d. "Aqiqa, Islamic Birth Ritual [Religious Text]." Edited by Susan Douglass. Accessed October 14, 2017. http://chnm.gmu.edu/cyh/items/show/252.

Clark, Andrew F. 1999. "The Ties that Bind: Servility and Dependency among the Fulbe of Bundu (Senegambia) c. 1930s–1980s." In *Slavery and Colonial Rule in Africa*, edited by Suzanne Miers and Martin Klein, 91–108. London: Frank Cass.

Cleland, John, Stan Berstein, Alex Ezeh, Anibal Faundes, Anna Glasier, and Jolene Innis. 2006. "Family Planning: The Unfinished Agenda." *Lancet* 368 (9549): 1810–27.

Coale, Ansley, and E. M. Hoover. 1958. *Population Growth and Economic Development in Low-Income Countries: A Case Study of India's Prospects.* Princeton, NJ: Princeton University Press.

Coale, A. J., and S. Cotts Watkins. 1986. *The Decline of Fertility in Europe.* Princeton, NJ: Princeton University Press.

Cockburn, Robert, Paul N. Newton, E. Kyeremateng Agyarko, Dora Akunyili, and Nicholas J. White. 2005. "The Global Threat of Counterfeit Drugs: Why Industry and Governments Must Communicate the Dangers." *PLOS Medicine* 2 (4): 302–8.

Cole, Jonathan. 2012. "Engendering Health: Pronatalist Politics and the History of Nursing and Midwifery in Colonial Senegal, 1914–1967." In *Routledge Handbook on the Global History of Nursing,* edited by Patricia D'Antonio, Julie A. Fairman, and Jean C. Whelan, 114–30. New York: Routledge.

Collignon, René, and Charles Becker. 1989. *Santé et population en Sénégambie, des origines à 1960.* Paris: INED.

Colls, Rachel, and Maria Fannin. 2013. "Placental Surfaces and the Geographies of Bodily Interiors." *Environment and Planning A* (45): 1087–1104.

Comaroff, Jean, and John Comaroff. 1991. *Of Revelation and Revolution, Vol. 1: Christianity, Colonialism, and Consciousness in South Africa.* Chicago, IL: University of Chicago Press.

Comaroff, John, and Jean Comaroff. 1997. *Of Revelation and Revolution, Vol. 2: The Dialectics of Modernity on a South African Frontier.* Chicago, IL: University of Chicago Press.

Conklin, Alice L. 1997. *A Mission to Civilize: The Republican Idea of Empire in France and West Africa, 1895–1930.* Stanford, CA: Stanford University Press.

———. 2002. "*Faire Naître v. Faire du Noir*: Race Regeneration in France and French West Africa, 1895–1940." In *Promoting the Colonial Idea: Propaganda and Visions of Empire in France,* edited by Tony Chafer and Amanda Sakur, 143–55. Basingstoke, UK: Palgrave MacMillan.

Connelly, Matthew. 2008. *Fatal Misconception: The Struggle to Control World Population.* Cambridge, MA: Harvard University Press.

Cooper, Barbara M. 1994. "Reflections on Slavery, Seclusion, and Female Labor in the Maradi Region of Niger in the Nineteenth and Twentieth Centuries." *Journal of African History* 35 (1): 61–78.

———. 1995. "The Politics of Difference and Women's Associations in Niger: Of 'Prostitutes,' the Public, and Politics." *Signs* 20 (4): 851–82.

———. 1997. *Marriage in Maradi: Gender and Culture in a Hausa Society in Niger, 1900–1989.* Portsmouth, NH: Heinemann.

———. 2001. "The Strength in the Song: Muslim Personhood, Audible Capital, and Hausa Women's Performance of the Hajj." In *Gendered Modernities: Ethnographic Perspectives,* edited by Dorothy L. Hodgson, 79–104. New York: Palgrave.

———. 2003. "Anatomy of a Riot: The Social Imaginary, Single Women and Religious Violence in Niger." *Canadian Journal of African Studies* 37 (2–3): 467–512.

———. 2006. *Evangelical Christians in the Muslim Sahel.* Bloomington: Indiana University Press.

———. 2007. "La rhétorique de la 'mauvaise mère.'" In *Niger 2005: Une catastrophe si naturelle,* edited by Xavier Crombé and Jean-Hervé Jézéquel, 199–228. Paris: Karthala.

———. 2009. "Chronic Malnutrition and the Trope of the Bad Mother." In *A Not-So Natural Disaster: Niger '05*, edited by Xavier Crombé and Jean-Hervé Jézéquel, 147–68. London: Hurst.

———. 2010a. "Secular States, Muslim Law, and Islamic Religious Culture: Gender Implications of Legal Struggles in Hybrid Legal Systems in Contemporary West Africa." *Droits et Culture* 59 (1): 97–120.

———. 2010b. "Injudicious Intrusions: Chiefly Authority and Islamic Judicial Practice in Maradi, Niger." In *Muslim Family Law in Colonial and Postcolonial Africa*, edited by Richard Roberts, Shamil Jeppie, and Ebrahim Moosa, 183–218. Amsterdam: Amsterdam University Press.

———. 2010c. "Engendering a Hausa Vernacular Christian Practice." In *Being and Becoming Hausa: Interdisciplinary Perspectives*, edited by Anne Haour and Benedetta Rossi, 257–77. Leiden: Brill.

———. 2011. "The Implications of Reproductive Politics for Religious Competition in Niger." In *Christianity and Public Culture in Africa*, edited by Harri Englund, 89–108. Athens: Ohio University Press.

———. 2013. "De quoi la crise démographique au Sahel est-elle le nom?" *Politique Africaine* 2 (130):69–88.

———. 2015. "Representing Adolescent Sexuality in the Sahel." In *Writing through the Visual and Virtual: Inscribing Language, Literature, and Culture in Francophone Africa and the Caribbean*, edited by Renee Larrier and Ousseina Alidou, 113–23. New York: Lexington Books.

———. 2016. "The Gender of Nutrition in French West Africa: Military Medicine, Intra-Colonial Marginality and Ethnos Theory in the Making of Malnutrition in Niger." In *Health and Difference: Rendering Human Variation in Colonial Engagements*, edited by Alexandra Widmer and Veronika Lipphardt, 149–77. Oxford: Berghan.

———. 2018a. "Maternal Health in Niger and the Evangelical Imperative: The Life of a Missionary Nurse in the Post-war Era." In *Transforming Africa's Religious Landscapes: The Sudan Interior Mission, Past and Present*, edited by Tim Geysbeek and Shobana Shankar. Trenton, NJ: Africa World Press.

———. 2018b. "Sahil in West African History." In *Oxford Research Encyclopedia of African History*, edited by Thomas Spear. Oxford: Oxford University Press.

———. (in press). "Traveling Companions: The Burial of the Placenta in Niger." *African Studies Review*.

Cooper, Frederick. 1996. *Decolonization and African Society: The Labor Question in French and British Africa*. Cambridge: Cambridge University Press.

———. 2003. "Industrial Man Goes to Africa." In *Men and Masculinities in Modern Africa*, edited by Lisa A. Lindsay and Stephan F. Miescher, 128–37. Portsmouth, NH: Heinemann.

Cournot, M. Louis. 1885. *Répression de l'infanticide: Audience solennelle de rentrée de cour d'appel d'Angers du 16 Oct. 1885*. Angers: A. Dedouvres, Imprimeur de la cour d'appel.

Coutumiers juridiques de l'AOF. 1939. 3 vols. Publications du Comité d'études historiques et scientifiques de l'Afrique Occidentale Française. Paris: Librairie Larose.

Cross, Nigel, and Rhiannon Barker. 1993. *At the Desert's Edge: Oral Histories from the Sahel*. London: Panos.

Cusson, Maurice, Nabi Youla Doumbia, and Henry Yebouet. 2017. *Mille homicides en Afrique de l'Ouest: Burkina Faso, Côte d'Ivoire, Niger et Sénégal*. Montréal: Presses de l'Université de Montréal.

d'Alix, Andrée. 1914. *La Croix-Rouge Française: Le rôle patriotique des femmes*. Paris: Perrin et cie. *Nineteenth Century Collections Online*. Accessed September 2, 2017. http://tinyurl.galegroup.com.proxy.libraries.rutgers.edu/tinyurl/5AG2J9.

David, Philippe. 2007. *Niger en transition, 1960–1965: Souvenirs et rencontres*. Paris: L'Harmattan.

Davison, Jean. 1989. *Voices from Mutira: Lives of Rural Gikuyu Women*. Boulder, CO: Lynne Rienner.

Defo, Barthélémy Kuate. 2014. "Demographic, Epidemiological, and Health Transitions: Are They Relevant to Population Health Patterns in Africa?" *Global Health Action* S6 (7): 1–39.

Delafosse, Maurice. (1912) 1972. *Haut Sénégal-Niger*. 3 vols. Paris: Maisonneuve & Larose. Originally Paris: Larose.

Delafosse, Maurice, Docteur Poutrin, and Alexandre Le Roy. 1930. *Enquête coloniale dans l'Afrique française, occidentale et équatoriale, sur l'organisation de la famille indigène, les fiançailles, le mariage, avec une esquisse générale des langues de l'Afrique*. Paris: Protat frères.

Deutsche Welle. 2016. "Niger: Sleepwalking into Huge Population Growth." January 3, 2016. Accessed June 18, 2017. http://www.dw.com/en/niger-sleepwalking-into-huge-population-growth/a-19084486.

Diarra, Marthe, and Marie Monimart. 2009. "De-feminization of Agriculture in Southern Niger: A Link with the Crisis?" In *A Not-So Natural Disaster: Niger 2005*, edited by Xavier Crombé and Jean-Hervé Jézéquel, 125–46. London: Hurst.

Diarra, S. 1979. "Les stratégies spatiales des éleveurs-cultivateurs peul du Niger central agricole." In *Maîtrise de l'espace agraire et développement en Afrique tropicale: Logique paysanne et rationalité technique. Actes du Colloque de Ouagadougou, 4–8 décembre 1978*, edited by Paul Pelissier, 87–91. Paris: Office de la recherche scientifique et technique outre-mer.

Diouf, Cheikhou. 1998. "Une relecture du statut de l'enfant naturel dans le droit musulman." *Revue sénégalaise de sociologie* 2–3: 265–74.

Djibo, Hadiza. 2001. *La participation des femmes africaines à la vie politique: Les exemples du Sénégal et du Niger*. Paris: L'Harmattan.

Domergue-Cloarec, Danielle. 1997. "La prévention dans la politique sanitaire de l'AOF." In *AOF: Réalités et héritages* Tome 2, edited by Charles Becker et al., 1228–39. Dakar: Direction des Archives du Sénégal.

Drabo, Colette, and Romial Toe. 2014. "Imam Ismael Tiendrebeogo à propos du test ADN en Islam: 'Dans le cadre d'une enquête policière, il n'y a aucun problème.'" *Le Pays (Burkina Faso)*, September 11, reposted to *Tamtaminfo*. Accessed August 4, 2016. http://www.tamtaminfo.com/imam-ismael-tiendrebeogo-a-propos-du-test-adn-en-islam-dans-le-cadre-dune-enquete-policiere-il-ny-a-aucun-probleme/#comments.

Dupire, Marguerite. 1962. *Peuls nomades. Étude descriptive des Wodaabe du Sahel nigérien*. Paris: Institut d'Ethnologie.

———. 1970. *Organisation sociale des Peul: Étude d'ethnographie comparée*. Paris: Plon.

Echard, Nicole. 1978. "La pratique religieuse des femmes dans une société d'hommes: Les Hausa du Niger." *Revue française de sociologie* 19: 551–62.

Echenberg, Myron. 1991. *Colonial Conscripts: The Tirailleurs Sénégalais in French West Africa, 1857–1960*. Portsmouth, NH: Heinemann.

Engels, Fredrick. (1884) 1909. *Origin of the Family, Private Property, and the State*. Translated by Ernest Untermann. Chicago, IL: Charles H. Kerr.

Eustace, Nicole, Eugenia Lean, Julie Livingston, Jan Plamper, William M. Reddy, and Barbara H. Rosenwein. 2012. "'AHR' Conversation: The Historical Study of Emotions." *The American Historical Review* 117 (5):1486–1531.

Fadlalla, Amal Hassan. 2007. *Embodying Honor: Fertility, Foreignness, and Regeneration in Eastern Sudan*. Madison: University of Wisconsin Press.

Fairhead, James, and Melissa Leach. 1996. *Misreading the African Landscape: Society and Ecology in a Forest-Savanna Mosaic*. Cambridge: Cambridge University Press.

Fairhead, James, Melissa Leach, and Mary Small. 2004. "Childhood Vaccination and Society in the Gambia: Public Engagement with Science and Delivery." Working Paper 218. Brighton: Institute for Development Studies.

Fargues, Philippe, and Ouaïdou Nassour. 1998. *Douze ans de mortalité urbaine au Sahel: Niveaux, tendances, saisons et causes de mortalité à Bamako 1974–1985*. Paris: INED.

Faulkingham, Ralph Harold. 1975. *The Spirits and Their Cousins: Some Aspects of Belief, Ritual, and Social Organization in a Rural Hausa Village in Niger*. Research report no. 15. Amherst: Department of Anthropology, University of Massachusetts.

Febvre, Lucien. 1973. "Sensibility and History: How to Reconstitute the Emotional Life of the Past." In *A New Kind of History*, edited by Peter Burke, 12–26. London: Harper Row.

Feldman-Savelsberg, Pamela. 1999. *Plundered Kitchens, Empty Wombs: Threatened Reproduction and Identity in the Cameroon Grassfields*. Ann Arbor: University of Michigan Press.

Foley, Ellen. 2010. *Your Pocket Is What Cures You: The Politics of Health in Senegal*. New Brunswick, NJ: Rutgers University Press.

Fordyce, Lauren, and Aminata Maraesa. 2012. *Risk, Reproduction, and Narratives of Experience*. Nashville, TN: Vanderbilt.

Fortier, Corinne. 2001. "Le lait, le sperme, le dos. Et le sang? Représentations physiologiques de la filiation et de la parente de lait en Islam Malékite et dans la société Maure," *Cahiers d'études africaines* 1 (161): 97–138.

Fuglestad, Finn. 1983. *A History of Niger, 1850–1960*. Cambridge: Cambridge University Press.

Gado, Boureima Alpha. 1993. *Une histoire des famines au Sahel: Études des grandes crises alimentaires (XIXe-XXe siècles)*. Paris: L'Harmattan.

Galy Kadir, Abdelkader. 2004. *Slavery in Niger: Historical, Legal and Contemporary Perspectives*. Niamey: Anti-Slavery International and Association Timidria.

Garba, M., M. Nayama, A. P. Alio, M .L. Holloway, B. S. Hamisu, and H. M. Salihu. 2011. "Maternal Mortality in Niger: A Retrospective Study in a High Risk Maternity," *African Journal of Medicine and Medical Science* 40 (4): 393–397.

Garnier, D., K. B. Simondon, and E. Benefice. 2005. "Longitudinal Estimates of Puberty Timing in Senegalese Adolescent Girls." *American Journal of Human Biology* 17 (6): 718–20.

Gauban, Octave. 1905. "De l'infanticide." PhD diss., l'Université de Bordeaux. Bordeaux: Imprimerie y Cadoret.

Geronimus, A. 1994. "The Weathering Hypothesis and the Health of African-American Woman and Infants: Implications for Reproductive Strategies and Policy Analysis." In *Power and Decision: The Social Control of Reproduction*, edited by G. Sen and R. C. Snow, 77–100. Cambridge, MA: Harvard University Press.

Gervais, Raymond R. 1997. "État colonial et savoir démographique en AOF." In *AOF: Réalités et héritages* 2, edited by Charles Becker, 961–80. Dakar: Direction des Archives du Sénégal.

Greenberg, Joseph. 1946. *The Influence of Islam on a Sudanese Religion*. Seattle: University of Washington Press.

Greene, Jeremy, Marguerite Thorp Basilico, Heidi Kim, and Paul Farmer. 2013. "Colonial Medicine and Its Legacies." In *Reimagining Global Health: An Introduction*, edited by Paul Farmer, Jim Yong Kin, Arthur Kleinman, and Matthew Basilico, 33–73. Berkeley: University of California Press.

Greenhalgh, Susan, ed. 1995. *Situating Fertility: Anthropology and Demographic Inquiry*. Cambridge: Cambridge University Press.

Grodos, Daniel. 2008. *Niamey Post: Lettres du Niger 2001-2004*. Paris: L'Harmattan.

Guillermet, Élise. 2009. "Droit Islamique et pratiques sociales, la question de l'orphelin: Étude de cas à Zinder au Niger." *Afrique contemporaine* 3 (231): 171–85.

Guyer, Jane I., and Samuel M. Eno Belinga. 1995. "Wealth in People as Wealth in Knowledge: Accumulation and Composition in Equatorial Africa." *Journal of African History* 36 (1): 91–120.

Gwarzo, Tahir Haliru. 2011. "Islamic Religious Leaders and Family Planning in Northern Nigeria: A Case Study of Zamfara, Sokoto and Niger States." *Journal of Muslim Minority Affairs* 31 (1): 143–51.

Haardt, Georges-Marie, and Louis Audouin-Dubreuil. 1924. *Across the Sahara by Motor Car from Touggout to Timbuctoo*. Translated by E. E. Fournier d'Albe. New York: D. Appleton.

———. 1927a. *La croisière noire*. Paris: Plon.

———. 1927b. *The Black Journey; Across Central Africa with the Citroen Expedition*. New York: Cosmopolitan Book Corporation.

Hall, Bruce S. 2011. *A History of Race in Muslim West Africa, 1600–1960*. Cambridge: Cambridge University Press.

Hartmann, Betsy, Banu Subramaniam, and Charles Zerner. 2005. *Making Threats: Biofears and Environmental Anxieties*. New York: Rowman and Littlefield.

Hashemi, Kamran. 2007. "Religious Legal Traditions, Muslim States and the Convention on the Rights of the Child: An Essay on the Relevant UN Documentation." *Human Rights Quarterly* 29: 194–227.

Haute Commissariat de l'Afrique Française. 1941. La Justice Indigène en Afrique Occidentale Française. Décret du 11 février 1941, instituant un code pénal indigène pour l'Afrique Occidentale Française; décret du 3 décembre 1931, réorganisant la Justice Indigène en Afrique Occidental Française avec les modifications intervenues jusqu'au décret inclus du 11 février 1941. Rufisque: Imprimerie du Haute Commissariat.

Heller, Alison. 2014. "Bedside Manner and the Invisible Patient: The Silence Surrounding Women's Gynaecological Health in Niger." *Anthropology Today* 30 (1): 20–23.

———. 2019. *Fistula Politics: Birthing Injuries and the Quest for Continence in Niger*. New Brunswick, NJ: Rutgers University Press.

Heller, Alison, and Anita Hannig. 2017. "Unsettling the Fistula Narrative: Cultural Pathology, Biomedical Redemption, and Inequities of Health Access in Niger and Ethiopia." *Anthropology and Medicine* 24 (1): 81–95.

Heward, Christine. 1999. "Introduction: The New Discourses of Gender, Education and Development." In *Gender, Education & Development: Beyond Access to Empowerment*, edited by Christine Heward and Sheila Bunwaree, 1–14. London: Zed Books.

Hill, Polly. 1977. *Population, Prosperity, and Poverty: Rural Kano, 1900–1970*. New York: Cambridge University Press.

Hiskett, Mervyn. (1973) 1994. *The Sword of Truth: The Life and Times of the Shehu Usman dan Fodio*. Evanston, IL: Northwestern University Press.

Hörbst, Viola. 2010. "Assisted Reproductive Technologies in Mali and Togo: Circulating Knowledge, Mobile Technology, Transnational Efforts." In *Medicine, Mobility, and Power in Global Africa: Transnational Health and Healing*, edited by Hansjörg Dilger, Abdoulaye Kane, and Stacey A. Langwick, 163–189. Bloomington: Indiana University Press.

Hunt, Nancy Rose. 1988. "'Le Bébé en Brousse': European Women, African Birth Spacing and Colonial Intervention in Breast Feeding in the Belgian Congo." *International Journal of African Historical Studies* 21 (3): 401–32.

———. 1999. *A Colonial Lexicon of Birth Ritual, Medicalization, and Mobility in the Congo*. Durham, NC: Duke University Press.

Hunwick, John. 1993. "Not Yet the Kano Chronicle: Kings Lists with and without Narrative Elaboration from Nineteenth Century Kano." *Sudanic Africa* 4: 95–130.

———. 2000. "Aḥmad Bābā on Slavery." *Sudanic Africa* 11: 131–139.

Hunwick, John, and Eve Troutt Powell. 2002. *The African Diaspora in the Mediterranean Lands of Islam*. Princeton, NJ: Markus Wiener.

Idrissa, Abdourahmane, and Samuel Decalo. 2012. *Historical Dictionary of Niger*, 4th ed. Lanham, MD: Scarecrow.

Iliffe, John. 1995. *Africans: The History of a Continent*. Cambridge: Cambridge University Press.

———. 2005. *Honour in African History*. Cambridge: Cambridge University Press.

Inhorn, Marcia. 1994. *Quest for Conception: Gender, Infertility, and Egyptian Medical Traditions*. Philadelphia: University of Pennsylvania Press.

———. 2002. "The 'Local' Confronts the 'Global': Infertile Bodies and New Reproductive Technologies in Egypt." In *Infertility around the Globe*, edited by Marcia C. Inhorn and Frank van Balen, 263–82. Berkeley: University of California Press.

———. 2003. "Global Infertility and the Globalization of New Reproductive Technologies: Illustrations from Egypt." *Social Science and Medicine* 56: 1837–51.

Institut National de la Statistique (INS). 1999. *Enquête démographique et de santé et à indicateurs multiples du Niger, 1998*. Calverton, MD: Macro International.

Institut National de la Statistique (INS) and ICF International. 2013. *Enquête démographique et de santé et à indicateurs multiples du Niger 2012: Rapport de synthèse*. Calverton, MD: INS and ICF International.

———. 2014. *Erratum*. Correction to INS 2013. Table 7.6: Taux de fécondité desirée. Released December 2, 2014. Calverton, MD: INS and ICF International.

Institut National de la Statistique (INS) and Macro International Inc. 2007. *Enquête démographique et de santé et à indicateurs multiples du Niger 2006*. Demographic and health surveys. Calverton, MD: INS and Macro International.

Institut National de la Statistique et des Études Économiques (INSEE). 1948. *Annuaire statistique des territoires d'outre-mer*. Paris: Imprimerie nationale.

Issaka Maga, H., and J. P. Guengant. 2017. "Countries with Very Slow or Incipient Fertility Transition." In *Africa's Population: In Search of a Demographic Dividend*, edited by Hans Groth and John F. May, 146–64. Heidelberg: Springer.

Issoufou, Mahamadou. 2015. "Address to the African Development Conference." *Transition* 118: 1–2. Accessed June 19, 2017. http://www.jstor.org/stable/10.2979/transition.118.1.

Jaffré, Yannick, and J-P. Olivier de Sardan. 2003. *Une médicine inhospitalière: Les difficiles relations entre soignants et soignés dans cinq capitales d'Afrique de l'Ouest*. Paris: Karthala.

Jaffré, Yannick, Yveline Diallo, Patricia Vasseur, and Chrystelle Grenier-Torres. 2009. *La bataille des femmes: Analyse anthropologique de la mortalité maternelle dans quelques services d'obstétrique d'Afrique de l'Ouest*. Arles: Éditions Faustroll.

Janzen, John, and William Arkinstall. (1978) 1982. *The Quest for Therapy: Medical Pluralism in Lower Zaire*. Berkeley: University of California Press.

Jeune Afrique. 2014. "'Usines à bébés': Une vingtaine de personnes arrêtées au Niger." June 26. Accessed August 3, 2016. https://www.jeuneafrique.com/51571.

Jhonel. 2014. *Niamey, cour commune: Slam*. Paris: L'Harmattan.

Johnson-Hanks, Jennifer. 2006a. *Uncertain Honor: Modern Motherhood in an African Crisis*. Chicago, IL: University of Chicago Press.

———. 2006b. "On the Politics and Practice of Muslim Fertility: Comparative Evidence from West Africa." *Medical Anthropology Quarterly* 20 (1): 12–30.

Joint Institute for the Study of the Atmosphere and Ocean (JISAO). 2016. "Sahel Precipitation Index (20-10N, 20W-10E), 1900–November 2016." Accessed March 18, 2017. https://doi.org/doi:10.6069/H5MW2F2Q.

Jones, L. L., P. L. Griffiths, S. A. Norris, J. M. Pettifor, and N. Cameron. 2009. "Age at Menarche and the Evidence for a Positive Secular Trend in Urban South Africa." *American Journal of Human Biology* 21 (1): 130–32.

Juompan-Yakam, Clarisse. 2014. "Niger, Benin, Nigeria . . . : Usines à bébés, le trafic de la honte." *Jeune Afrique*, July 28, 2014. Accessed June 18, 2017. http://www.jeuneafrique.com/47941.

Kaler, Amy. 2003. *Running After Pills: Politics, Gender, and Contraception in Colonial Zimbabwe*. Portsmouth, NH: Heinemann.

Kang, Alice J. 2015. *Bargaining for Women's Rights: Activism in an Aspiring Muslim Democracy*. Minneapolis: University of Minnesota Press.

Kanya-Forstner, Alexander Sydney. 1969. *The Conquest of the Western Sudan: A Study in French Military Imperialism*. Cambridge: Cambridge University Press.

Keenan, J. D., R. L. Bailey, S. K. West, A. M. Arzika, J. Hart, J. Weaver, K. Kalua, et al. 2018. "Azithromycin to Reduce Childbood Mortality in Sub-Saharan Africa." *New England Journal of Medicine* 378 (17): 1583–92.

Kéita, Aoua. 1975. *Femme d'Afrique: La vie d'Aoua Kéita racontée par elle-même*. Paris: Presénce Africaine.

Kelley, Thomas. 2008. "Unintended Consequences of Legal Westernization in Niger: Harming Contemporary Slaves by Reconceptualizing Property." *American Journal of Comparative Law* 56 (4): 999–1038.

Kimbà, Idrissa A. 1993. "L'impôt de capitation: Les abus du régime de surtaxation et la résistance des populations." *African Economic History* 21: 97–111.

King, Noel, ed. 1995. *Ibn Battuta in Black Africa*. Translated by Said Hamdun. Princeton, NJ: Markus Wiener.

Kirk, Dudley. 1996. "Demographic Transition Theory." *Population Studies* 50: 361–87.

Klausen, Susanne. 2015. *Abortion under Apartheid: Nationalism, Sexuality and Women's Reproductive Rights in South Africa*. New York: Oxford University Press.

Klein, Martin A. 1998. *Slavery and Colonial Rule in French West Africa*. Cambridge: Cambridge University Press.

———. 2005. "The Concept of Honour and the Persistence of Servility in the Western Soudan." *Cahiers d'études africaines* 45 (179–180): 831–51.

Labouret, H. 1933. "L'Alimentation des indigènes en Afrique Occidentale Française." In *L'Alimentation indigène dans les colonies françaises, protectorats et territoires sous mandat*, edited by G. Hardy and C. Richet, 138–54. Paris: Vigot Frères.

Lachenal, Guillaume. 2013. "Médecine, comparaisons et échanges inter-impériaux dans le mandat camerounais: Une histoire croisée franco-allemande de la mission Jamot." *Canadian Bulletin of Medical History* 30 (2): 23–45.

Lancy, David. 2015. *The Anthropology of Childbood: Cherubs, Chattel, Changelings*. 2nd ed. Cambridge: Cambridge University Press.

Landau, Paul. 1995. *The Realm of the Word*. Portsmouth, NH: Heinemann.

Last, D. M., and M. A. Al-Hajj. 1965. "Attempts at Defining a Muslim in Nineteenth-Century Hausaland and Bornu." *Journal of the Historical Society of Nigeria* 3 (2): 231–40.

Last, Murray. 1967. *The Sokoto Caliphate*. London: Longmans, Green.

———. 1976. "The Presentation of Sickness in a Community of Non-Muslim Hausa." In *Social Anthropology and Medicine*, edited by J. B. Loudon, 104–49. London: Academic Press.

———. 1980. "Historical Metaphors in the Kano Chronicle." *History in Africa* 7: 161–78.

———. 1991. "Spirit Possession as Therapy: Bori among Non-Muslims in Nigeria." In *Women's Medicine: The Zar-Bori Cult in Africa and Beyond*, edited by I. M. Lewis, 49–63. Edinburgh: Edinburgh University Press.

———. 1993. "History as Religion: De-constructing the Magians 'Maguzawa' of Nigerian Hausaland." In *L'invention religieuse en Afrique: Histoire et religion en Afrique noire*, edited by Jean-Pierre Chrétien, Claude-Helene Perrot, Gérard Prunier, and Françoise Raison-Jourde, 267–96. Paris: Karthala.

———. 2004. "Hausa." In *Encyclopedia of Medical Anthropology: Health and Illness in the World's Cultures*, Vol. 2, edited by C. Ember and M. Ember, 718–29. New York: Klewer Academic.

Lawrance, Benamin, and Richard Roberts. 2012. *Trafficking in Slavery's Wake: Law and the Experience of Women and Children*. Athens: Ohio University Press.

Leach, Melissa, and James Fairhead. 2007. *Vaccine Anxieties: Global Science, Child Health and Society*. New York: Earthscan.

Lefebvre, Camille. 2011. "Science et frontière en équation: Le terrain de la Mission Tilho entre Niger et Tchad (1906–1909)." In *Territoires impériaux: Une histoire spatiale du fait colonial*, edited by Hélène Blais, Florence Deprest, and Pierre Singaravélou, 109–38. Paris: Sorbonne.

———. 2015. *Frontières de sable, frontières de papier*. Paris: Sorbonne.

Leroux, Henri. 1948. "Animisme et Islam dans la subdivision de Maradi (Niger)." *Bulletin de l'IFAN* 10. PhD diss., University of Paris. Dakar: IFAN.

Levtzion, Nehemia, and Randall L. Pouwels. 2000. "Introduction: Patterns of Islamization and Varieties of Religious Experience among Muslims of Africa." In *The History of*

Islam in Africa, edited by Nehemia Levtzion and Randall L. Pouwels, 1–18. Athens: Ohio University Press.

Lewis, I. M. 1971. *Ecstatic Religion*. London: Penguin.

Livingston, Julie. 2003. "Pregnant Children and Half-Dead Adults: Modern Living and the Quickening Life Cycle in Botswana." *Bulletin of the History of Medicine* 77 (1): 133–62.

———. 2008. "Disgust, Bodily Aesthetics and the Ethic of Being Human in Botswana." *Africa* 78 (2): 288–307.

———. 2012. *Improvising Medicine: An African Oncology Ward in an Emerging Cancer Epidemic*. Durham, NC: Duke University Press.

Locoh, Thérèse, and Yara Makdessi. 1996. "Politique de population et baisse de la fécondité en Afrique Sub-Saharienne." *Les dossiers du CEPED* 44. Paris: CEPED.

Loftsdóttir, Kristín. 2007. "Bounded and Multiple Identities." *Cahiers d'études africaines* 185: 65–92.

Lovejoy, Paul E. 1978. "Plantations in the Economy of the Sokoto Caliphate." *Journal of African History* 19 (3): 341–68.

———. 2011. *Transformations in Slavery: A History of Slavery in Africa*. Cambridge: Cambridge University Press.

Lovejoy, Paul E., and Stephen Baier. 1975. "The Desert-Side Economy of the Central Sudan." *International Journal of African Historical Studies* 8 (4): 551–81.

Lovejoy, Paul, and Jan S. Hogendorn. 1993. *Slow Death for Slavery: The Course of Abolition in Northern Nigeria, 1897–1936*. Cambridge: Cambridge University Press.

Luneau, René. (1981) 2010. *Chants de femmes au Mali*. Paris: Karthala.

Lunn, Joe. 1999. "'Les Races Guerrières': Racial Preconceptions in the French Military about West African Soldiers during the First World War." *Journal of Contemporary History* 34 (4): 517–36.

Luxereau, Anne. 1984. *Rapport d'enquête sur les systèmes thérapeutiques traditionnels existant à Maradi*. Bordeaux: Groupe de Recherche Interdisciplinaire pour le Développement.

———. 1991. *Croissance urbaine et santé à Maradi (Niger): Préserver sa santé: Représentations de la personne en santé, de la maladie, des recours thérapeutiques*. Bordeaux: Groupe de Recherche Interdisciplinaire pour le Développement.

Lydon, Ghislaine. 1997. "The Unraveling of a Neglected Source: Women in Francophone West Africa in the 1930s." *Cahiers d'études africaines* 147 (37): 555–84.

Lyons, Marynez. 1992. *The Colonial Disease: A Social History of Sleeping Sickness in Northern Zaire, 1900–1940*. New York: Cambridge University Press.

Mahmood, Saba. 2005. *Politics of Piety: The Islamic Revival and the Feminist Subject*. Princeton, NJ: Princeton University Press.

Malik, ibn Anas. n.d. "Aqiqa, Islamic Birth Ritual [Al-Muwatta Hadith 26:7]." In *Children and Youth in History*, annotated by Susan Douglass. Accessed May 26, 2015. https://chnm.gmu.edu/cyh/primary-sources/252.

Malthus, Thomas. 1798. *An Essay on the Principle of Population, as It Affects the Future Improvement of Society with Remarks on the Speculations of Mr. Godwin, M. Condorcet, and Other Writers*. London: St. Paul's Church-Yard.

Maman, Ali. 2014. "Journée mondiale de lutte contre la drépanocytose/Message du ministre de la Santé publique : 'L'accès aux soins permanents de qualité pour chaque drépanocytaire' thème retenu." *Le Sahel* June 19. Accessed December 14, 2018. https://www.nigerdiaspora.net/index.php/politique-archives/item/67455.

Manchuelle, François. 1989. "Slavery, Emancipation and Labour Migration in West Africa: The Case of the Soninke." *Journal of African History* 30 (1): 89–106.

———. 1997. *Willing Migrants: Soninke Labor Diasporas, 1848–1960*. Athens: Ohio University Press.

Mangin, Charles. 1910. *La force noire*. Paris: Hachette.

Mangin, Gilbert. 1997. "Les institutions judiciaires de l'AOF." In *AOF: Realites et heritages*, edited by Charles Becker, Saliou Mbaye, and Ibrahima Thioub, 139–52. Dakar: Direction des Archives du Sénégal.

Mann, Gregory. 2009. "What Was the *Indigénat*?: The 'Empire of Law' in French West Africa." *Journal of African History* 50: 331–53.

Mann, Kristin, and Richard Roberts. 1991. *Law in Colonial Africa*. Portsmouth, NH: Heinemann.

Masquelier, Adeline. 1995. "Consumption, Prostitution, and Reproduction: The Poetics of Sweetness in 'Bori.'" *American Ethnologist* 22 (4): 883–906.

———. 2001a. "Behind the Dispensary's Prosperous Facade: Imagining the State in Rural Niger." *Public Culture* 13 (2): 267–91.

———. 2001b. *Prayer Has Spoiled Everything: Possession, Power and Identity in an Islamic Town of Niger*. Durhamm, NC: Duke University Press.

———. 2008. "When Spirits Start Veiling: The Case of the Veiled She-Devil in a Muslim Town of Niger." *Africa Today* 54 (3): 39–64.

———. 2009. *Women and Islamic Revival in a West African Town*. Bloomington: Indiana University Press.

———. 2012. "Public Health or Public Threat? Polio Eradication Campaigns, Islamic Revival, and the Materialization of State Power in Niger." In *Medicine, Mobility, and Power in Global Africa*, edited by Hansjörg Dilger, Abdoulaye Kane, and Stacey A. Langwick, 213–40. Bloomington: Indiana University Press.

Meillassoux, Claude. 1991. *The Anthropology of Slavery: The Womb of Iron and Gold*. Chicago, IL: University of Chicago Press.

Miers, Suzanne, and Richard Roberts. 1988. *The End of Slavery in Africa*. Madison: University of Wisconsin Press.

Moore, Henrietta. 1988. *Feminism and Anthropology*. Cambridge: Polity.

Moore, Henrietta, and Meghan Vaughan. 1994. *Cutting Down Trees: Gender, Nutrition, and Agricultural Change in the Northern Province of Zambia, 1890–1990*. Portsmouth, NH: Heinemann.

Moumouni, A. 2000. "Conceptions et pratiques de l'avortement en pays Songhay-Zarma." *Reseau anthropologie de la santé en Afrique* 1 (April): 104–9.

Mounkaila, Fatimata. 2008. *Anthologie de la littérature orale Songhay-Zarma: Tome 2 Chants d'intégration sociale*. Paris: L'Harmattan.

Moussa, Hadiza. 2012. *Entre absence et refus d'enfant: Socio-anthropologie de la gestion de la fécondité féminine à Niamey, Niger*. Paris: L'Harmattan.

Musallam, B. F. 1983. *Sex and Society in Islam*. Cambridge: Cambridge University Press.

Nast, Heidi. 2005. *Concubines and Power: Five Hundred Years in a Northern Nigerian Palace*. Minneapolis: University of Minnesota Press.

Ndao, Mor. 2008. "Colonisation et politique de santé maternelle et infantile au Sénégal (1905–1960)." *French Colonial History* 9: 191–211.

Nguyen, Thuy Linh. 2016. *Childbirth, Maternity, and Medical Pluralism in French Colonial Vietnam, 1880–1945*. Rochester, NY: Rochester University Press.

Nicolas, Guy. 1975. *Dynamique sociale et appréhension du monde au sein d'une société Hausa.* Paris: Institut d'Ethnologie.

Nicolas, Jacqueline. 1967. *Les juments des dieux: Rites de possession et condition féminine en pays Hausa (Valle de Maradi, Niger).* Niamey: IFAN.

Nisbett, Nicolas, Mara van den Bold, Stuart Fillespie, Purnima Menon, Peter Davis, Terry Roopnaraine, Halie Kampman, Neha Kohli, Akriti Singh, and Andrea Warren. 2017. "Community-Level Perceptions of Drivers of Change in Nutrition: Evidence from South Asia and sub-Saharan Africa." *Global Food Security* 13: 74–82.

Nogue, Madame Maurice. 1923. "Les sages-femmes auxiliaires de l'Afrique Occidentale Française." *Bulletin de la Comité des Études Historiques et Scientifiques de l'AOF* 1: 429–70.

Notestein, F. W. 1945. "Population: The Long View." In *Food for the World*, edited by E. Schultz, 36–57. Chicago, IL: University of Chicago Press.

Olivier de Sardan, Jean-Pierre. 1984. *Les sociétés Songhay-Zarma (Niger-Mali): Chefs, guerriers, esclaves, paysans.* Paris: Karthala.

Olivier de Sardan, J. P., A. Moumouni, and A. Souley. 2001. "'L'accouchement, c'est la guerre': Grossesse et accouchement en milieu rural nigérien." *Études et Travaux du Laboratoire d'Etudes et de Recherche sur les Dynamiques Sociales et le Développement Local* No. 1. Accessed December 17, 2018. http://www.lasdel.net/images/etudes_et_travaux/L _accouchement_c_est_la_guerre.pdf.

Omran, Abdel Rahim. 1984. *Family Planning for Health in Africa.* Chapel Hill, NC: Carolina Population Center/USAID.

———. 1992. *Family Planning in the Legacy of Islam.* New York: United Nations Population Fund/Routledge.

Onwuejeogwu, Michael. 1969. "The Cult of the Bori Spirits among the Hausa." In *Man in Africa*, edited by Mary Douglas and Phyllis Kaberry, 279–305. London: Tavistock.

Painter, Thomas M. 1988. "Migrations among the Zarma of Niger." *Africa: Journal of the International African Institute* 58 (1): 87–100.

Palmer, H. R. (1928) 1967. "The Kano Chronicle." *Sudanese Memoirs* 3: 92–132.

Patil, Vrushali. 2008. "Population Control." *Encyclopedia of Gender and Society*, edited by Jodi O'Brien. Thousand Oaks, CA: Sage.

Pelckmans, Lotte. 2015. "Stereotypes of Past-Slavery and 'Stereo-styles' in Post-Slavery: A Multidimensional, Interactionist Perspective on Contemporary Hierarchies." *International Journal of African Historical Studies* 48 (2): 281–301.

Pettigrew, Erin. 2016. "The Heart of the Matter: Interpreting Bloodsucking Accusations in Mauritania." *Journal of African History* 57 (3): 417–35.

———. 2017. "Politics and Affiliations of Enchantment among the Ahel Guennar of Southern Mauritania." In *Culture et Politique dans L'Ouest Saharien*, edited by Sébastien Boulay and Francisco Freire, 293–318. Paris: Étrave.

Poitou, Danielle. 1978. *La délinquance juvénile au Niger*, no. 41. Niamey: Études Nigériennes.

Powloski, L. R. 2002. "Growth and Development of Adolescent Girls from the Segou Region of Mali (West Africa)." *American Journal of Physical Anthropology* 117 (4): 364–72.

Pradervand, Pierre. 1992. "A Visit to the Village of Saye." *People and the Planet* 1: 1–2.

Pratt, Mary Louise. 1992. *Imperial Eyes: Travel Writing and Transculturation.* New York: Routledge.

Prentice, S., Antony J. Fulford, Landing Jarjou, Gail Goldberg, and Ann Prentice. 2010. "Evidence for a Downward Secular Trend in Age of Menarche in a Rural Gambian Population." *Annals of Human Biology* 37 (5): 717–21.

Rabain, Jacqueline. (1979) 1994. *L'enfant du lignage du sevrage à la classe d'âge*. Paris: Éditions Payot ar Rives.

Rain, David. 1999. *Eaters of the Dry Season: Circular Labor Migration in the West African Sahel*. Boulder, CO: Westview Press.

Randall, Sara. 2011. "Fat and Fertility, Mobility and Slaves: Long-Term Perspectives on Tuareg Obesity and Reproduction." In *Fatness and the Maternal Body: Women's Experiences of Corporeality*, edited by May Unnithan-Kumar and Soraya Tremayne, 43–70. New York: Berghahn.

Renne, Elisha P. 1996. "Perceptions of Population Policy, Development, and Family Planning Programs in Northern Nigeria." *Studies in Family Planning* 27 (3): 127–36.

———. 2010. *The Politics of Polio in Northern Nigeria*. Bloomington: Indiana University Press.

République du Niger. 1966. *Étude démographique et économique en milieu nomade: Démographie, budgets, et consommation*. Paris: INSEE.

———. 1985. *Recensement général de la population 1977: Résultats définitifs. Rapport d'Analyse*. Niamey: Ministère du Plan Direction de la Statistique et de l'Informatique.

République du Niger, Coordination Intersectorielle de Lutte Contre Les IST/VIH/SIDA (CISLS). 2014. "Rapport d'activités 2014 sur la Riposte au SIDA au Niger." Niamey: Système National d'Information Sanitaire (SNIS).

République du Niger, Ministère de la Santé Publique. 2015. *Annuaire des statistiques sanitaires du Niger année 2014*. Niamey: Système National d'Information Sanitaire (SNIS).

République du Niger, Mission Démographique du Niger. 1962. *Étude démographique du Niger le fascicule, données collectives*. Paris: INSEE.

Retel-Laurentin, Anne. 1963. "Fécondité en pays Nzakara." *La vie médicale* (Noël): 55–103.

———. 1974. *Infécondité en Afrique noire: Maladies et conséquences sociales*. Paris: Masson et Cie.

Riesman, Paul. 1992. *First Find Your Child a Good Mother: The Construction of Self in Two African Communities*, edited by David Szanton, Lila Abu-Lughod, Sharon Hutchinson, Paul Stoller, and Carol Trosset with a prologue by Suzanne Riesman. New Brunswick, NJ: Rutgers University Press.

Roberts, Richard. 1996. *Two Worlds of Cotton: Colonialism and the Regional Economy in the French Soudan, 1800–1946*. Stanford, CA: Stanford University Press.

———. 2005. *Litigants and Households: African Disputes and Colonial Courts in the French Soudan, 1895–1912*. Portsmouth, NH: Heinmann.

Roberts, Richard, and Martin Klein. 1980. "The Banamba Slave Exodus of 1905 and the Decline of Slavery in the Western Sudan." *Journal of African History* 21 (3): 375–94.

Robertson, Claire, and Martin Klein, eds. 1983. *Women and Slavery in Africa*. Madison: University of Wisconsin Press.

Rodet, Marie. 2007. *Les migrantes ignorées du Haut-Sénégal (1900–1946)*. Paris: Karthala.

———. 2015. "Escaping Slavery and Building Diasporic Communities in French Soudan and Senegal, ca. 1880–1940." *International Journal of African Historical Studies* 48 (2): 363–86.

Romaniuk, Anatole. 1980. "Increase in Natural Fertility during the Early Stages of Modernization: Evidence from an African Case Study, Zaire." *Population Studies* 34 (2): 293–310.

———. 2011. "Persistence of High Fertility in Tropical Africa: The Case of the Democratic Republic of the Congo." *Population and Development Review* 37 (1): 1–28.

Ronsin, Francis. 1980. *La grève des ventres: Propagande néo-malthusienne et baisse de la natalité française (XIXe-XXe siècles)*. Paris: Aubier Montaigne.

Rossi, Benedetta. 2010. "Tuareg Trajectories of Slavery: Preliminary Reflections on a Changing Field." In *Tuareg Society within a Globalized World: Saharan Life in Transition*, edited by Ines Kohl and Anja Fischer, 89–108. London: I. B. Tauris.

Roth, Cassia. 2017. "From Free Womb to Criminalized Woman: Fertility Control in Brazilian Slavery and Freedom." *Slavery and Abolition* 38 (2): 269–86.

Rothmaler, Eva. 2012. "Cuisine as Health Factor: Some Aspects of Nutrition in Western Africa." In *Man and Health in the Lake Chad Basin*, edited by Eva Rothmaler, Rémi Tchokothe, and Henry Tourneux, 151–68. Koln: Rüdiger Köppe Verlag.

Rutstein, Shea O., and Iqbal H. Shah. 2004. "Infecundity, Infertility, and Childlessness in Developing Countries." *DHS Comparative Reports*, no. 9. Calverton, MD: ORC Macros and the World Health Organization.

Said-Mohamed, Rihlat, John M. Pettifor, and Shane A. Norris. 2018. "Life History Theory Hypotheses on Child Growth: Potential Implications for Short and Long-Term Child Growth, Development and Health." *American Journal of Physical Anthropology* 165: 4–19.

Saidou, Issaka. 2012. "Hommage posthume à Gorges [sic] Mahamane Condat: L'ancien président de l'Assemblée territorial du Niger n'est plus." *NigerDiaspora*, October 30, 2012. Accessed October 30, 2016. https://nigerdiaspora.net/index.php/societe -archives/item/40388-hommage-posthume-%C3%A0-gorges-mahamane-condat -l%E2%80%99ancien-pr%C3%A9sident-de-l%E2%80%99assembl%C3%A9e-territoriale -du-niger-n%E2%80%99est-plus.

Salamone, Frank A. 1974. *Gods and Goods in Africa: Persistence and Change in Ethnic and Religious Identity in Yauri Emirate, North-Western State, Nigeria*. New Haven, CT: Human Relations Area Files.

Salau, Mohammed Bashir. 2011. *The West African Slave Plantation: A Case Study*. New York: Palgrave Macmillan.

Salvaing, Bernard. 1994. *Les missionnaires à la rencontre de l'Afrique au XIXe siècle*. Paris: L'Harmattan.

Sassens, Saskia. 2001. *Mediating Means and Fate: A Socio-Political Analysis of Fertility and Demographic Change in Bamako, Mali*. Leiden: Brill.

Savineau, Denise Moran. (1938) 2007. *La famille en A.O.F. condition de la femme*, edited by Claire H. Griffiths. Paris: L'Harmattan.

Schmidt, Elizabeth. 2007. *Cold War and Decolonization in Guinea, 1946–1958*. Athens: Ohio University Press.

Schneider, William. 1990. *Quality and Quantity: The Quest for Biological Regeneration in Twentieth Century France*. Cambridge: Cambridge University Press.

Seignette, N. (1898) 1911. *Code musulman par Khalil: Rite Malékite—statut réel. Texte arabe [Mukhtaṣar fī al-fiqh] et traduction française*. Paris: Nouvelle édition.

Shabana, Ayman. 2012. "Paternity between Law and Biology: The Reconstruction of the Islamic Law of Paternity in the Wake of DNA Testing." *Zygon: Journal of Religion and Science* 47 (1): 214–39.

Shipton, Parker. 2007. *The Nature of Entrustment: Intimacy, Exchange, and the Sacred in Africa*. New Haven, CT: Yale University Press.

———. 2009. *Mortgaging the Ancestors: Ideologies of Attachment in Africa*. New Haven, CT: Yale University Press.

Shouse, Eric. 2005. "Feeling, Emotion, Affect," *M/C Journal of Media and Culture* 8 (6). Accessed June 19, 2017. http://journal.media-culture.org.au/0512/03-shouse.php.

Simmons, Dana. 2015. *Vital Minimum: Need Science, and Politics in Modern France*. Chicago, IL: University of Chicago Press.

Slobodkin, Yan. 2018. "Famine and the Science of Food in the French Empire, 1900–1939." *French Politics, Culture and Society* 36 (1): 52–75.

Smith, Mary F. (1954) 1981. *Baba of Karo: A Woman of the Muslim Hausa*. London: Faber and Faber.

Smith, M. G. 1967. "A Hausa Kingdom: Maradi under Dan Baskore, 1854–75." In *African Kingdoms in the Nineteenth Century*, edited by Daryll Forde and Phyllis Kaberry, 93–122. London: Oxford University Press.

———. 1984. "The Kano Chronicle as History." In *Studies in History of Kano*, edited by Bawuro M. Barkindo, 31–58. Kano: Department of History, Bayero University.

Smythe, Kathleen. 2006. *Fipa Families: Reproduction and Catholic Evangelization in Nkansi, Ufipa, 1880–1960*. Portsmouth, NH: Heinemann.

Sokol, E., V. Aguayo, and D. Clark. 2007. *Protecting Breastfeeding in West and Central Africa: 25 Years Implementing the International Code of Marketing of Breastmilk Substitutes*. New York: UNICEF.

Souley, Aboubacar. 2003. "Maladie héréditaires et maladies du contact en milieu hausa (Niger)." In *Les maladies de passage*, edited by Doris Bonnet and Yannick Jaffre, 61–76. Paris: Karthala.

Stilwell, Sean. 2000. "Power, Honour and Shame: The Ideology of Royal Slavery in the Sokoto Caliphate." *Africa: Journal of the International African Institute* 70 (3):394–421.

Stoller, Paul. 1994. "Embodying Colonial Memorie." *American Anthropologist* 96 (3): 634–48.

———. 1995. *Embodying Colonial Memories: Spirit Possession, Power and the Hauka in West Africa*. New York: Routledge.

Super User. 2012. "Fait divers: Un clou enfoncé dans un foetus de huit mois." *Tamtaninfo*. October 24, 2012. Accessed August 3, 2016. http://www.tamtaminfo.com/fait-divers -un-clou-enfonce-dans-un-foetus-de-huit-mois/.

Sutherland-Addy, Esi, and Aminata Diaw, eds. 2005. *Women Writing Africa*. Vol. 2, *West Africa and the Sahel*. New York: The Feminist Press.

Thiénot, Dorothée. 2015. "Nigeria: Bébés à tout prix, un scandale Ouest-Africain." *Jeune Afrique*, May 11, 2015. Accessed August 4, 2016. https://www.jeuneafrique.com/231033.

Thomas, Lynn M. 2003. *Politics of the Womb: Women, Reproduction, and the State in Kenya*. Berkeley: University of California Press.

———. 2007. "Gendered Reproduction: Placing Schoolgirl Pregnancies in African History." In *Africa after Gender?*, edited by Catherine M. Cole, Takyiwaa Manuh, and Stephan F. Miescher, 48–62. Bloomington: Indiana University Press.

Tilho, Jean. 1910. *Documents scientifiques de la mission Tilho 1906–1909*. 2 vols. Paris: Imprimerie nationale.

———. 1928. "Variations et disparition possible du Tchad." *Annales de Géographie* 37: 238–60.

Traoré, Dominique. 1965. *Médecine et magie africaines*. Paris: Présence Africaine.

Tremearne, Arthur John Newman. (1913) 1970. *Hausa Superstitions and Customs: An Introduction to the Folk-Lore and the Folk*. London: Frank Cass.

———. (1914) 1968. *The Ban of the Bori: Demons and Demon-Dancing in West and North Africa*. London: Frank Cass.

Triaud, Jean-Louis. 2014 "Giving a Name to Islam South of the Sahara: An Adventure in Taxonomy." *Journal of African History* 55 (1): 3–15.

Turshen, Meredeth. 1999. *Privatizing Health Services in Africa*. New Brunswick, NJ: Rutgers University Press.

Ullmann, Manfred. 1978. *Islamic Medicine*. Edinburgh, UK: Edinburgh University Press.

UN Committee on the Elimination of Discrimination against Women. 2015. "Consideration of Reports Submitted by States Parties under Article 18 of the CEDAW Convention: Combined Third and Fourth Periodic Reports of States Parties due in 2012, Niger, 13 August 2015." New York: United Nations.

United Nations Development Programme (UNDP). 2016. *Human Development Report 2016: Human Development for Everyone*. New York: United Nations.

United Nations Population Division (UNPD). 2003. *Fertility, Contraception and Population Policies*. New York: United Nations.

United Nations Population Division (UNPD). 2015. "World Population Prospects: The 2015 Revision, Key Findings and Advance Tables." Working Paper No. ESA/P/WP.241.

United Nations Population Fund (UNFPA). n.d. "Education à la vie familiale." *Les risques liés aux comportements sexuels chez l'adolescent*. Dakar: UNFPA.

U.S. Department of State. 2007. "Niger: Country Reports on Human Rights Practices, 2006. Released by the Bureau of Democracy, Human Rights, and Labor, March 6, 2007.

van de Walle, Etienne, and Francine van de Walle. 1988. "Birthspacing and Abstinence in Sub-Saharan Africa." *International Family Planning Perspectives* 14 (1):25–26.

———. 1989. "Postpartum Sexual Abstinence in Tropical Africa." *PSC African Demography Working Paper Series* 17.

van Walraven, Klaas. 2013. *The Yearning for Relief: A History of the Sawaba Movement in Niger*. Leiden: Brill.

Vaughan, Megan. 1991. *Curing Their Ills: Colonial Power and African Illness*. Stanford, CA: Stanford University Press.

Villarosa, Linda. 2018. "Why America's Black Mothers and Babies Are in a Life-or-Death Crisis." *New York Times Magazine*, April 11, 2018. Accessed April 27, 2018. https://www.nytimes.com/2018/04/11/magazine/black-mothers-babies-death-maternal-mortality.html.

von Maydell, H. J. 1990. *Trees and Shrubs of the Sahel: Their Characteristics and Uses*. Weikersheim: Josef Margraf Verlag.

Walentowitz, Saskia. 2011. "Women of Great Weight: Fatness, Reproduction and Gender Dynamics in Tuareg Society." In *Fatness and the Maternal Body: Women's Experiences of Corporeality and the Shaping of Social Policy*, edited by Maya Unnithan-Kumar and Soraya Tremayne, 71–97. New York: Berghahn Books.

Ware, Rudolph T. III. 2014. *The Walking Qur'an: Islamic Education, Embodied Knowledge, and History in West Africa*. Chapel Hill: University of North Carolina Press.

Wiley, Diana. 2001. *Starving on a Full Stomach: Hunger and the Triumph of Cultural Racism in Modern South Africa*. Charlottesville: University of Virginia.

Wilks, Ivor. 2000. "The Juula and the Expansion of Islam into the Forest." In *The History of Islam in Africa*, edited by Nehemia Levtzion and Randall L. Pouwels, 93–116. Athens: Ohio University Press.

Wilson-Haffenden, James Rhodes. (1927) 1967. *The Red Men of Nigeria: An Account of a Lengthy Residence among the Fulani*. Oxford: Taylor and Francis.

Women Living Under Muslim Laws (WLUML). 2006. *Knowing Our Rights: Women, Family, Laws and Customs in the Muslim World*. Nottingham, UK: Russell.

World Health Organization. 2015. "Trends in Maternal Mortality: 1990 to 2015. Estimates by WHO, UNICEF, UNFPA, the World Bank and the United Nations Population Division."

Wynd, Shona. 1999. "Education, Schooling and Fertility in Niger." In *Gender, Education & Development: Beyond Access to Empowerment,* edited by Christine Heward and Sheila Bunwaree, 101–16. London: Zed Books.

Zorn, Jean-François. 1993. *Le Grand Siècle d'une mission Protestante: La Mission de Paris de 1822 à 1914.* Paris: Karthala.

Unpublished Papers, Theses, Memoirs and Dissertations

Abdou, Salamatou. 2007. "Causes et conséquences de l'avortement clandestine en milieu scolaire: Cas des Lycées Korombe et Kassai de Niamey." Thèse de diplôme d'État d'assistante sociale. ENSP, Niamey, Niger. 118/2007M.

Adamou, Rikiatou Djibo. 2001. "Causes et conséquences sociales de l'infanticide à Niamey: Cas des femmes incarcères pour infanticide à la maison d'arrêt et de réinsertion sociale de Niamey." Mémoire de fin d'études diplôme d'État de technicien supérieur de l'action social. ENSP, Niamey, Niger. 19/2001S.

Allio, Mahaman. 2001. "Une révolution avortée: Le code de la famille au Niger: Traditions, pratiques religieuses et justice au Niger." Second symposium of the Islamic law in Africa project, Dakar, June 29–July 1, 2001.

Amedome, Noutsougan. 2010. "La réinsertion des enfants mendiants à Niamey: Situation et perspectives." CERAH working paper/Memoir MAS Université de Genève.

Aougui, Mainassara Rassiratou. 2008. "Causes et conséquences du phénomène de l'abandon d'enfant: Cas de la commune IV de Niamey 2004–2007." Mémoire diplôme d'État de technicien supérieur de l'action sociale. ENSP, Niamey, Niger. 11/2008S.

Bogosian [Ash], Catherine Mornane. 2002. "Forced labor, resistance and memory: The deuxième portion in the French Soudan, 1926–1950." PhD diss., University of Pennsylvania.

Boubey, Oumarou Mariama. 2008. "Causes des infanticides en milieu urbain: Cas des filles mères incarcérées à la maison d'arrêt de Niamey." Mémoire de fin d'études diplôme d'État de technicien supérieur de l'action sociale. ENSP, Niamey, Niger. 68/2008S.

Boulel, Hore Hamma Aissa. 1987. "Evolution et mobiles de l'infanticide dans le département de Niamey au cours de la période quinquennale 1982–1986." Travail de fin d'études, diplôme d'État de technicienne supérieure de l'action sociale. ENSP, Niamey, Niger. 109/1987S.

Family Care International. 1998. "Rapport d'enquête sur les attitudes et pratiques en genre et santé de la reproduction au Niger."

Issoufou, Aichatou Tounkara. 2006. "Raisons et conséquences sociales des grossesses hors mariage en milieu urbain: Cas des filles-mères des quartiers Gawaye et Kirkissoye de la commune Niamey V." Mémoire de fin d'études diplôme d'État de technicien supérieur de l'action social. ENSP, Niamey, Niger. 53/2006S.

Maliki, Mariama, and Rabi Moussa. 1980. "Étude des taches et des problèmes professionnels rencontres en milieu rural par une jeune sage-femme, Madaoua." Cahier de mémoire. ENSP, p. 5.

Mamane, Idi Hadiza. 2003. "Problématique de la non-reconnaissance des grossesses hors mariage: Cas des adolescents âgées de 14 à 20 ans au niveau du service social de la justice commune II du 1 jan. 2000 au 30 avril 2003." Mémoire de fin d'études diplôme d'État de technicien supérieur de l'action social. ENSP, Niamey, Niger. 6/2003S.

Mounkaila, Fatouma, and Hamsatou Oumarou. 1980. "Soins et surveillance pre-peri et post nataux dans la pratique de l'obstétrique traditionnelle en milieu rural." Mémoire de fin d'études. ENSP 1979–1980. Pp. 34–35.

Palès, Léon. 1929. "État actuel de la paléopathologie: Contribution à l'étude de la pathologie comparative." Thèse de médecine de Bordeaux, 1929–1930, no. 76, 1929.

Pettigrew, Erin. 2014. "Muslim Healing, Magic, and Amulets in the Twentieth-Century History of the Southern Sahara." PhD diss., Stanford University.

Salamatou, Oumarou Cisse, Nana Aichatou Maiga Idrissa, and Rabi Zakari Tchemogo. 2008. "Étude sur les femmes fistuleuses hébergées dans le centre de l'ONG Dimol." Mémoire en vue de l'obtention du Diplôme d'État d'Assistantes Sociales. ENSP, Niamey, Niger. 123/2008M.

Schoultz, Kristan Kay. 1998. "Understanding Social Vulnerability: Gender and Sexually Transmitted Infection in Niamey, Niger." PhD diss., Brown University.

Seyni, Soumaila Haoua. 2001. "La femme en milieu carcéral: Conditions de détention et resocialisation. Cas de la Prison Civile de Niamey." Mémoire de fin d'études diplôme d'État de technicien supérieur de l'action social. ENSP, Niamey, Niger. 10/2001S.

Twagira, Laura Ann. 2013. "Women and Gender at the Office du Niger (Mali): Technology, Environment, and Food c. 1900–1985." PhD diss., Rutgers University.

Walentowitz, Saskia. 2003. "'Enfant de soi, enfant de l'autre': La construction symbolique et sociale des identités à travers une étude anthropologique de la naissance chez les Touaregs (Kel Eghlal et Ayttawari de l'Azawagh, Niger)." Thèse EHESS anthropologie social et ethnologie. Dir. de thèse Pierre Bonte. Lille: Atelier national de reproduction des thèses.

Primary Sources

Niger

ARCHIVES DU MINISTÈRE DE SANTÉ PUBLIQUE, RÉPUBLIQUE DU NIGER (AMSP)

AMSP Direction de la Planification Familiale Centre National de Santé Familiale. 1989. "Rapport du Séminaire National en Techniques de Planification Familiale Tenu au CNSF, Niamey du 18–28 Septembre 1989."

AMSP FNUP/République du Niger Ministère de la Santé. Diallo, Dr. Boubacar. 2000. Évaluation; 4ᵉ Programme de population et Développement: Sous-Programme santé en matière de Reproduction.

AMSP UNESCO/FNUP/Ministère de l'éducation nationale et de la recherché. 1993. "Introduction de l'éducation à la vie familiale et en matière de population à l'école: Résultats et Recommandations du Projet." FMR/BREDA/93 Niger, Niamey 1993.

ARCHIVES NATIONALES DU NIGER (ANN)

Fonds Colonial

Rapports de tournée

14.3.59 Moncoucut. 1941. "Rapport de tournée effectuée par l'élève administrateur MONCOUCUT dans l'est et le nord de la subdivision de Maradi du 28 août au 12 septembre 1941."

14.3.62 Author unknown. 1941. "Compte rendu de tournée effectuée du 3 au 18 août dans le cercle de Maradi."

14.3.63 Yobi. 1941. "Compte rendu de tournée effectuée du 19 septembre au 30 octobre 1941 dans le Gober [Gobir] par l'instituteur Hama Yobi."

14.3.65 Richert. 1942. "Rapport de la tournée effectuée du 20 novembre au 2 décembre 1942 par l'administrateur-adjoint Richert dans les cantons de Gober et de Maradi."

14.3.80 Paumelle. 1945. "Compte-rendu de tournée de recensement effectuée par l'administrateur adjoint Paumelle Jean dans le Gober."

14.3.97 Leroux. 1946. "Rapport de tournée de recensement effectuée par Monsieur LEROUX Henri, stagiaire de l'administration coloniale dans le canton de Djirataoua du 3 au 11 et du 22 au 28 juillet 1946."

14.3.98 Cunin. 1946. "Rapport sur le recensement du village de Maradi juillet-août-sept 1946 par M. CUNIN, Camille, administrateur-adjoint des colonies."

École Coloniale
3 ECOL 115 5 Guemas, Marc. 1953. "Condition juridique et sociale des Iklane Soudanais et Nigériens" 1952–53.

Affaires politiques
1 E 10 30 Author unknown. 1926. Maradi Peulhs, "Rapport de tournée (subdivision de Maradi) recensement des peulhs."

1 E 10 35 Pambrun. 1927. Tillabéry, "Rapport de tournée effectuée par M. Pambrun de 5 août au 6 septembre dans le canton de Dargol."

1 E 10 68 Perrault, P. C. C. 1928. Zinder Canton de Gangara, "Rapport d'une tournée effectuée de 13 au 27 mai 1928 dans le canton de Gangara," September 13.

1 E 10 73 Pambrun. 1928. Tillabéry, "Rapport sur la tournée effectuée du 16 novembre inclus [*sic*] dans le canton de Kokoro par M. Pambrun," January 10.

1 E 16 35 Author unknown. 1934. Tillabéry (Ouallam), "Rapport de la tournée de recensement effectuée le 5 janvier au 4 février 1934 dans le canton de Ouallam."

1 E 16 55 Vincens, Georges, commis des services financiers et comptables. 1934. Zinder, "Rapport de la tournée de recensement du canton de Guidimouni Mazamni effectuée de 12 au 28 décembre 1934," January 2.

1 E 16 71 Quint, lieutenant, adjoint au commandant de cercle d'Agadez. 1934. Agadez (Air), "Rapport de la tournée de recensement effectuée du 15 juin au 16 juillet 1934 en Air nord-ouest et sud-ouest; du 2 au 17 mars inclus dans le nord-est du cercle."

5 E 2 5 Author unknown. 1938. Questions des Bellas, enquête sur les serviteurs des populations nomads 1927–51. Enquête 1938, Dori, July 22.

5 E 2 5 Author unknown, inspecteur du cercle Tillabéry. 1943. Questions des Bellas, enquête sur les serviteurs des populations nomads 1927–51 "Rapport de l'inspecteur, Touareg et Bella de Tillabéry 1931–37."

5 E 2 5 Bourgine, Maurice, lieutenant-gouverneur of Niger. 1933. Questions des Bellas, letter to the gouverneur général de l'AOF Jules Brevié, Niamey, September 16.

5 E 2 5 Chapelle, commandant de cercle d'Agadez chef de Bataillon. n.d. Questions des Bellas, "Justice en zone nomade: Rapport de sur l'application du code pénal dans la zone nomade."

5 E 2 5 Chevet, Paul, haute commissaire de la république en AOF. 1949. Questions des Bellas, letter to the gouverneurs de Mauritanie, Soudan, Niger 730 INT/AP2, "Politique nomade question des serviteurs, émancipation des Bellas," Dakar, August 17.

5 E 2 5 Gerber, P. G., commandant de cercle de Maradi. 1950. Questions des Bellas, letter to gouverneur du Niger Jean Toby, July 21.

5 E 2 5 Louveau, Edmond, administrateur en chef des colonies p.i. du Soudan Français. 1949. Questions des Bellas, letter marked "Confidentiel" to Monsieur le gouverneur du Niger Jean Toby, Bamako, March 22.

5 E 2 5 Urfer, Paul, chef de subdivision Filingué. 1949. Questions des Bellas, report to commandant de cercle de Niamey, "Politique nomade au Soudan 1949," November 14.

5 E 2 5 Reeb, Capitaine, chef de subdivision nomade de Tahoua. 1947. Questions des Bellas, enquête sur les serviteurs des populations nomades 1927–51, "Les Iklan ou les Touareg Noirs," mémoire pour l'admission au centre des hautes études musulmanes.

Police et sureté

1 F 2 20 Barthes, R. 1946. Prostitution, circulaire to police services of Dakar, December 5.

1 F 2 20 Bocce, médecin-capitaine médecin-chef de la police de Niamey, infirmerie de Garnison de Niamey. 1952. Prostitution, letter to médecin lieutenant-colonel Lorre, August 12.

1 F 2 20 Cassagnaud, lieutenant-colonel commandant de la bataillon autonome du Niger-Ouest. 1952. Prostitution, letter to médecin lieutenant-colonel Lorre, August 13.

1 F 2 20 Chiramberro, J., chef des services de police au Niger Prostitution. 1952. Report, "Enquête sur la prostitution" sent to monsieur le directeur des services de sécurité de l'AOF in Dakar, October 30.

1 F 2 20 de Boisboissel, commandant de cercle de Niamey. 1952. Prostitution, confidential letter from to gouverneur du Niger, objet: "Prostitution et maladies vénériennes," September 25.

1 F 2 20 Espitalier, chef de la sureté du Niger. 1950. Prostitution, letter to monsieur le gouverneur du Niger, Niamey, objet: "Prostitution." February 28.

1 F 2 20 Lorre, le médecin-lieutenant-colonel, directeur local de la santé publique du Niger. 1951. Prostitution, "Rapport de présentation—action antisyphilitique: nouveau traitement de la syphilis à la pénicilline," September 29.

1 F 2 20 Mathurin, le médecin-capitaine Mathurin, service général d'hygiène et prophylaxie groupement Djerma-Sonrai. 1951. "Compte-rendu de la visite des prostituées à Niamey," May 10.

1 F 3 1 Author unknown, 1952. Condition juridique de la femme, "Questionnaire concernant la condition juridique et le traitement de la femme: Droits de la famille," territoire du Niger.

1 F 5 8 Tresse, P., le commissaire de police. 1952. "Rapport 1951" January 14.

2 F 1 Extrait du registre d'écrou, cercle de Niamey 1er trimestre 1929.

Études générales, monographies, thèses

(École Normale William Ponty and École Normale Frédéric Assomption de Katibougou)

1 G 4 3 Bakary Djibo, "L'alimentation indigène au Niger" 1939.

1 G 4 5 Dankane Ouddou, "L'alimentation indigène, subdivision de Filingue" 1938–39.

1 G 4 6 Condat Georges Mahamane, "Rite funéraires dans les cercles de Maradi et Zinder" (Niger) 1938–39.

1 G 4 7 Garba Labo, "Alimentation indigène dans le cercle de Maradi" (Niger) 1938–39.

1 G 4 8 Kano Ibra, "Alimentation indigène au Manga" (Niger) 1938–39.

Services sanitaires

1 H 2 10 Maternité: Actes officiels, arrêté no. I.I41/SS gouvernement général de l'AOF, colonie du Niger, bureau des finances règlementant l'utilisation par le service de santé des femmes indigènes dites "Matrones."

1 H 2 10 Rapenne, lieutenant-gouverneur Jean. 1939. Maternité actes officiels: Correspondance général, 1934–39; Letter to commandants de cercles (Niger) Niamey, April 13.

1 H 2 23 Court, lieutenant-gouverneur. 1937. Dossier concernant la syphilis: 1936–52. Letter to gouverneur général Marcel de Coppet de l'AOF AS: "Traitement de syphilis: AMI 'en profondeur,'" July 8.

1 H 3 9 Boisson, gouverneur général Pierre. 1940. Correspondance diverse: 1940–54. Letter to gouverneurs des colonies du Groupe, "Réorganisation de l'assistance rurale" Dakar, September 17.

1 H 3 12 Saliceti, 1942. Le médecin lieutenant-colonel Saliceti, chef de service de santé du Niger "Rapport de tournée d'inspection dans les postes médicaux," January 21, 1942.

1 H 3 25 Commandant de cercle Fada. 1946. Déclaration des maladies vénériennes 1945–46. Telegram to gouverneur Toby in Niamey n. 324 8.

1 H 3 25 Toby, Gouverneur du Niger. 1946. Déclaration des maladies vénériennes 1945–46. Telegram [Urgent] to commandant de cercle Fada n. 1244.

1 H 29 26 Ricou, le médecin général inspecteur, directeur général de la santé publique et directeur du service de santé des troupes en AOF. 1943. "Les maladies vénériennes en Afrique Occidentale Française," December.

2 H 1 37 Court, lieutenant-gouverneur of Niger, Joseph. 1937. Questions des métis. Draft letter to gouverneur général de l'AOF Marcel de Coppet, dated 8 April.

Justice indigène

M 5 15 Notices des actes d'instruction. Extrait du registre d'écrou Zinder, December 31, 1937.

M 6 16 Justice indigène. Relations avec le Parquet. Letter from the officier du ministère publique près le tribunal colonial d'appel du Niger Segealon to the procureur général of the AOF, December 27, 1934.

M 6 16 Justice indigène. Relations avec le Parquet. Letter from the officier du ministère publique près le tribunal d'appel du Niger to the procureur général près la cour d'appel de l'AOF à Dakar, October 17, 1935.

FONDS MODERNES

ANN C3351 "Séminaire national sur population et développement: Formulation d'un plan d'action," Kollo, July 1986.

Senegal

INSTITUT FONDAMENTAL D'AFRIQUE NOIRE (DAKAR, SÉNÉGAL) (IFAN)

Fonds Cahiers ENWP

École Normale William Ponty (Lycée Ponty) or École Normale Frédéric Assomption de Katibougou

C 3 Fanne Fodé, "L'enfant dans le milieu familial Peul" (Sénégal) 1949.

C 3 Kane Bousra, "L'enfant dans le milieu familial" (Sénégal) n.d.

C 3 Kebe Babacar, "L'enfant dans le milieu familial" (Sénégal) 1949.

C 3 N'Diaye Mody Diabe Maurice, "L'enfant dans le milieu familiale Bambara" (Sénégal) 1948-49.

C 3 Sarr Alioune, "L'enfant dans le milieu familiale Diola" (Sénégal) 1949.

C 3 Toure Alpha, "L'enfant dans le milieu familial Sine-Saloum" (Sénégal) n.d.

C 13 Gaston Dory, "Niger: Boissons Gourma" (Niger—Fada N'Gourma) 1943.

C 13 Oualy Michel, "Niger: Boissons Gourmantche" (?) n.d.

C 14 Ba Habibou, "Éducation traditionelle Fouta" (Guinée) n.d.

C 14 Barry Mamadou Aliou, "L'enfant dans le milieu familial" (Guinée) 1949.

C 14 Caba Sory, "Système d'éducation d'une société Kissienne" (Guinée) 1949.

C 14 Couyate Karamoko, "Formation morale de l'enfant" (Guinée) n.d.

C 14 Diakite Mamadou, "Éducation du garçon et de la fille" (Guinée) École Normale Frédéric Assomption de Katibougou, 1945.

C 14 Gayego Leopold, "Éducation de l'enfant noire" (Haute-Volta) n.d.

C 14 Pascal L. Macos, "L'enfant dans le milieu familial" (Guinée) 1949.

C 14 Sagno Mamady, "Mémoire" cercle de N'Zerikori (Guinée) 1948–1949.

C 14 Sow Ibrahima, "Type d'éducation Foulah" (?) n.d.

C 24 Kalapo Issa, "Les Bozos" (Niger) n.d.

C 30 Amadou Badiane, "L'enfant dans le milieu familial" Diourou (Sénégal) 1949.

C 30 Diallo Seydou, "L'enfant dans le milieu familial Lebou" (Sebikotane, Sénégal) 1949.

C 30 Diouck Sanor, "L'enfant dans le milieu familial [Wolof]" (Sénégal) 1949.

C 30 Elhadji Diouf, "L'enfant dans le milieu familial" (Saloum, Sénégal) 1949

C 30 Magatte Fall, "Savoir vivre de l'enfant les règles de politesse enfantine" (Saint Louis, Sénégal) 1949.

C 30 Oumar Diouf, "L'enfant dans le milieu familial Lebou" (Petite Côte, Sénégal) 1949.

C 30 Seydou Cissoko, "L'enfant dans le milieu familial Sarakolle" Bakel, (Sénégal) 1949.

C 33 Diallo Mamadou Dioudia, "L'autorité du chef de famille autrefois et aujourd'hui" (Katibougou Guinée) n.d.

C 33 Samoura Sinkoun, "La Famille Diallonke" (?) n.d.

C 53 Koke Issaka, "Les Rêves" (Niger) n.d.

C 53 Mossi Adamou, "Les Rêves" (Niger) 1944–45.

C 53 Soumana Gouro, "Les Rêves ou 'andiris'" (Niger) n.d.

C 71 Jean-Louis Méon, "Une peuplade du Haute-Niger français, les Djermas" (Niger) n.d.

ARCHIVES NATIONALES DU SÉNÉGAL (ANS)

Services sanitaires

1 H 2 23 Court, 1937. Dossier concernant la syphilis: 1936–52. Letter from lieutenant-gouverneur Court to the gouverneur général de l'AOF AS: "Traitement de syphilis: AMI 'en profondeur,'" le 8 juillet 1937.

1 H 102 versement 162, Kervingant, médecin lieutenant-colonel. 1950. Protection maternelle et infantile: Organisation I "Assistance Social 'Protection Maternelle et Infantile,'" Niamey, March 23.

1 H 102 versement 162, Peltier, le médecin général inspecteur. 1948. Protection maternelle et infantile: Organisation I "Documentation sur la protection de l'enfance du 1er janvier au 31 décembre 1946," July 13.

1 H 102 versement 162, Queinnec, le médecin lieutenant-colonel. 1950. Protection maternelle et infantile: Organisation I "Assistance Social 'Protection Maternelle et Infantile' Territoire de la Haute-Volta," February 27.

1 H 102 versement 163, Brevié, Jules, gouverneur général de l'AOF. 1934. Protection maternelle et infantile: Organisation I. "Mesures législatives et administratives—œuvres concernant l'enfance en AOF," report submitted to the ministre des Colonies, Dakar, March 30.

1 H 102 versement 163, Cayla, Léon, inspection général des services sanitaires et médicaux. 1940. Protection maternelle et infantile: Organisation I. "Instructions sur la lutte contre la mortalité infantile et les maladies endemo-epidemiques," June 1.

1 H 122 versement 163, Author unknown. 1953. La répartition des sexes à la naissance dans les populations de l'Afrique Noire Française et de Madagascar. Démographie 1933–58.

1 H 122 versement 163, Campunaud, médecin lieutenant-colonel. 1939. Démographie 1933–58, "Rapport de présentation de l'enquête démographique demandée aux médecins de la Côte d'Ivoire, 1939," March 16.

1 H 122 versement 163, Cazanove and Lasnet. 1930. Démographie 1933–58 Clipping: "Essai de Démographie des Colonies Françaises," Extrait du supplément au *Bulletin mensuel, office international d'hygiène publique* 1 XXII (8), August.

1 H 122 versement 163, Dechambenoit, Paul, médecin auxiliaire principal de 4ᵉ classe, 1938. Démographie 1933–58, "Enquête démographique sur les causes de la non progression de la population dans le cercle de Kindia," December.

1 H 122 versement 163, Geismar, Léon, gouverneur général p.i. de l'AOF. 1938. Démographie 1933–58 Letter to gouverneurs des colonies du Group AS: "Enquête démographique en AOF," August 2.

1 H 122 versement 163, Jardon, médecin colonel. 1939. Démographie 1933–58, "Enquête démographique à Dakar," March 13.

1 H 122 versement 163, Lefrou, médecin lieutenant-colonel, 1938. Démographie 1933–58, "Contribution à une enquête démographique en AOF: Le problème démographique en Pays Mossi," December 26.

2 H 6 versement 26, Bertillon, Jacques, president du comité, n.d. Organisation de la "Journée des mères de familles nombreuses en AOF 1920–23," manifeste du comité

2 H 6 versement 26, Mayet, L., secrétaire général trésorerie de l'AOF for the gouverneur général de l'AOF. 1922. Organisation de la "Journée des mères de familles nombreuses en AOF 1920–23," letter to trésorerie du comité de la Journée des mères de familles nombreuses, April 3.

2 H 6 versement 26, Merlin, Martial, gouverneur général of the AOF. 1921. Organisation de la "Journée des mères de familles nombreuses en AOF 1920–23," note from Merlin to the comité de la Journée des mères

2 H 6 versement 26, "Situation actuel du service de l'assistance médicale aux indigènes." 1920. Réorganisation des cadres, June 12.

Justice indigène

M 89 Letter from lieutenant-gouverneur Haut-Sénégal et Niger in Kayes to the gouverneur général de l'AOF, January 10, 1907.

M 89 Letter from procureur général to gouverneur général de l'AOF, March 29, 1907.

M 89 Letter from lieutenant-gouverneur Haut-Sénégal et Niger in Kayes to gouverneur général de l'AOF, July 24, 1907.

M 89 Lieutenant-colonel Lamolle, commandant le territoire militaire du Niger. 1906. Note de service N 32A, September 1.

M 119 État des jugements rendus en matière civile et commercial pour le tribunal de province de Niamey pendant le 2ᵉ trimestre 1906.

M 119 État des jugements rendus en matière correctionnelle par le tribunal de province de Niamey, 2ᵉ trimestre 1906, May 14, June 11.

M 119 État des jugements rendus sur appel en matière civile et commercial, tribunal de cercle de Niamey, 2ᵉ trimestre 1906, June 18, June 26.

M 119 Région de Zinder, cercle de Tahoua, Jugements rendus en matière criminelle 2ᵉ trimestre 1906, May 11.

M 119 Région de Zinder, cercle de Tahoua, Jugements rendus en matière criminelle 2ᵉ trimestre 1905, June 22.

M 123 Conventions entre indigènes, 1914.

M 123 Letter reporting on the functioning of la justice indigène in the territoire militaire du Niger 1ᵉʳ trimestre 1912 from procureur général de l'AOF to the gouverneur général de l'AOF, March 27, 1912.

M 123 Letter reporting on the functioning of la justice indigène in the territoire militaire du Niger 3ᵉ trimestre 1911 from procureur général de l'AOF to the gouverneur général de l'AOF, February 27, 1912.

3 M 11 Rapport sur le fonctionnement de la justice indigène pendant l'année 1930.

3 M 11 Rapport sur le fonctionnement de la justice indigène pendant l'année 1932.

3 M 20 Rapport sur le fonctionnement de la justice indigène pendant l'année 1933.

3 M 20 Rapport sur le fonctionnement de la justice indigène pendant l'année 1934.

3 M 109 Affaires connues par le tribunal de Niamey (Niger) et expédiées au procureur général pour contrôle 1933. Arrêt no. 50.

3 M 109 Notice d'arrêt 1925.

3 M 109 Notices des arrêts 1933.

3 M 109 Notices des arrêts 1934.

3 M 109 Letter from procureur général to lieutenant-gouverneur du Niger, affaire Kanni, July 28, 1934.

3 M 109 Letter from procureur général to lieutenant-gouverneur du Niger, October 15, 1934.

3 M 117 184 Arrêt chambre d'accusation, #32, novembre 1939.

3 M 117 184 Notice des arrêts rendus par la chambre d'accusation, réquisition 12, March 1940.

France

AIX-EN-PROVENCE: ARCHIVES NATIONALES D'OUTRE-MER (ANOM)

Afrique Occidentale Française

17 G 381 Mme Savineau, Rapport 3 De Ségou à Mopti et Bandiagara, December 27, 1937.

17 G 381 Mme Savineau, Rapport 4 Goundam-Timbuktu-Gao, January 16, 1938.

17 G 381 Mme Savineau, Rapport 5 Le Niger Occidental, March 9, 1938.

17 G 381 Mme Savineau Rapport 8, Ouagadougou, April 3, 1938.

17 G 381 Mme Savineau, Rapport 15 Fouta Djallon, April 16 to May 10, 1938.

22 G 20 Statistiques de la population des colonies de l'AOF pour les années 1905–1908, "Sénégal 1908."

22 G 20 Statistiques de la population des colonies de l'AOF pour les années 1905–1908, "Table: Colonies composant le gouvernement général de l'Afrique Occidental Française 1905."

22 G 20 Statistiques de la population des colonies de l'AOF pour les années 1905–1908, draft letter from the gouverneur-général de l'AOF to the office colonial AS: "Statistiques de la population du Sénégal en 1905," n.d.

22 G 20 Statistiques de la population des colonies de l'AOF pour les années 1905–1908, Chef du bureau militaire, "Organisation des forces de l'Afrique Occidentale Française à la date du 1er Janvier 1906."

22 G 20 Statistiques de la population des colonies de l'AOF pour les années 1905–1908, lieutenant-gouverneur Clozel, "Envoie statistiques 1908 Haute-Sénégal Niger."

22 G 20 Statistiques de la population des colonies de l'AOF pour les années 1905–1908, lieutenant-gouverneur Clozel, "Envoie statistiques 1908 territoire militaire du Niger."

22 G 20 Statistiques de la population des colonies de l'AOF pour les années 1905–1908, télégramme 163 1er mai, 1907.

FONDS MINISTÉRIELS

Agence économique de la France d'outre-mer

FM AGEFOM 382 Carde, gouverneur général. 1928. Travail obligatoire, circulaire to the lieutenant gouverneurs des colonies and Dakar AS: "Régime appliqué aux travailleurs indigènes employés sur les chantiers de travaux publics," Dakar, January 1.

FM AGEFOM 382 Carde, gouverneur général p.i. 1929. Travail obligatoire, circulaire to the lieutenant-gouverneurs du Group AS: "Travail indigène," Paris, October 11.

FM AGEFOM 382 Travail obligatoire, journal officiel Soudan Français [clipping] 1927. Arrête du lieutenant-gouverneur réglementant les conditions d'exercice du travail des indigènes engagés par l'administration.

FM AGEFOM 384 Assistance médical indigène 1926.

FM AGEFOM 395 "Divers."

FM AGEFOM 395 8bis Brévié, Jules, lieutenant-gouverneur. 1926. Immigration/Émigration: letter to gouverneur général de l'AOF Jules Carde, AS: "Mouvement de population entre le Niger et la Nigeria," June 23.

Affaires politiques

FM 1AFFPOL 541 De Coppet, gouverneur général de l'Afrique Occidentale Française. 1936. "Discours prononcé par le gouverneur général de l'Afrique Occidentale Française à l'ouverture de la session du conseil du gouvernement, December 1936."

FM 1AFFPOL 591 Bourgine, lieutenant-gouverneur du Niger. 1934. Niger 1916–30 "Rapport politique annuel colonie du Niger, 1933" March 22.

FM 1AFFPOL 591 Court, lieutenant-gouverneur du Niger. 1937. "Rapport économique année 1937 Niger."

FM 1AFFPOL 591 Lefebvre, lieutenant-colonel chargé de l'expédition des affaires du territoire militaire du Niger. 1918a. Niger 1916–1930, "Rapport politique 1er trimestre 1918," August 6.

FM 1AFFPOL 591 Lefebvre, lieutenant-colonel chargé de l'expédition des affaires du territoire militaire du Niger. 1918b. Niger 1916–1930, "Rapport politique 3ᵉ trimestre 1918," n.d.

FM 1AFFPOL 591 Lefebvre, lieutenant-colonel chargé de l'expédition des affaires du territoire militaire du Niger. 1919. Niger 1916–1930, "Rapport 3ᵉ trimestre 1919," November 17.

FM 1AFFPOL 591 Mourin, chef de bataillon. 1915. Niger 1916–1930, "Rapport politique 3ᵉ trimestre 1915," November 11.

FM 1AFFPOL 591 Sarraut, Albert, ministre des Colonies. 1933. Niger 1916–30. Instructions to gouverneurs général of the AOF, AEF, Madagascar, Togo and Cameroon AS: "Mesures à prendre en vue d'éviter les crises alimentaires," July 25.

FM 1AFFPOL 591 Tellier, lieutenant-gouverneur du Niger. 1932. Letter to gouverneur général de l'AOF Brévié in Dakar AS: "Crise alimentaire," June 23.

FM 1AFFPOL 592 Commission d'enquête. n.d. Crise alimentaire 1931–1932. "Commission d'enquête et d'information sur la famine au Niger en 1931."

FM 1AFFPOL 592 Sol, M. Bernard, inspecteur des colonies. n.d. Crise alimentaire 1931–1932 "Rapport concernant la situation alimentaire de la colonie du Niger en 1931–1932."

FM 1AFFPOL 3058 Merly, inspecteur des colonies. 1926. "Mission d'inspection de l'AOF" Letter to monsieur le ministre des colonies AS: "Service du personnel," March 30.

FM 1 AFFPOL 3058 Table effectifs des diverses sections de l'école de médecine 1921–1926.

PARIS: CENTRE POPULATION ET DÉVELOPPEMENT (CEPED)

CEPED 14512 "Rapport général, conférence sur les politiques de population du Sahel Ndjamena 5–10 décembre 1989," communication du Niger: Présentation de la politique de population du Niger.

PARIS: CENTRE DES ARCHIVES ÉCONOMIQUES ET FINANCIÈRES (CAEF)

CEAF B 0057552/ 2 Groupes de travail sur problèmes démographiques en Afrique 1962–1968, "Le Caire, rapport cycle d'études des problèmes démographiques en Afrique 29 Oct–10 Nov. 1962."

CAEF B 0057552/ 3 Réunion des chefs de service de la statistique de l'ouest africain "Rapport de monsieur Ficatier, administrateur de l'INSEE, chef du service de la coopération: réunion à Niamey 19–23 octobre 1964."

CAEF B 0057553 Conférence africaine sur la population, Ghana, 1971, "Report of the economic commission for Africa sessions II and XI."

CAEF B-0057576/ 2 Afrique Occidentale Française (AOF), dénombrements de 1926–1937.

CAEF B 0057576/ 2 Dossiers opérationnels communs a des groups de territoires. "Remarques sur l'utilisation statistique des actes de l'État-Civil en AOF," May 19, 1951.

CAEF B-0057578/ 1 Enseignement, statistiques scolaires en AOF, letter from ministère de la France d'outre-mer, objet: orientation scolaire et universitaire, September 20, 1955.

CAEF B-0057586/ 2 Niger 1948–1959, "Enseignement situation en 1948."

PARIS: MUSÉE DU QUAI BRANLY (MQB)

"Mission Citroën Centre-Afrique (1924-1925)" Territoire du Niger. Photographie de l'album "Expédition centre Afrique," 1924–1925:

Vol. 2, 148 image dated November 25, 1924, PA000115.157.
Vol. 2, 159 image dated November 27, 1924, PA000115.202.
Vol. 2, 162 image dated November 27, 1924, PA000115.211.
Vol. 2, 196 image dated December 5, 1924, PA000115.315.
Vol. 2, 197 image dated December 6, 1924, PA000115.321.
Vol. 3, 201 image dated December 6, 1924, PA000001.2.
Vol. 3, 248, image dated December 16, 1924, PA000001.174.
Vol. 3, 262 image dated December 17, 1924, PA000001.214.
Vol. 3, 264, image dated December 17, 1924, PA000001.220.

MARSEILLE: INSTITUT DE MÉDECINE TROPICALE DU SERVICE DE SANTÉ DES ARMÉES (ANTENNE IRBA DE MARSEILLE) (PHARO). (IMTSSA)

IMTSSA 62 Author unknown. 1956. "Rapport médical année 1955, territoire du Niger, 2ᵉ partie."

IMTSSA 62 Guillaume, médecin lieutenant-colonel. 1940. "Rapport médical année, colonie du Niger, année 1939, partie administrative."

IMTSSA 62 Kervingant, médecin lieutenant-colonel. 1948. "Rapport médical année 1947, colonie du Niger, partie médicale."

IMTSSA 62 Kervingant, médecin lieutenant-colonel. 1949. "Rapport médical année 1948, colonie du Niger, partie médicale."

IMTSSA 62 Lorre, médecin lieutenant-colonel. 1951. "Rapport médical année 1950, territoire du Niger, partie médicale."

IMTSSA 62 Lorre, médecin lieutenant-colonel. 1952. "Rapport médical année 1951, partie administrative."

IMTSSA 62 Morvan, médecin lieutenant-colonel. 1946. "Rapport médical année 1945, colonie du Niger, partie médicale."

IMTSSA 62 Morvan, médecin lieutenant-colonel. 1947. "Rapport médical année 1946, colonie du Niger, partie médicale."

IMTSSA 62 Saliceti, médecin lieutenant-colonel. 1941. "Rapport médical, colonie du Niger, année 1940."

IMTSSA 62 Saliceti, médecin lieutenant-colonel. 1943. "Rapport médical année 1942, colonie du Niger."

IMTSSA 162 Mayer, André. 1954. "Préface," in L. Palès, *L'Alimentation en AOF.*

IMTSSA 162 Palès, médecin colonel L. 1945. "Rapport préliminaire sur les travaux de l'organisme d'enquête pour l'étude anthropologique des populations indigènes de l'AOF. (Alimentation-Nutrition)."

IMTSSA 162 Palès, médecin colonel L. 1954. "L'Alimentation en AOF: Milieux, enquêtes, techniques, rations."

IMTSSA 398 Auffret, pharmacien commandant C. and le pharmacien commandant F. Tanguy. 1947. "Vitamine A et carotène dans le sang de femmes indigènes de la région de Dakar au moment de l'accouchement" in *Rapport* no. 3: Guinée Occidentale, Dakar, Sénégal et Soudan, AOF.

IMTSSA 398 Bergouniou, médecin commandant J. L. 1951. "AOF: Problème alimentaire et nutritionnel."

IMTSSA 398 Palès, médecin colonel L. 1948. "Le bilan de la mission anthropologique de l'AOF 1946–1948."

IMTSSA 398 Palès, médecin colonel L. avec le concours de Mlle Tassin de Saint-Péreuse. 1949. "Raciologie comparative des populations de l'AOF: I parallèle anthropométrique succinct (stature) des militaires et des civils."

BORDEAUX: UNIVERSITÉ DE BORDEAUX MAISON DES SUDS (CENTRE DE DOCUMENTATION) (MS)

Collection Claude Raynaut, Carton "Enquête 100 Villages."

United States

SIM INTERNATIONAL ARCHIVES, FORT MILL, SOUTH CAROLINA (SIM)

Niger Station Records—Galmi (SRG)
SR 28 Galmi Station Records 1970–1992. Harry Enns, "An Evaluation of the Galmi Village Health Project" presented to Mr. Fernand Turcotte for the course Intervention in Public Health MNG. Laval University MBA Studies 1988.

Papers of Elizabeth R. Chisholm (ERC)
ERC 1/A 3 Letters to Family. 1953. March 30, 1953, Tsibiri, "Dear Folks."
ERC 1/A 3 Letters to Family. 1953. April 19, 1953, Tsibiri, "Dear Folks."
ERC 1/A 3 Letters to Family. 1953. May 18, 1953, Tsibiri, "Dear Folks."
ERC 1/A 3 Letters to Family. 1953. Aug. 9, 1953, Tsibiri, "Dear Folks."
ERC 1/A 3 Letters to Family. 1953. Aug. 14, 1953, Tsibiri, "Dear Folks."
ERC 1/A 3 Letters to Family. 1953. Sept. 2, 1953, Tsibiri, "Dear Folks."
ERC 1/A 3 Letters to Family. 1953. Dec. 13, 1953, Tsibiri, "Dear Barbara."
ERC 1/A 3 Letters to Family. 1954. July 12, 1954, Tsibiri, "Dear Folks."
ERC 1/A 3 Letters to Family. 1954. Dec. 31, 1954, Tsibiri, "Dear Friends."
ERC 1/A 7 Letters to Family. 1955. July 11, 1955, Tsibiri, "Dear Folks."
ERC 1/A 7 Letters to Family. 1955. Sept. 27, 1955, Tsibiri, "Dear Friends."
ERC 1/A 17 Letters to Family. 1960. Nov. 17, 1960, Tsibiri, "Dear Dad."
ERC 1/B 21 Letters to Family. 1964. Dec. 25, 1964, Guescheme, "Dear Folks."
ERC 1/B 23 Letters to Family. 1966. July 5, 1966 Guescheme, "Dear Mom and Dad."
ERC 1/B 28 Letters to Family. 1970. April 20, 1970, Guesheme "Dear Mom and Aunt Mae."
ERC 2/ 1 Prayer Letters. 1972–1973. Aug/Sept 1972, Guescheme, "Dear Mom & Ruth."
ERC 1/B 30 Letters to Family. 1975. Jan. 30, 1975, Guescheme, "Dear Friends."
ERC 1/B 30 Letters to Family. 1975. Feb. 9, 1975, Guescheme "Dear Friends"
ERC 1B/ 30 Letters to Family. 1975. Prayer Letter February 1975.
ERC 1/B 31 Letters to Family. 1977. Aug. 26, 1977, Guescheme, "Dear Mom & Ruth."
ERC 1/B 31 Letters to Family. 1977. Nov. 20, 1977, Guescheme, "Dear Friends."
ERC 1/B 32 Letters to Family. 1980–1983. Prayer Letter January 1982, Galmi.

INTERVIEWS

A'i Kyau (Maradi) April 25, 1989.
Ali Buzu, Secretaire Général, Timidria, June 6, 2014.
Elizabeth Chisholm (Sebring, FL USA) November 16, 1990.

Gidan Kakan Hawa (Niamey) January 15, 2014.

Gidan Mallamai (Niamey) January 12, 2014.

Habsou I. Institut pratique de santé publique (Niamey) May 31, 2014.

Hadiza I. Institut pratique de santé publique (Niamey) May 31, 2014.

Hajjiya Agaani (Maradi) April 12, 1989.

Hajjiya Rakiya Kanta, association de sage-femmes du Niger (Niamey) June 4, 2014.

Hajjiya Ta Mai Raga (Maradi) February 18, 1989.

Hawa Almajira (Maradi) March 15, 1989.

Mariama (Niamey) June 10, 2014.

Monsieur A. (Niamey) May 29, 2014.

Madame A. (Niamey) January 3, 2013.

Madame B. and Madame F. ORTN (Niamey) January 3, 2013.

Madame Bonkano. Secretaire permanante de l'AFN (Niamey) June 4, 2014.

Madame D. (Niamey) June 2, 2014.

Madame H. F. Assistante Sociale (TSAS) (Niamey) June 12, 2014.

Madame M. Sage-femme (Niamey) May 28, 2014.

Madame N., Hajjiya, Buzu, and Madame A. Z. (Union de femmes musulmanes du Niger) (Niamey) June 18, 2014.

Madame S. (Niamey) January 4, 2013.

Magistrate B. A. (Niamey) June 11, 2014.

Mai Bauri (Niamey) Marché Katako, January 23, 2014.

Mai Talla (Niamey) June 9 2014.

Mallama O. Association de femmes musulmanes du Niger (Niamey) June 12, 2014.

R. S. Lycée CLAB (Niamey) May 25, 2014.

Rabi and Indo (Niamey) January 9, 2014.

Rahilatou I. Institut pratique de santé publique (Niamey) May 31, 2014.

Rigu (Maradi) October 11, 1989.

S.S. Lycée CLAB (Niamey) May 25, 2014.

Sa'a Ta Wainiya (Niamey) January 10, 2014, June 10, 2014.

Ta Konni (Niamey) January 11, 2014.

Tsofuwa Ta Zarmaganda (Niamey), January 11, 2014.

INDEX

Numbers in italics refer to illustrations.

abolition of slavery, 12, 14, 17–19, 297; attempts to control Bella, 81–82, 140; captives recast as "wives," 18, 70, 72–73, 206; competition between wives and captives, 25, 64–65, 91; continuation after abolition, 89, 124, 170; debt as means to retain former slaves, 87; fertility and status of women, 292; forced labor, 130; former slaves and agricultural settlements, 16; French gradualism, 18, 24, 87; illegitimacy as akin to slavery, 108; increased reproductive burden on wives, 99, 298; inversion of relations, 18, 24, 170; male assertion of free status through acquisition of wife and rights to offspring, 80, 81; male labor migration, 97; marking status difference post abolition, 17, 18–19, 26, 171–72; military service, 131; redemption fee as marriage payment, 81; sexual availability, 73, 76, 77, 115, 157; shame and honor, 27, 28, 76, 82, 108; shifting labor onto wives, 87, 104; "traditional" labor tribute, 17, 140

abortion, 109, 154, 220, 262, 269, 287, 299; acceptable reasons for, 221; assertions of universal danger of, 257; in context of birth spacing, 137, 286; and decline of marital abstinence, 286; self-induced, 286; versus infanticide, 236, 261

abstinence. *See* contraception

abuse: child, 279; emotional 66, 110, 299; human rights, 224; sexual, 244

acceptability of withdrawal. See *al-azl*

adolescent, 32, 101; girls and demographic data, 205–6, 216; and marital sex, 244; menarche, 228; puberty and marriage, 221; sexuality, 105, 151, 154, 255–58; sexual training, 240

adoption, 258, 292, 294, 295

adultery, xii, 52, 95, 100, 103, 105, 106, 151, 162, 234, 235

affect, 27; affective determinants of fertility, 28, 299; joy (or happiness) of successful childbirth, 77, 292, 293, 298, 299–300, 305; repugnancy in French colonial law, 26; revulsion for bastard, 235; revulsion toward public displays of affection, 238. *See also arziki*; contempt; envy; fear; resentment; shame

age at first marriage, 290–91, 299; and first pregnancy, 221; and fistula, 248; popular resentment at government intrusion in, 246–47

al-azl (acceptability of withdrawal), xi, 157, 159, 256–57, 285, 290

animist. See *kafiri*

arziki, 37, 39, 41–45, 77, 298. *See also* compositional wealth

assesseur, xi, 87–88, 93, 95–99

Baba of Karo, 51–52, 60, 154–55, 157–59, 163

baby trafficking, 293–94

Bambara, 10, 74, 94, 96, 98, 160–61, 234, 263, 292

baptême. *See* naming ceremony

bauri. See weaning

Bella, xi, 10, 16–17, 81–83, 136, 140, 170–71, 206, 238, 249–52

birth spacing, 264, 268, 222; and conjugal abstinence, 251; contempt for failure to space well, 137, 157–59, 229–30, 283–84; conjugal abstinence while nursing, 281; God's will, 252; husbands and failure of birth spacing, 229–31, 281–82; ideal spacing, 282–83; and weaning, 285–86

bori. See spirit possession

breastfeeding. *See* nursing
Buzu. *See* Bella

contempt, 137, 157–59, 229–30, 283–84
cas pratique (case studies in medical
    context): Habsou, 267; Rahilatou, 266;
    Hadiza, 270–71
childbirth, 23; age at first birth, 52;
    anticipating dangers of, 28; in clinic or
    maternity, 185–86, 300; description by
    Aoua Kéita, 164–66; description by Baba,
    163–64; description by Jean-Louis Méon,
    149–50; laboring alone, 164–66, only in
    marriage, 50; presumption of adultery
    in long labor, 179; preferred positions,
    183; perception of increased difficulty of,
    251–52; returning home to deliver, 181,
    268, 281. *See also* placenta; reproductive
    mishaps
Chisholm, Elizabeth, 22, 190–93, 199n15
Christian missions, 54, 99, 147, 176–77,
    179–80, 188, 191, 210. *See also* Sudan
    Interior Mission
Citroën mission. *See croisière noire*
compositional wealth (wealth through the
    accumulation of diversity), 9; in persons,
    8–9, in spiritual forces, 39–40, 45–46; in
    seeds, 9, 11, 37, 40, 43, 44–45, 49, 50, 156,
    279, 300, 302–4
conception, 48
conjugal abstinence. *See* contraception
contraception, viii, 33, 262, 264, 271–73,
    278, 299; acceptability of withdrawal
    (*al-azl*), 255–57; among Catholic
    women in Cameroon 7; collapse of
    early opening toward 223–25; condoms
    and association with prostitution and
    HIV/AIDS prevention 273–74; conjugal
    abstinence, 159–60, 229–31, 281–82;
    discourse of overpopulation, 202, 203,
    208–9; education as contraception, 255;
    fertility control, 202; foreign intrusion, 7,
    214; under Kountché, 217–21; lactational
    amenorrhea, 262, 275, 280, 285; Muslim
    acceptance in context of marriage, 209,
    212–13; oral contraception, 218, 252, 271–73,

286, 290; politics of early independence
    era, 202; political volatility surrounding,
    23; "race suicide" in France, 217; rhythm
    method, 22, 290; source of debauchery
    among unmarried girls, 252; traditional
    methods, 284–85; weighing danger of
    pregnancy against danger of illiteracy,
    253; withdrawal and slavery, 256
corvée (forced labor), xi, 129–30, 170
Coutumiers juridiques, 52, 88, 94, 95, 98
croisière noire, 25, 62; in Madaroumfa, 67; in
    N'Guigmi, 70–71, *71*; in Niamey, 63–66,
    67–69; in Tessawa, 67, *68*, 70; in Zinder,
    66–67

demography, 115–16; colonial compulsion to
    collect flawed data, 117; data collection and
    taxation 117; demographic competition,
    2, 298; demographic dividend, 254–55;
    demographic impact of shortened
    conjugal abstinence, 230; demographic
    studies, 205, 207, 215–16; demographic
    transition, 4; failure of existing models of
    transition, 277; insufficiency of colonial
    administrative staff, 29, 117–18, 138;
    limits of data collection within national
    boundaries, 3; perception of population
    stagnation or decline, 128; population
    equilibrium, 118; post-independence
    debates, 203; pronatalism, 115–16, 124–25;
    proportion of women married by age
    eighteen, 245; proximate determinants of
    fertility, 299; relative size of populations
    of Tuareg and Bella, 140, 206–7; school
    assignment on, 120, 150; underpopulation
    and venereal disease, 141. *See also*
    infertility; overpopulation
Diola, 162, 164, 282
drought, 22–23, 213–14

École des Sage-Femmes, 178, 182
Ecole William Ponty, 28, 34n12, 85, 100,
    113n33, 113n34, 114n35; essays of students,
    28–29, 44–45, 86, 100, 122, 149–50, 152
education, 299; Christian schooling and
    readiness for marriage, 21, 254–55; and

civil registry, 203; danger of sexuality of schoolgirls, 171–72, 219–20, 233, 236, 241–42, 245–46, 252–53, 276, 290; after decolonization, 23, 36; evangelical rejection of emphasis on schooling, 35; French resistance to mission education, 20, 24, 189–90; French Niger's lag behind British Nigeria, 188–89; interviews with contemporary female students, 32, 249; investment by kin, 268, 288–89, 304; Islamic schooling, 224, 250; leaders of women's associations, 218; medical school in Dakar, 125–26, 176–79; *métisses*, 68, 77, 172; mode of social mobility for women and servile classes, 18, 24; resentment of government promotion of girls schooling, 246–47; syphilis cases, 142; theses by students in public health, 210–12; training to become *sage-femme*, 166. *See also* sexual education

eggs, 168, 217, 291, 293

emotion. *See* affect

entourage, xi, 17, 45, 65, 72, 110, 122, 160, 211, 240, 271

entrustment, 1, 8, 169, 298, 304–5

envy, 28, 29, 120, 160–61; counterpart to shame, 28; danger to milk, 158; evil eye, 7, 28, 51, 161, 279; and family code, 219; reproductive competition, 6, 28, 53–54, 70, 191, 265; witchcraft accusations, 91

excision. *See* genital cutting

famine, 124, 131–33, 134, 140, 178, 193, 202; food shortage, 15–16, 168, 193, 202, 276, 277

fear, 27–28; of illegitimate pregnancy, 233, 298; of infertility, 298; *la hantise* (dread or obsession), 233; of sexuality of schoolgirls, 171–72, 219–20, 233, 236, 241–42, 245–46, 252–53, 276, 290. *See also* affect

fistula, 247–49, 252

fostering, 7, 263, 292, 304

Fulani, xi, 10, 12, 16–17, 26–28, 46–47, 68, 72, 78, 90, 91, 106, 128, 134, 144, 146, 153, 155, 159, 167, 170–71, 173n4, 250. *See also* RimaiBe

Fulfulde. *See* Fulani

genetics, 257, 288–89; DNA testing for paternity, 243, 294

genital cutting, 103, 152; female genital cutting, 96, 103–4, 105, 137, 151–53, 155, 183, 248; male circumcision, 102, 103, 155; and personhood, 96, 108

Haardt, Georges-Marie, 25, 62–71, 77

Hausa, xi, 2, 8–10, 12, 15–17, 25–28, 32, 36–61, 63, 65–67, 72, 74, 77, 80, 90–91, 101, 108, 118, 131, 136, 143, 154–55, 158–62, 189–91, 204, 227, 240, 243, 250, 262, 264, 278, 282, 284, 291, 301, 303–4

hens, 59, 217

Iacovleff, Alexander, 25, 62, 70–71, *71*

infant and child mortality, 7, 48, 52, 53, 95, 125, 126, 133, 137, 139, 167, 168, 174–76, 191, 198, 202, 221, 231, 242, 262, 280, 299; and naming, 167–68

infanticide, 95–111; versus abortion, 236; court cases, 91–92; in *Coutumiers juridiques*, 93; in French law, 93; and Islam, 84; judicial records, 24; and moral constraint, 85; presumption of guilt in cases of miscarriage, 111

infertility, 37, 291–95, 206, 211; and *bori* cult, 53–54, 57, 58, 191; and co-wives, 265; feigning to escape unwelcome marriage, 291; and piety, 263; and population, 174; protections from, 302–3; remedies offered by male spiritual figures, 59, 60; sense of responsibility, 7, 8, 22; skepticism about contraception, 202, 262; work of Hadiza Moussa, vii, 1–3, 6, 31

inheritance: of capacity to feel shame 75–79; cousin marriage and land, 289; exclusion of foster and adopted child from, 292–93; exclusion of illegitimate child from, 94, 108, 153, 204, 219, 243; family code, 219, 234; under Islamic law, 18, 80, 219; property, 14, 18, 24, 42; patrilineal, 79–81; of spirits, 39, 53

Indigenous therapies, 7, 43, 46, 49, 50, 51, 53–56, 57, 59, 60, 91, 106, 119, 162, 166, 167, 279–80, 284–85, 293, 303; mistrust of *boka*, 59. *See also* weaning: *bauri*

Islam, 45–47, 63; *Islam noir*, 15; medicine, 46, 55–59; jihadists of nineteenth century, 45–47, 57–60; Salafi reformists, 23, 60, 203; Sufi counter-reform, 224–25

jealousy. *See* envy
jiki, 48, 53, 58, 304
justice indigène, xi, 89, 92, 124, 141

kadi. *See* qadi
kafiri, xi, 38, 56, 66, 102, 160, 227, 280, 281
Kanuri, xi, 10, 17, 26, 27, 72, 74, 91, 136
Kéita, Aoua, 164, 165–66
Kel Tamasheq. *See* Bella; Tuareg
Képine, Hawa, viii, 32–33, 243, 250, 252, 264, 266–67, 268, 271, 286–87, 288
Kountché, Seyni, 22–23, 198, 214–25, 230, 238
kunya, xi, 27–28, 74, 77, 85, 230. *See also* shame
kurwa, 43, 47–49, 51, 59

La croisière noire (film), 25, 62
lactational amenorrhea. *See* nursing
law, 30–31; British poor laws 3, 5; colonial, 86; customary law 88, 99; efforts to reform family law, 234–35, 258; French law, 90, 93, 204; *indigénat*, 87, 89, 124, 143; Islamic, 14, 24, 29, 80, 62, 95; *justice indigène*, 90, 124; post-independence, 22, 110; Tribuneaux, xii, 86. See also *Coutumiers juridiques*

Malthusian model, 3–4, 5, 36–37, 214
marital abstinence. *See* contraception
masculinity, 63, 81, 102–3, 160, 164, 171, 230, 247
maternal mortality, 106, 162, 177, 247, 258, 299
matrone, xii, 126, 145n5, 180, 211; and abortion 287; and discretion, 148; *fille de salle*, 271; inadequacy, 186–87, 211–12; medical training, 182; necessity in absence of more *sage-femmes*, 211; occult skills, 148, 160–62, 179, 287; placenta burial, 300–5; revulsion toward bastard, 235; Toko, 149–50; vigilance needed, 164, 183

Métis/métisse, xii, 67–68, 69, 136, 145n2, 170, 172, 176, 180, 181
military, 13, 17, 115, 214–18, 297; and administrative structures, 121, 122–23; indigenous military training, 108; and law, 124; military allure of *croisière noire*, 62; military medical officers, 21, 30, 125–27, 138, 142, 184, 191, 194; military recruitment, 130–31, 152, 163; Niger as military territory, 20, 25, 88, 89, 128, 130; power and military display, 63, 66, 72; and prostitution, 142–45, 170, 177, 185; social mobility, 24; soldiers as index of nutritional well-being, 194; Tirailleurs, 121, 138, 171
milk, 12; "bad" milk 157–58, 159, 280, 285; colostrum 190, 150; female wealth as "living milk," 81; gavage, 82; milk cow and marriage, 77; "milk draws milk," 275, 276, 279; milk kinship, 73, 165; milk as tribute, 169; mother's milk, 37, 160, 163, 175, 191, 195, 197, 228, 230, 280, 284; powdered, 184, 228, 230, 276, 278; Solani 288; substitute milk for baby, 105, 150, 175, 191, 230, 285
miscarriage, 54, 93, 97, 111, 119, 131, 141, 143, 162, 220, 237, 285, 299
monstrosity, 6, 27, 84, 95, 96, 106, 115, 119, 162, 168, 169, 235–36; and difficult labor, 149
Moussa, Hadiza, viii, 31, 240, 263, 286, 302

naming ceremony, 3, 107–8, 203, 210, 265, 282, 291; and bastardy of former slaves, 82; for recognition of child, 107–8, 162, 243–44
Nana Asma'u, 57–59
nursing (infant), 57, 74, 148, 153, 165, 175, 195, 197, 198; and abortion, 221; bad milk, 159, 285; and *bauri*, 278–80; conjugal sex while, 137, 156, 158, 229–31, 262, 281, 286; and contraception, 231, 256, 268, 272, 286, 303; and lactational amenorrhea, 249, 280, 285, 299; and polygamy, 15, 158, 160; and pregnancy, 156–60, 264, 280, 282; wet nurse, 165; and weaning, 251, 272, 274–76
nutrition 30, 193–98, 211; exclusive breastfeeding, 275; judgment of mothers, 3, 6, 277–78; onset of menses, 228;

ORANA, 194–97; promotion of *bouilli*, 278; women's health, 198, 175, 275–77, 290. *See also* indigenous medicine

ORANA. *See* nutrition

overpopulation, 202–3; population control, 22, 208, 209, 212–13; dependency ratios, 5, 205, 208, 216; population policy, 214–15

pagan. See *kafiri*

pain, training in endurance of, 103–4, 148, 151–52; enduring pain of childbirth, 152, 164

Palès, Léon, 194–97, 200n16

paternity disputes, 234, 236, 241–42; and sexual abuse, 243

personhood, 6–7, 27, 29, 84, 94, 99, 109, 151, 235–36, 259, 298, 299; and illegitimacy, 106, 227, 292; and legal reform, 235, 259; naming day as marker of, 107–8. *See also* monstrosity; placenta

placenta: burial, 27, 50, 187, 300–5; expulsion, 212, 269, 300; personhood, 302

polygamy, 6, 54, 101, 141, 159–60, 191, 245–46, 264–66, 268, 274, 299, 302

pregnancy, 26; consequences outside of marriage, 85, 97–98, 99, 101, 154, 233–34, 253; crime of feigning pregnancy, 293; danger of jealousy, 28; decision to avoid, 225, 240, 249; difficulty of nutritional studies, 197; and female education, 255; increased exposure to, 231; interior experience, 48; learning how to avoid through self-discipline, 153; in medicine of the Prophet, 57; nuances of the timing of, 155–58, 268; and nutrition, 228; and overwork, 141; pre-marital, 52, 257; and protection of fetus, 120, 162, 168; protective charms, 57; ruptured tubal pregnancy, 192; and self-discipline, 7, 50, 106, 168, 263, 283–85; shame leading to infanticide, 108–11, 235. *See also* nursing

prostitution: association with medical personnel, 185; conjugal abstinence and prostitution, 137; *croisière noire* photographs, 68; and demobilization,

143–45; driven from Nigeria, 273; food insecurity and, 220; medical surveillance in Niger, 142–43; military field bordellos, 143; policing in Dakar, 141–42; and sexuality of female health workers, 183; and soldiers, 170; and visiting nurses, 139. *See also* sexual exchange

qadi (kadi), xii, 89–90

rape: of child captives post-abolition, 104; as cause of incarceration for delinquents, 220; of female captives, 90; and incest, 258; as justification for abortion, 258; reasons for early marriage of girls, 247; and vulnerability of domestic workers, 257

reproductive mishaps, interpretation of, 50, 161–62, 166, 168, 282

reproductive restraint, 3, 7, 104, 105, 115, 148, 151, 153, 154, 156, 157, 165, 214, 215, 229–30, 262, 283–85, 298

resentment, 12, 23, 66, 91, 120, 204, 230, 273, 282. *See also* affect

RimaiBe, xi, 17, 170–71

sage-femme, xii, 32, 125–27, 131, 139, 145n5, 148, 164, 165, 223, 270–73, 278, 287, 300; in colonial health system, 179–83, 184; and Islamist milieu, 251; postcolonial situation and overwork, 210, 248; relations with *matrones*, 186; reticence to talk about sex, 240; sense of embattlement, 270; students, 266; suitable training, 211; training of, 175–79

Sahel, 3, 9–13, 277; bilad al-sudan 11; family life in, 100–7, 202, 292; French colonial interest in, 13–14, 297; importance of naming ceremony throughout, 107; perception of, 213–14, subfertility in, 216; visual inventory of, 62

Savineau, Denise Moran Report, 3; and conjugal abstinence, 160; on family life, 85; and girl children, 167; on infanticide 94–96, 99, 183; on *matrones*, 164; on military echoes in health interventions, 186; on resistance to schooling for girls,

Savineau (*cont.*)
171; on slave status, 170; on uneven medical services, 181–83
schooling. *See* education
seduction, 1, 42–44, 49, 64
sentiment. *See* affect
sexual education, 238, 240, 246, 249, 252, 253, 257–58
sexual exchange: association of condom with, 273; debates about girls and prostitution, 252; by schoolgirls, 220, 242
shame, vii, xi, 6–8, 12, 148, 299; as attribute of good Muslim, 75–76; and child abandonment, 259; and consumption of food, 67, 168; contraception and shame, 223, 249; and dangers of schooling for girls, 255; distribution of gifts, 75; enacted or performed, 75; and enslavement, 26, 72, 124, 297; as female correlate of male honor, 72; and female sexual self-restraint, 74, 104–5, 153, 227; honorable death is better than life with shame, 26, 74; as indigenous concept, 74; and infanticide, 108–10, 261; infertility and emotional abuse, 299; in-law avoidance, 75; and jealousy, 28, 64; as marker of noble status, 74, 297; necessity of response to violation of honor, 75; and obligation to reproduce, 298; and personhood, 27; policing of female sexuality, 106; semantic range, 27, 74; sexual abuse, 244; sexual vulnerability and shamelessness, 76; shamelessness and male failure to observe sexual restraint, 230, 262; shamelessness and wifely behavior, 171, 274; shamelessness of spirits, slaves, and casted groups, 76; as sign of breeding, 75; as sign of respect, 75; silence in childbirth, 27–28, 148, 164–66; and timing of pregnancy, 156–59, 229–30, 281–84, 286. *See also* affect
slavery: and compositional wealth, 9; distribution of female slaves to attract male dependents, 79; enslaveability in Islam, xi, 11, 12, 15, 26; necessary for conducting trade, 11; necessary for marking status, 165; offspring belong to owner of the womb, 78;

personhood and, 6, 84; settled agricultural slaves, 12; sexual vulnerability of female slaves, 76–78, 156, 256–57; skills of female slaves, 11; slave armies, 11, 79; as trade goods, 12; war captives 12, 26; wet nurses, 165. *See also* abolition
Songhai. *See* Zarma
songs: Bambara lamentation on womanhood, 263; celebration of virgin bride, 227; Diola song, "Torments of Labor," 281–82; "Grandmother Is Dead," 161; Jhonel song, "Niamey, Our Common Courtyard," 261–62; Kouli-Kouta song, 64, 65; Mairam's song, 70–71, 71; as sites of license, 263; song linking infertility to piety, 263; Zarma insult song, 284
spirits: and ancestors, 161; appeasement of, 161; Arna spirits, 39–40; Atacourma, 118; black (malevolent) spirits, 54, 119, 150; *bori*, 39, 52–54, 59–60; Death, 118; djinns, 39, 41, 118–20, 161, 167; elaboration of ideas about, 40–41; fear of women who die in childbirth, 162; possession and infertility, 53–54, 191; Uwar Dawa Baka, 38; Uwar Gona, 37
stillbirth, 106, 111, 119, 128, 143, 162, 168, 220, 264, 269
Sudan Interior Mission (SIM), 21–22, 226; maternal and infant health services, 188–93; use of *matrones*, 211–12
suicide, 170, 237, 287
supposition d'enfant (the crime of feigning pregnancy to lay claim to a child), 293

taxation: colonial census and, 117, 124, 129, 133, 134, 144; and 1930s economic depression, 92, 97; evading census, 120–22; and famine, 124, 132, 140; financing for "civilizing mission," 298; forced labor as tax, 130; and free status, 81, 140; incentives to large families, 137; and *indigénat*, 124; Islamic, 27, 29, 47; as malevolent colonial presence, 121; military and, 122, 163; *prestation*, xii, 130–31; of slaves, 9, 12, 16; units of, 123, 134
Tirailleurs. *See* military

Toubou. *See* Tubu

Tuareg, x, xi, 12, 14, 16, 63, 66, 77–79, 81, 82, 134, 140–41, 154, 164–65, 171, 206, 252. *See also* Bella

Tubu, x, xi, 10, 137

virginity, 50, 104, 153, 227

virility, 57, 293

wealth. *See arziki*; compositional wealth

weaning, 139, 175, 196, 229, 262; in anticipation of pregnancy, 273; and *bauri*, 280; and conjugal abstinence, 148, 229–30; and infant mortality, 167, 251; and malnutrition, 277–78; and mother's diet, 276; in response to a pregnancy, 157, 280, 285; weaning foods, 210, 230, 278. *See also* birth spacing, indigenous medicine

wet nurse, 105, 165

witchcraft, 48, 59, 91, 119, 150, 187, 282, 287, 302–3. *See also* envy

withdrawal. See *al-azl*

Wolof, 10, 11, 14, 94, 153, 164

womb, 8, 48, 49, 50, 53, 78–79, 80, 119, 165, 168, 265, 284–85, 301–2

Zarma/Songhai, ix, xi, 10, 11, 15, 17, 26, 27, 63, 66, 72, 74, 79, 91–92, 94, 101, 103, 118, 119, 121, 132, 137, 149, 152, 154, 164, 170, 171, 180, 220, 221, 224, 234, 235, 240, 242, 254, 263, 268, 269, 275–76, 279, 282, 283, 284, 303

zina. *See* adultery

BARBARA M. COOPER is Professor of History at Rutgers University (New Brunswick). She is the author of *Marriage in Maradi: Gender and Culture in a Hausa Society in Niger* and *Evangelical Christians in the Muslim Sahel*, which was awarded the Herskovits Prize for the best book published in African studies.